HEALTH AND HUMAN DEVELOPMENT

CANCER MANAGEMENT IN LATIN AMERICA II

MELANOMA TO COST-EFFECTIVENESS

HEALTH AND HUMAN DEVELOPMENT

JOAV MERRICK - SERIES EDITOR

NATIONAL INSTITUTE OF CHILD HEALTH AND HUMAN DEVELOPMENT,
MINISTRY OF SOCIAL AFFAIRS, JERUSALEM

Cancer Management in Latin America II: Nasopharyngeal to Renal Cancer
Maurício F Silva, Gustavo Nader Marta, Luis CM Antunes, Fiona Lim, Bo Angela Wan, Beatriz Amendola, Joav Merrick (Editors)
2020. ISBN: 978-1-53616-735-1 (Hardcover)
2020. ISBN: 978-1-53616-736-8 (eBook)

Cancer Management in Latin America I: Nasopharyngeal to Renal Cancer
Maurício F Silva, Gustavo Nader Marta, Luis CM Antunes, Fiona Lim, Bo Angela Wan, Beatriz Amendola, Joav Merrick (Editors)
2020. ISBN: 978-1-53616-733-7 (Hardcover)
2020. ISBN: 978-1-53616-734-4 (eBook)

Alternative Medicine Research Yearbook 2017
Joav Merrick (Editor)
2018. ISBN: 978-1-53613-726-2 (Hardcover)
2018. ISBN: 978-1-53613-727-9 (eBook)

Clinical Art Psychotherapy with War Veterans
Alexander Kopytin and Alexey Lebedev
2018. ISBN: 978-1-53612-975-5 (Softcover)
2017. ISBN: 978-1-53612-976-2 (eBook)

Cancer and Exercise
Leila Malek, Fiona Lim, Bo Angela Wan, Patrick L Diaz, Edward Chow, Joav Merrick (Editors)
2018. ISBN: 978-1-53612-747-8 (Hardcover)
2018. ISBN: 978-1-53612-748-5 (eBook)

Brennan Healing Science: An Integrative Approach to Therapeutic Intervention
Nina Koren, Muriel Moreno and Joav Merrick (Editors)
2018. ISBN: 978-1-53612-825-3 (Hardcover)
2018. ISBN: 978-1-53612-826-0 (eBook)

Palliative Care: Oncology Experience from Hong Kong
Louisa Cheuk-Yu Lui, Kam-Hung Wong, Rebecca Yeung, Joav Merrick (Editors)
2017. ISBN: 978-1-53612-397-5 (Softcover)
2017. ISBN: 978-1-53612-430-9 (eBook)

Psychosocial Needs: Success in Life and Career Planning
Daniel TL Shek, Janet TY Leung, Tak Y Lee and Joav Merrick (Editors)
2017. ISBN: 978-1-53611-951-0 (Hardcover)
2017. ISBN: 978-1-53611-971-8 (eBook)

Cannabis: Medical Aspects
Blair Henry, Arnav Agarwal, Edward Chow, Hatim A Omar, and Joav Merrick (Editors)
2017. ISBN: 978-1-53610-510-0 (Hardcover)
2017. ISBN: 978-1-53610-522-3 (eBook)

Palliative Care: Psychosocial and Ethical Considerations
Blair Henry, Arnav Agarwal, Edward Chow, and Joav Merrick (Editors)
2017. ISBN: 978-1-53610-607-7 (Hardcover)
2017. ISBN: 978-1-53610-611-4 (eBook)

Oncology: The Promising Future of Biomarkers
Anthony Furfari, George S Charames, Rachel McDonald, Leigha Rowbottom, Azar Azad, Stephanie Chan, Bo Angela Wan, Ronald Chow, Carlo DeAngelis, Pearl Zaki, Edward Chow and Joav Merrick (Editors)
2017. ISBN: 978-1-53610-608-4 (Hardcover)
2017. ISBN: 978-1-53610-610-7 (eBook)

Public Health Yearbook 2016
Joav Merrick (Editor)
2017. ISBN: 978-1-53610-947-4 (Hardcover)
2017. ISBN: 978-1-53610-956-6 (eBook)

Alternative Medicine Research Yearbook 2016
Joav Merrick (Editor)
2017. ISBN: 978-1-53610-972-6 (Hardcover)
2017. ISBN: 978-1-53611-000-5 (eBook)

Pain Management Yearbook 2016
Joav Merrick (Editor)
2017. ISBN: 978-1-53610-949-8 (Hardcover)
2017. ISBN: 978-1-53610-959-7 (eBook)

Medical Cannabis: Clinical Practice
Shannon O'Hearn, Alexia Blake, Bo Angela Wan, Stephanie Chan, Edward Chow and Joav Merrick (Editors)
2017. ISBN: 978-1-53611-907-7 (Softcover)
2017. ISBN: 978-1-53611-927-5 (eBook)

Cancer: Treatment, Decision Making and Quality of Life
Breanne Lechner, Ronald Chow, Natalie Pulenzas, Marko Popovic, Na Zhang, Xiaojing Zhang, Edward Chow, and Joav Merrick (Editors)
2016. ISBN: 978-1-63483-863-4 (Hardcover)
2015. ISBN: 978-1-63483-882-5 (eBook)

Cancer: Bone Metastases, CNS Metastases and Pathological Fractures
Breanne Lechner, Ronald Chow, Natalie Pulenzas, Marko Popovic, Na Zhang, Xiaojing Zhang, Edward Chow, and Joav Merrick (Editors)
2016. ISBN: 978-1-63483-949-5 (Hardcover)
2015. ISBN: 978-1-63483-960-0 (eBook)

Cancer: Spinal Cord, Lung, Breast, Cervical, Prostate, Head and Neck Cancer
Breanne Lechner, Ronald Chow, Natalie Pulenzas, Marko Popovic, Na Zhang, Xiaojing Zhang, Edward Chow and Joav Merrick (Editors)
2016. ISBN: 978-1-63483-904-4 (Hardcover)
2015. ISBN: 978-1-63483-911-2 (eBook)

Cancer: Survival, Quality of Life and Ethical Implications
Breanne Lechner, Ronald Chow, Natalie Pulenzas, Marko Popovic, Na Zhang, Xiaojing Zhang, Edward Chow and Joav Merrick (Editors)
2016. ISBN: 978-1-63483-905-1 (Hardcover)
2015. ISBN: 978-1-63483-912-9 (eBook)

Cancer: Pain and Symptom Management
Breanne Lechner, Ronald Chow, Natalie Pulenzas, Marko Popovic, Na Zhang, Xiaojing Zhang, Edward Chow, and Joav Merrick (Editors)
2016. ISBN: 978-1-63483-905-1 (Hardcover)
2015. ISBN: 978-1-63483-881-8 (eBook)

Alternative Medicine Research Yearbook 2015
Joav Merrick (Editor)
2016. ISBN: 978-1-63484-511-3 (Hardcover)
2016. ISBN: 978-1-63484-542-7 (eBook)

Public Health Yearbook 2015
Joav Merrick (Editor)
2016. ISBN: 978-1-63484-511-3 (Hardcover)
2016. ISBN: 978-1-63484-546-5 (eBook)

Quality, Mobility and Globalization in the Higher Education System: A Comparative Look at the Challenges of Academic Teaching
Nitza Davidovitch, Zehavit Gross, Yuri Ribakov, and Anna Slobodianiuk (Editors)
2016. ISBN: 978-1-63484-986-9 (Hardcover)
2016. ISBN: 978-1-63485-012-4 (eBook)

Alternative Medicine Research Yearbook 2014
Joav Merrick (Editor)
2015. ISBN: 978-1-63482-161-2 (Hardcover)
2015. ISBN: 978-1-63482-205-3 (eBook)

Pain Management Yearbook 2014
Joav Merrick (Editor)
2015. ISBN: 978-1-63482-164-3 (Hardcover)
2015. ISBN: 978-1-63482-208-4 (eBook)

Public Health Yearbook 2014
Joav Merrick (Editor)
2015. ISBN: 978-1-63482-165-0 (Hardcover)
2015. ISBN: 978-1-63482-209-1 (eBook)

Forensic Psychiatry: A Public Health Perspective
Leo Sher and Joav Merrick (Editors)
2015. ISBN: 978-1-63483-339-4 (Hardcover)
2015. ISBN: 978-1-63483-346-2 (eBook)

Leadership and Service Learning Education: Holistic Development for Chinese University Students
Daniel TL Shek, Florence KY Wu and Joav Merrick (Editors)
2015. ISBN: 978-1-63483-340-0 (Hardcover)
2015. ISBN: 978-1-63483-347-9 (eBook)

Mental and Holistic Health: Some International Perspectives
Joseph L Calles Jr, Donald E Greydanus, and Joav Merrick (Editors)
2015. ISBN: 978-1-63483-589-3 (Hardcover)
2015. ISBN: 978-1-63483-608-1 (eBook)

India: Health and Human Development Aspects
Joav Merrick (Editor)
2014. ISBN: 978-1-62948-784-7 (Hardcover)
2014. ISBN: 978-1-62948-794-6 (eBook)

Alternative Medicine Research Yearbook 2013
Joav Merrick (Editor)
2014. ISBN: 978-1-63321-094-3 (Hardcover)
2014. ISBN: 978-1-63321-144-5 (eBook)

Health Consequences of Human Central Obesity
Kaushik Bose and Raja Chakraborty (Editors)
2014. ISBN: 978-1-63321-152-0 (Hardcover)
2014. ISBN: 978-1-63321-181-0 (eBook)

Public Health Yearbook 2013
Joav Merrick (Editor)
2014. ISBN: 978-1-63321-095-0 (Hardcover)
2014. ISBN: 978-1-63321-097-4 (eBook)

Public Health: Improving Health via Inter-Professional Collaborations
Rosemary M Caron and Joav Merrick (Editors)
2014. ISBN: 978-1-63321-569-6 (Hardcover)
2014. ISBN: 978-1-63321-594-8 (eBook)

Textbook on Evidence-Based Holistic Mind-Body Medicine: Holistic Practice of Traditional Hippocratic Medicine
Søren Ventegodt and Joav Merrick
2013. ISBN: 978-1-62257-105-5 (Hardcover)
2012. ISBN: 978-1-62257-174-1 (eBook)

Textbook on Evidence-Based Holistic Mind-Body Medicine: Healing the Mind in Traditional Hippocratic Medicine
Søren Ventegodt and Joav Merrick
2013. ISBN: 978-1-62257-112-3 (Hardcover)
2012. ISBN: 978-1-62257-175-8 (eBook)

Textbook on Evidence-Based Holistic Mind-Body Medicine: Sexology and Traditional Hippocratic Medicine
Søren Ventegodt and Joav Merrick
2013. ISBN: 978-1-62257-130-7 (Hardcover)
2012. ISBN: 978-1-62257-176-5 (eBook)

Health and Happiness from Meaningful Work: Research in Quality of Working Life
Søren Ventegodt and Joav Merrick (Editors)
2013. ISBN: 978-1-60692-820-2 (Hardcover)
2009. ISBN: 978-1-61324-981-9 (eBook)

Conceptualizing Behavior in Health and Social Research: A Practical Guide to Data Analysis
Said Shahtahmasebi and Damon Berridge
2013. ISBN: 978-1-60876-383-2 (Hardcover)
2013. ISBN: 978-1-53611-212-2 (eBook)

Adolescence and Sports
Dilip R Patel, Donald E Greydanus, Hatim Omar and Joav Merrick (Editors)
2013. ISBN: 978-1-60876-702-1 (Hardcover)
2010. ISBN: 978-1-61761-483-5 (eBook)

Pediatric and Adolescent Sexuality and Gynecology: Principles for the Primary Care Clinician
Hatim A Omar, Donald E Greydanus, Artemis K. Tsitsika, Dilip R. Patel and Joav Merrick (Editors)
2013. ISBN: 978-1-60876-735-9 (Softcover)

Human Development: Biology from a Holistic Point of View
Søren Ventegodt, Tyge Dahl Hermansen and Joav Merrick
2013. ISBN: 978-1-61470-441-6 (Hardcover)
2011. ISBN: 978-1-61470-541-3 (eBook)

Building Community Capacity: Case Examples from Around the World
Rosemary M Caron and Joav Merrick (Editors)
2013. ISBN: 978-1-62417-175-8 (Hardcover)
2013. ISBN: 978-1-62417-176-5 (eBook)

Managed Care in a Public Setting
Richard Evan Steele
2013. ISBN: 978-1-62417-970-9 (Softcover)
2013. ISBN: 978-1-62417-863-4 (eBook)

Bullying: A Public Health Concern
Jorge C Srabstein and Joav Merrick (Editors)
2013. ISBN: 978-1-62618-564-7 (Hardcover)
2013. ISBN: 978-1-62618-588-3 (eBook)

Bedouin Health: Perspectives from Israel
Joav Merrick, Alean Al-Krenami and Salman Elbedour (Editors)
2013. ISBN: 978-1-62948-271-2 (Hardcover)
2013: ISBN: 978-1-62948-274-3 (eBook)

Health Promotion: Community Singing as a Vehicle to Promote Health
Jing Sun, Nicholas Buys and Joav Merrick (Editors)
2013. ISBN: 978-1-62618-908-9 (Hardcover)
2013: ISBN: 978-1-62808-006-3 (eBook)

Public Health Yearbook 2012
Joav Merrick (Editor)
2013. ISBN: 978-1-62808-078-0 (Hardcover)
2013: ISBN: 978-1-62808-079-7 (eBook)

Alternative Medicine Research Yearbook 2012
Joav Merrick (Editor)
2013. ISBN: 978-1-62808-080-3 (Hardcover)
2013: ISBN: 978-1-62808-079-7 (eBook)

Advanced Cancer: Managing Symptoms and Quality of Life
Natalie Pulenzas, Breanne Lechner, Nemica Thavarajah, Edward Chow, and Joav Merrick (Editors)
2013. ISBN: 978-1-62808-239-5 (Hardcover)
2013: ISBN: 978-1-62808-267-8 (eBook)

Treatment and Recovery of Eating Disorders
Daniel Stein and Yael Latzer (Editors)
2013. ISBN: 978-1-62808-248-7 (Softcover)

Health Promotion: Strengthening Positive Health and Preventing Disease
Jing Sun, Nicholas Buys and Joav Merrick (Editors)
2013. ISBN: 978-1-62257-870-2 (Hardcover)
2013: ISBN: 978-1-62808-621-8 (eBook)

Pain Management Yearbook 2011
Joav Merrick (Editor)
2013. ISBN: 978-1-62808-970-7 (Hardcover)
2013: ISBN: 978-1-62808-971-4 (eBook)

Pain Management Yearbook 2012
Joav Merrick (Editor)
2013. ISBN: 978-1-62808-973-8 (Hardcover)
2013: ISBN: 978-1-62808-974-5 (eBook)

Suicide from a Public Health Perspective
Said Shahtahmasebi and Joav Merrick
2013. ISBN: 978-1-62948-536-2 (Hardcover)
2014: ISBN: 978-1-62948-537-9 (eBook)

Food, Nutrition and Eating Behavior
Joav Merrick and Sigal Israeli (Editors)
2013. ISBN: 978-1-62948-233-0 (Hardcover)
2013: ISBN: 978-1-62948-234-7 (eBook)

Public Health Concern: Smoking, Alcohol and Substance Use
Joav Merrick and Ariel Tenenbaum (Editors)
2013. ISBN: 978-1-62948-424-2 (Hardcover)
2013. ISBN: 978-1-62948-430-3 (eBook)

Mental Health from an International Perspective
Joav Merrick, Shoshana Aspler and Mohammed Morad (Editors)
2013. ISBN: 978-1-62948-519-5 (Hardcover)
2013. ISBN: 978-1-62948-520-1 (eBook)

Adolescence and Chronic Illness. A Public Health Concern
Hatim Omar, Donald E Greydanus, Dilip R Patel and Joav Merrick (Editors)
2012. ISBN: 978-1-60876-628-4 (Hardcover)
2010. ISBN: 978-1-61761-482-8 (eBook)

Child and Adolescent Health Yearbook 2009
Joav Merrick (Editor)
2012. ISBN: 978-1-61668-913-1 (Hardcover)
2012. ISBN: 978-1-62257-095-9 (eBook)

Child and Adolescent Health Yearbook 2010
Joav Merrick (Editor)
2012. ISBN: 978-1-61209-788-6 (Hardcover)
2012. ISBN: 978-1-62417-046-1 (eBook)

Child Health and Human Development Yearbook 2010
Joav Merrick (Editor)
2012. ISBN: 978-1-61209-789-3 (Hardcover)
2012. ISBN: 978-1-62081-721-6 (eBook)

Public Health Yearbook 2010
Joav Merrick (Editor)
2012. ISBN: 978-1-61209-971-2 (Hardcover)
2012. ISBN: 978-1-62417-863-4 (eBook)

Alternative Medicine Yearbook 2010
Joav Merrick (Editor)
2012. ISBN: 978-1-62100-132-4 (Hardcover)
2011. ISBN: 978-1-62100-210-9 (eBook)

The Astonishing Brain and Holistic Consciousness: Neuroscience and Vedanta Perspectives
Vinod D Deshmukh
2012. ISBN: 978-1-61324-295-7

Health Risk Communication
Marijke Lemal and Joav Merrick (Editors)
2012. ISBN: 978-1-62257-544-2 (Hardcover)
2012. ISBN: 978-1-62257-552-7 (eBook)

Translational Research for Primary Healthcare
Erica Bell, Gert P Westert and Joav Merrick (Editors)
2012. ISBN: 978-1-61324-647-4 (Hardcover)
2012. ISBN: 978-1-62417-409-4 (eBook)

Our Search for Meaning in Life: Quality of Life Philosophy
Søren Ventegodt and Joav Merrick
2012. ISBN: 978-1-61470-494-2 (Hardcover)
2011. ISBN: 978-1-61470-519-2 (eBook)

Randomized Clinical Trials and Placebo: Can You Trust the Drugs are Working and Safe?
Søren Ventegodt and Joav Merrick
2012. ISBN: 978-1-61470-067-8 (Hardcover)
2011. ISBN: 978-1-61470-151-4 (eBook)

Building Community Capacity: Minority and Immigrant Populations
Rosemary M Caron and Joav Merrick (Editors)
2012. ISBN: 978-1-62081-022-4 (Hardcover)
2012. ISBN: 978-1-62081-032-3 (eBook)

Applied Public Health: Examining Multifaceted Social or Ecological Problems and Child Maltreatment
John R Lutzker and Joav Merrick (Editors)
2012. ISBN: 978-1-62081-356-0 (Hardcover)
2012. ISBN: 978-1-62081-388-1 (eBook)

Treatment and Recovery of Eating Disorders
Daniel Stein and Yael Latzer (Editors)
2012. ISBN: 978-1-61470-259-7 (Hardcover)
2012. ISBN: 978-1-61470-418-8 (eBook)

Human Immunodeficiency Virus (HIV) Research: Social Science Aspects
Hugh Klein and Joav Merrick (Editors)
2012. ISBN: 978-1-62081-293-8 (Hardcover)
2012. ISBN: 978-1-62081-346-1 (eBook)

AIDS and Tuberculosis: Public Health Aspects
Daniel Chemtob and Joav Merrick (Editors)
2012. ISBN: 978-1-62081-382-9 (Softcover)
2012. ISBN: 978-1-62081-406-2 (eBook)

Public Health Yearbook 2011
Joav Merrick (Editor)
2012. ISBN: 978-1-62081-433-8 (Hardcover)
2012. ISBN: 978-1-62081-434-5 (eBook)

Alternative Medicine Research Yearbook 2011
Joav Merrick (Editor)
2012. ISBN: 978-1-62081-476-5 (Hardcover)
2012. ISBN: 978-1-62081-477-2 (eBook)

Building Community Capacity: Skills and Principles
Rosemary M Caron and Joav Merrick (Editors)
2012. ISBN: 978-1-61209-331-4 (Hardcover)
2012. ISBN: 978-1-62257-238-0 (eBook)

Textbook on Evidence-Based Holistic Mind-Body Medicine: Basic Principles of Healing in Traditional Hippocratic Medicine
Søren Ventegodt and Joav Merrick
2012. ISBN: 978-1-62257-094-2 (Hardcover)
2012. ISBN: 978-1-62257-172-7 (eBook)

Textbook on Evidence-Based Holistic Mind-Body Medicine: Basic Philosophy and Ethics of Traditional Hippocratic Medicine
Søren Ventegodt and Joav Merrick
2012. ISBN: 978-1-62257-052-2 (Hardcover)
2013. ISBN: 978-1-62257-707-1 (eBook)

Textbook on Evidence-Based Holistic Mind-Body Medicine: Research, Philosophy, Economy and Politics of Traditional Hippocratic Medicine
Søren Ventegodt and Joav Merrick
2012. ISBN: 978-1-62257-140-6 (Hardcover)
2012. ISBN: 978-1-62257-171-0 (eBook)

Behavioral Pediatrics, 3rd Edition
Donald E Greydanus, Dilip R Patel, Helen D Pratt and Joseph L Calles, Jr (Editors)
2011. ISBN: 978-1-60692-702-1 (Hardcover)
2009. ISBN: 978-1-60876-630-7 (eBook)

Rural Child Health: International Aspects
Erica Bell and Joav Merrick (Editors)
2011. ISBN: 978-1-60876-357-3 (Hardcover)
2011. ISBN: 978-1-61324-005-2 (eBook)

International Aspects of Child Abuse and Neglect
Howard Dubowitz and Joav Merrick (Editors)
2011. ISBN: 978-1-60876-703-8 (Hardcover)
2010. ISBN: 978-1-61122-049-0 (Softcover)
2010. ISBN: 978-1-61122-403-0 (eBook)

Environment, Mood Disorders and Suicide
Teodor T Postolache and Joav Merrick (Editors)
2011. ISBN: 978-1-61668-505-8 (Hardcover)
2011. ISBN: 978-1-62618-340-7 (eBook)

Positive Youth Development: Evaluation and Future Directions in a Chinese Context
Daniel TL Shek, Hing Keung Ma and Joav Merrick (Editors)
2011. ISBN: 978-1-60876-830-1 (Hardcover)
2011. ISBN: 978-1-62100-175-1 (Softcover)
2010. ISBN: 978-1-61209-091-7 (eBook)

Understanding Eating Disorders: Integrating Culture, Psychology and Biology
Yael Latzer, Joav Merrick and Daniel Stein (Editors)
2011. ISBN: 978-1-61728-298-0 (Hardcover)
2011. ISBN: 978-1-61470-976-3 (Softcover)
2011. ISBN: 978-1-61942-054-0 (eBook)

Advanced Cancer Pain and Quality of Life
Edward Chow and Joav Merrick (Editors)
2011. ISBN: 978-1-61668-207-1 (Hardcover)
2010. ISBN: 978-1-61668-400-6 (eBook)

Positive Youth Development: Implementation of a Youth Program in a Chinese Context
Daniel TL Shek, Hing Keung Ma and Joav Merrick (Editors)
2011. ISBN: 978-1-61668-230-9

Social and Cultural Psychiatry Experience from the Caribbean Region
Hari D Maharajh and Joav Merrick (Editors)
2011. ISBN: 978-1-61668-506-5 (Hardcover)
2010. ISBN: 978-1-61728-088-7 (eBook)

Narratives and Meanings of Migration
Julia Mirsky
2011. ISBN: 978-1-61761-103-2 (Hardcover)
2010. ISBN: 978-1-61761-519-1 (eBook)

Self-Management and the Health Care Consumer
Peter William Harvey
2011. ISBN: 978-1-61761-796-6 (Hardcover)
2011. ISBN: 978-1-61122-214-2 (eBook)

Sexology from a Holistic Point of View
Soren Ventegodt and Joav Merrick
2011. ISBN: 978-1-61761-859-8 (Hardcover)
2011. ISBN: 978-1-61122-262-3 (eBook)

Principles of Holistic Psychiatry: A Textbook on Holistic Medicine for Mental Disorders
Soren Ventegodt and Joav Merrick
2011. ISBN: 978-1-61761-940-3 (Hardcover)
2011. ISBN: 978-1-61122-263-0 (eBook)

Clinical Aspects of Psychopharmacology in Childhood and Adolescence
Donald E Greydanus, Joseph L Calles, Jr, Dilip P Patel, Ahsan Nazeer and Joav Merrick (Editors)
2011. ISBN: 978-1-61122-135-0 (Hardcover)
2011. ISBN: 978-1-61122-715-4 (eBook)

Climate Change and Rural Child Health
Erica Bell, Bastian M Seidel and Joav Merrick (Editors)
2011. ISBN: 978-1-61122-640-9 (Hardcover)
2011. ISBN: 978-1-61209-014-6 (eBook)

Rural Medical Education: Practical Strategies
Erica Bell, Craig Zimitat and Joav Merrick (Editors)
2011. ISBN: 978-1-61122-649-2 (Hardcover)
2011. ISBN: 978-1-61209-476-2 (eBook)

Advances in Environmental Health Effects of Toxigenic Mold and Mycotoxins
Ebere Cyril Anyanwu
2011. ISBN: 978-1-60741-953-2
2011. ISBN: 978-1-53611-209-2

Public Health Yearbook 2009
Joav Merrick (Editor)
2011. ISBN: 978-1-61668-911-7 (Hardcover)
2011. ISBN: 978-1-62417-365-3 (eBook)

Child Health and Human Development Yearbook 2009
Joav Merrick (Editor)
2011. ISBN: 978-1-61668-912-4

Alternative Medicine Yearbook 2009
Joav Merrick (Editor)
2011. ISBN: 978-1-61668-910-0 (Hardcover)
2011. ISBN: 978-1-62081-710-0 (eBook)

The Dance of Sleeping and Eating among Adolescents: Normal and Pathological Perspectives
Yael Latzer and Orna Tzischinsky (Editors)
2011. ISBN: 978-1-61209-710-7 (Hardcover)
2011. ISBN: 978-1-62417-366-0 (eBook)

Drug Abuse in Hong Kong: Development and Evaluation of a Prevention Program
Daniel TL Shek, Rachel CF Sun and Joav Merrick (Editors)
2011. ISBN: 978-1-61324-491-3 (Hardcover)
2011. ISBN: 978-1-62257-232-8 (eBook)

Chance Action and Therapy: The Playful Way of Changing
Uri Wernik
2010. ISBN: 978-1-60876-393-1 (Hardcover)
2011. ISBN: 978-1-61122-987-5 (Softcover)
2011. ISBN: 978-1-61209-874-6 (eBook)

Bone and Brain Metastases: Advances in Research and Treatment
Arjun Sahgal, Edward Chow and Joav Merrick (Editors)
2010. ISBN: 978-1-61668-365-8 (Hardcover)
2010. ISBN: 978-1-61728-085-6 (eBook)

Challenges in Adolescent Health: An Australian Perspective
David Bennett, Susan Towns, Elizabeth Elliott and Joav Merrick (Editors)
2009. ISBN: 978-1-60741-616-6 (Hardcover)
2009. ISBN: 978-1-61668-240-8 (eBook)

Obesity and Adolescence: A Public Health Concern
Hatim A Omar, Donald E Greydanus, Dilip R Patel and Joav Merrick (Editors)
2009. ISBN: 978-1-60692-821-9 (Hardcover)
2009. ISBN: 978-1-61470-465-2 (eBook)

Poverty and Children: A Public Health Concern
Alexis Lieberman and Joav Merrick (Editors)
2009. ISBN: 978-1-60741-140-6 (Hardcover)
2009. ISBN: 978-1-61470-601-4 (eBook)

Living on the Edge: The Mythical, Spiritual, and Philosophical Roots of Social Marginality
Joseph Goodbread
2009. ISBN: 978-1-60741-162-8 (Hardcover)
2013. ISBN: 978-1-61122-986-8 (Softcover)
2011. ISBN: 978-1-61470-192-7 (eBook)

Alcohol-Related Cognitive Disorders: Research and Clinical Perspectives
Leo Sher, Isack Kandel and Joav Merrick (Editors)
2009. ISBN: 978-1-60741-730-9 (Hardcover)
2009. ISBN: 978-1-60876-623-9 (eBook)

Children and Pain
Patricia Schofield and Joav Merrick (Editors)
2009. ISBN: 978-1-60876-020-6 (Hardcover)
2009. ISBN: 978-1-61728-183-9 (eBook)

Complementary Medicine Systems: Comparison and Integration
Karl W Kratky
2008. ISBN: 978-1-60456-475-4 (Hardcover)
2008. ISBN: 978-1-61122-433-7 (eBook)

Pain in Children and Youth
Patricia Schofield and Joav Merrick (Editors)
2008. ISBN: 978-1-60456-951-3 (Hardcover)
2008. ISBN: 978-1-61470-496-6 (eBook)

Adolescent Behavior Research: International Perspectives
Joav Merrick and Hatim A Omar (Editors)
2007. ISBN: 1-60021-649-8

HEALTH AND HUMAN DEVELOPMENT

CANCER MANAGEMENT IN LATIN AMERICA II

MELANOMA TO COST-EFFECTIVENESS

MAURÍCIO F SILVA
GUSTAVO NADER MARTA
LUIS CM ANTUNES
FIONA LIM
BO ANGELA WAN
BEATRIZ AMENDOLA
AND
JOAV MERRICK
EDITORS

nova
Medicine & Health
New York

NOTICE TO THE READER

Library of Congress Cataloging-in-Publication Data

Names: Silva, Maurício F. (Maurício Fraga), editor. | Marta, Gustavo Nader, editor. | Antunes, Luís C. M. (Luís Carlos Moreira), editor. | Lim, Fiona, editor. | Wan, Bo Angela, editor. | Amendola, Beatriz E., editor. | Merrick, Joav, 1950- editor.
Title: Cancer management in Latin America / [edited by Maurício F. Silva, Gustavo Nader Marta, Luis C.M. Antunes, Fiona Lim, Bo Angela Wan, Beatriz Amendola, Joav Merrick].
Description: New York : Nova Science Publishers, Inc., [2019-] | Series: Health and human development | Includes bibliographical references and index. | Contents: I. Nasopharyngeal to renal cancer -- |
Identifiers: LCCN 2019051794 (print) | LCCN 2019051795 (ebook) | ISBN 9781536167351 (hardcover) | ISBN 9781536167344 (adobe pdf)
Subjects: LCSH: Cancer--Treatment--Latin America.
Classification: LCC RC279.L29 C36 2019 (print) | LCC RC279.L29 (ebook) | DDC 362.19699/40098--dc23
LC record available at https://lccn.loc.gov/2019051794
LC ebook record available at https://lccn.loc.gov/2019051795

Published by Nova Science Publishers, Inc. † New York

Contents

INTRODUCTION

In: Cancer Management in Latin America II
Editors: Maurício F Silva et al.
ISBN: 978-1-53616-735-1

Chapter 1

CANCER MANAGEMENT IN LATIN AMERICA: MELANOMA TO COST-EFFECTIVENESS

Maurício F Silva[1,2,3]*, MD, PhD, Gustavo Nader Marta[4,5], MD, PhD, Luis CM Antunes[6,7], MD, PhD, Fiona Lim[8], MBBS, Bo Angela Wa[9], MPhil, Beatriz Amendola[4], MD and Joav Merrick[10-13], MD, MMedSci, DMSc

[1]Radiation Oncology Department, Santa Maria Federal University,Santa Maria, Brazil
[2]Radiation Oncology Unit, Hospital de Caridade Astrogildo de Azevedo, Santa Maria, Brazil
[3]Latin America Cooperative Oncology Group, Porto Alegre, Brazil
[4]Radiation Oncology Unit, Hospital Sírio Libanes, São Paulo, Brazil
[5]Instituto do Cancer do Estado de São Paulo, São Paulo, Brazil
[6]Clinica Viver, Santa Maria, Brazil
[7]Clinical Oncology Department, Santa Maria Federal University, Santa Maria, Brazil
[8]Department of Oncology, Princess Margaretti Hospital, Hong Kong, Chona
[9]Odette Cancer Centre, Sunnybrook Health Science Centre, Toronto, Canada
[10] National Institute of Child Health and Human Development, Jerusalen, Israel
[11]Department of Pediatrics, Mt Scopus Campus, Hadassah, Hebrew University Medical Center, Jerusalem, Israel
[12]Kentucky Children's Hospital, University of Kentucky, Lexington, Kentucky, United States
[13]Center for Healthy Development, School of Public Health, Georgia StateUniversity, Atlanta,United States

* Corresponding Author's Email: mauricio.f.silva@ufsm.br.

ABSTRACT

In book two, we continue our discussion of cancer in Latin America, first through management of Melanomas and sarcomas, followed by pediatric malignancies, gliomas, and lymphomas. After this, we focus on topics surrounding end-of-life care and quality of life, including metastases, cancer emergencies, and pain. Finally, this two-volume series will end on the cost-effectiveness of cancer care in Latin America We hope that this book will serve as a valuable resource of information to the health care professional and policy makers of Latin America.

INTRODUCTION

In book two, we continue our discussion of cancer in Latin America, first through management of Melanomas and sarcomas, followed by pediatric malignancies, gliomas, and lymphomas. After this, we focus on topics surrounding end-of-life care and quality of life, including metastases, cancer emergencies, and pain. Finally, this two-volume series will end on the cost-effectiveness of cancer care in Latin America in considering the topic as a whole.

Some exciting developments in the treatment of cancers include the utilization of targeted therapy through an understanding of the molecular signaling that drives abnormal cellular proliferation. For example, in melanomas, BRAF inhibitors like vemurafenib, and MEK inhibitors like trametinib significantly improve survival in this notoriously aggressive disease. The mainstay of treatment for non-Hodgkin lymphomas is chemotherapy with possible addition of rituximab, a monoclonal antibody against the cellular marker CD20. Recent development of targeted therapies and immunotherapies has allowed huge improvements in survival for non-Hodgkin lymphomas. Even in situations without cure, many patients can now expect to have normal life expectancies and will likely die from other causes, living with lymphoma as a chronic condition. This is likely the direction for many other types of cancer, with numerous clinical trials assessing the efficacy of targeted therapies and immunotherapies.

Improvements have also been made in improving morbidity. In general, targeted therapies have less side effects compared to chemotherapy. In addition, radiotherapy techniques are also being employed to reduce morbidity. In soft tissue sarcomas, radiation improves functional outcome by avoiding the need for amputations. Discussion of pediatric cancers largely focuses on the role of radiotherapy in enhancing disease control while limiting treatment-related toxicity. Radiotherapy is now part of the standard treatment for cure in Hodgkin's disease, with current investigations focusing on treatment deintensification to minimize toxicity.

Even in the face of incurable disease, there is a role for cancer management through the symptom palliation and pain relief. One such tool is radiotherapy, which is utilized in the acute setting to manage cancer emergencies such as spinal cord compression, and in reducing pain thorough treatment of bone metastases. In the latter half of this volume, we discuss management of end-stage cancer and various cancer symptoms.

Some of the common challenges in facing management these malignancies in Latin America include high costs of newer therapies, and a healthcare system with insufficient resources. Further development of more advanced therapies will need the support of a healthcare system capable of delivering it to the population in Latin America. We hope our book series can provide the oncologist with some insight as to the epidemiology, treatment conventions, and unique challenges on managing cancer in Latin America.

SECTION ONE: CANCER MANAGEMENT

In: Cancer Management in Latin America II
Editors: Maurício F Silva et al.
ISBN: 978-1-53616-735-1

Chapter 2

MANAGEMENT OF MELANOMA

Luís Carlos Moreira Antunes[1], MD, PhD, Adriano Teston[2,3], MD, PhD, Lucas Feijó Pereira[4], MD, Fiona Lim[5], MD, Bo Angela Wan[6], MD and Mauricio F Silva[2,3,7], MD, PhD

[1]Hematology and Oncology Service, Santa Maria University Hospital, Federal University of Santa Maria, Santa Maria, Brazil
[2]Radiation Oncology Unit, Hospital de Caridade Dr. Astrogildo de Azevedo, Santa Maria, Brazil
[3]Radiation Oncology Unit, Santa Maria University Hospital, Federal University of Santa Maria, Santa Maria, Brazil
[4]Department of Surgery, Santa Maria University Hospital, Federal University of Santa Maria, Brazil
[5]Department of Oncology, Princess Margaret Hospital, Hong Kong, PR China
[6]Odette Cancer Centre, Sunnybrook Health Sciences Centre, University of Toronto, Toronto, Canada
[7]Latin America Cooperative Oncology Group, Porto Alegre, Brazil

ABSTRACT

In recent decades, melanoma has increased incidence rates in Brazil and worldwide, besides, this tumor has a high capacity to generate metastases, resulting in high mortality rates. The success of early-stage treatment is dependent on surgical resection of the lesion, where compliance with the principles of oncologic surgery is essencial. When in advanced stages, overall survival is extremely low and until recently the response to cytotoxic chemotherapy, interferon and interleukin immunotherapy, or combination of these, was considered poor. Advances in the elucidation of the cellular and immunological mechanisms involved in the origin and progression of melanoma allowed the development of new therapies in both the adjuvant and the metastatic stages. However, new therapies also have limitations on response rates, disease control, toxicity, and cost. The latter limitation becomes more relevant when it comes to patients who rely, for the most part, on a public health system with insufficient resources.

INTRODUCTION

Except in Australia, melanoma incidence in moderate to high-risk populations has been increased at more than 3% annualy and is projected to continue rising (1, 2). According to the American Cancer Society, the US estimate for 2018 was 55,150 new cases of melanoma in men and 36,120 in women, with a total of 9,320 deaths in both sexes (3). There was an increase in the incidence rates of 1.8% in males and 2.3% in females between 2010 and 2014 (3). The highest incidence in the world occurs in Oceania, with melanoma occupying the fourth position among malignant neoplasms in Australia (4). In Brazil, the estimate for 2018 was 2,920 new cases in men and 3,340 in women, with estimated rates for Rio Grande do Sul, the southermoust state, of 8.02/100,000 for males and 7.09/100,000 for females (5). Publications in Latin America and/or Brazil are limited to data on icidence and mortality or reports of isolated institutions with a low number of patients (6). In Brazil, the largest country in Latin America, the main source of epidemiological data is from the Brazilian Population Based Cancer Registries.

With a much greater frequency in Caucasians than in blacks, the main risk factors for melanoma are: family history, multiple benign or atypical nevi, previous melanoma, immunosuppression, sensitivity to the sun, exposure to ultraviolet (UV) radiation, phenotypic characteristics including hair, light eyes and skin, and predisposition to the appearance of freckles (7, 8). The effect of exposure to UV light is the result of variations in specific genes (polymorphisms) that affect the skin's defensive response to UV light and, consequently, increase the risk of melanoma (7). There is damage to skin immune function, an increase in local production of growth factors, and the induction of the formation of reactive oxygen species that damage DNA (7). Interestingly, in Brazil that has an extensive area located between the equator and the tropic of capricorn, the highest incidence of melanoma is not concentrated in this region, but in areas with lower rates of ultraviolet radiation. These are located in the south and southeast and have, in turn, a higher concentration of European descendants (9-12).

Genetic alterations have been identified in both benign and melanoma nevi, suggesting a role in the initial stages of melanoma development (13, 14). These changes include *BRAF, NRAS, c-KIT, GNAQ, PTEN* and *MITF* (15-25).

In 25-40% of cases of familial melanoma, which represents 10% of melanomas, the *CDKN2A* locus is lost by deletion of a portion of chromosome 9 (25). This locus encodes proteins that act as tumor suppressors, such as *p16* (*INK4A*) and *p19* (25). Germline mutations in *CDKN2A* can be detected in 5% to 72% of cases, depending on the selection criteria used for the research and the geographic region (26). In Latin America, the mutation in *CDKN2A* has a frequency of 24% in families with a predisposition to melanoma (27). In the South of Brazil, the *CDKN2Ap.A148T* variant was identified as an allele of susceptibility, mainly in the descendants of Europeans (28).

In cases of non-familial or sporadic melanoma, *BRAF* mutation is present in about 50% of cases of cutaneous melanoma, especially in areas of skin without chronic solar damage (16, 17). Between 15% and 25% of cases of cutaneous melanoma occurs mutation of the *NRAS*, mainly in photo-exposed areas of skin (16, 29). These mutations in the *BRAF* and *NRAS* genes are mutually exclusive and cause the constitutive activation of serine-threonine kinases in the ERK-MAPK pathway stimulating growth in melanoma cells (14, 30-34). The *KIT* mutation is most frequent in melanomas of the mucosa (15 to 22%), acral and of areas of the body with chronic solar damage, and in these patients the *BRAF* mutation is not present (35-38).

PREVENTION

Access to dermatologists and other facilities that help in the early diagnosis of melanoma is very limited for the vast majority of the population that relies solely on public healthcare assistance in Latin America. On the other hand, it is worth noting the measure adopted in Brazil of prohibiting the use of sunbeds as of 2009. In 2014, the Brazilian consensus of photo protection was published by the Brazilian Society of Dermatology, taking into account the peculiarities of the Brazilian territory and its population (39). This consensus adopted the UVI scale and WHO general recommendation for photoprotection, as intensive protection (avoid sun exposure near noon, and use of T-shirts, sunscreen, sunglasses and hat) for UVI 6-10 (39). Protection with T-shirts, sunscreen and hat is also required for 3-4 UVIs (39).

CLINICAL STAGING

In the early stages (in situ, I, II and low-risk IIIA) laboratory exams (hemogram, hepatic function, lactate dehydrogenase) and imaging, can be done only for baseline staging and to evaluate specific signs and symptoms. In stage 0 (in situ) the routine imaging and lab tests is not recommended.

In patients with high-risk III-A, III-B and IIIC stages, ie, patients with at least 4-mm invasion depth, are evaluated with CT or MRI to exclude distant metastatic spread. Patients with clinical stage III (macroscopic lymph node metastasis), PET-CT has a rate of detection of distant metastasis up to 30% more than CT. The findings suggestive of metastases in patients with stages I to III should be confirmed by biopsy (40).

Stage IV evaluation should include magnetic resonance imaging (MRI), and PET-CT, especially when resection of single metastatic disease is planned.

According to the Brazilian Society of Nuclear Medicine, access to PET in Brazil is asymmetric and deficient. Only recently, in 2014, PET began to be offered by the SUS for patients with non-small cell lung cancer, colorectal cancer and lymphomas. In supplementary health, the coverage range is higher, and it can be used in the evaluation of patients with melanoma, however, half the number of devices are located in the southeastern region of the country (41).

SURGICAL TREATMENT OF CUTANEOUS MELANOMA

Cutaneous melanoma is a potential aggressive skin cancer. Prognosis and treatment depends on stage at presentation. Despite the arising of new clinical treatments for advanced stages, surgery still as the most important part of the treatment and diagnosis to majority of cases. The surgical treatment starts with an oriented biopsy of a suspicious pigmented lesion (42).

Biopsy

Table 1. Recommended margins

Thickness (breslow)	**Surgical margins**
In situ or lentigo maligna	0.5-1cm
≤1.0mm	1cm
1.01mm-≤2.0mm	1-2cm
>2.0mm	2cm

The biopsy is the initial part of the treatment of cutaneous melanoma. If possible, it should be done a totally excisional biopsy with narrow margins (between 1-3mm) and oriented parallel to lymphatics (longitudinal orientation on the extremities) to not interfere with lymphatic mapping. When it is impossible to make an excisional biopsy (including face, large lesions, plantar lesions), incisional or punch full-thickness biopsies should be done providing accurate micro-staging. Wide resection margins should be avoided to preserve correct lymphatic mapping (43). Figure 1 shows some principles of biopsy.

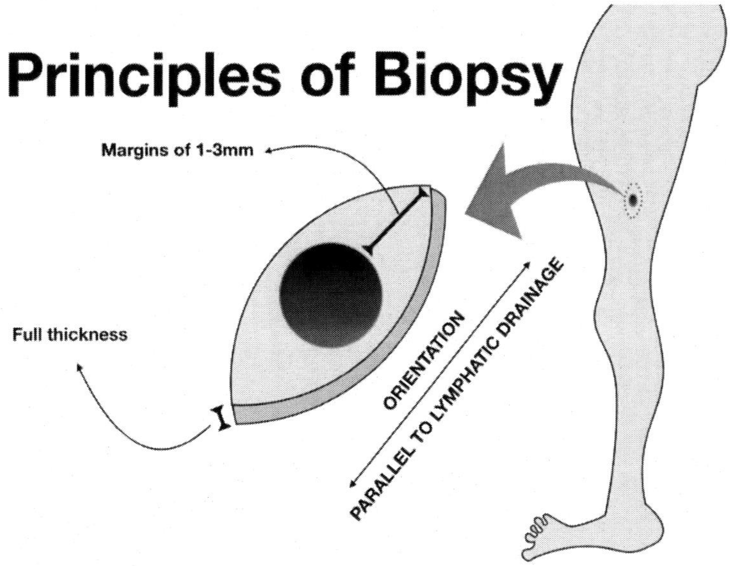

Figure 1.

Surgical wide resection

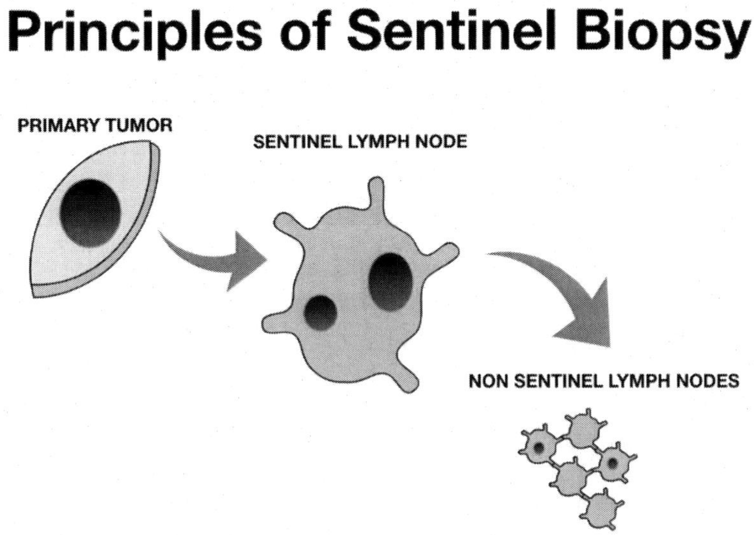

Figure 2.

The surgical resection is the base of cutaneous melanoma treatment. The surgical margins necessary for cutaneous melanoma are defined based on the thickness (Breslow level) of the primary tumor obtained after appropriated biopsy (see Table 1). Several trials have been conducted to define optimal surgical margins for primary melanoma. These trials did not show any benefit for margins larger than two cm, even for thicker melanomas. If the patient is not clinical fit for resection in cases of in situ melanoma or *lentigo maligna*, there are some studies showing high rates of response at least in short follow-up using topic Imiquimode® or radiation. But surgical resection is still the treatment of choice.

Sentinel lymph node biopsy (SLNB)

SLNB is a minimally invasive staging procedure developed to further risk-stratify patients with clinical stage I-II melanoma according to the presence or absence of subclinical nodal metastases (see Figure 2). Patients with positive SLNB are at higher risk of recurrence, and might be candidates for complete lymph node dissection (CLND) and/or adjuvant systemic therapy (44).

The sentinel lymph node biopsy is indicated in cases where melanoma is thicker than 0.8 mm or ulcerated (stage Ib) and there is not clinical positive lymph node. The propose of this procedure is determined if there is lymph node metastasis of cutaneous melanoma. There isn't indication for sentinel lymph node biopsy for *in situ* melanomas, *lentigo maligna* melanomas or stage Ia melanomas, because the risk of lymph node metastasis for this population is extremely low.

Sentinel lymph node biopsy is associated with increased melanoma-specific survival (i.e., survival until death from melanoma) among patients with node-positive intermediate-thickness melanomas (1.2 to 3.5 mm). The value of completion lymph node dissection for patients with sentinel node metastases is not clear (45).

The procedure is performed using nuclear medicine contrast (technetium 99m – ^{99m}Tc) or dye blue contrast. The accuracy is bigger when both modalities are performed simultaneously. The technique for SLNB consists of preoperative dynamic lymphoscintigraphy, intraoperative identification using isosulfan blue or methylene blue dye, and a gamma probe to detect radiolabeled lymph nodes (46-50). Many studies have reported high rates of successful SLN detection using this robust technique (>95%) (46-51).

Positive sentinel lymph node

Depending on a variety of factors described below, 5-40% of patients undergoing SLNB will be upstaged from clinical stage I-II to pathologic stage III, based on subclinical micrometastatic disease in the SLN (46-50, 52-58). Multivariate analyses have identified factors independently predictive of a positive SLN. The correlation between increased primary tumor thickness and SLN positivity is well established. Due in part to the low probability of finding a positive sentinel node in patients with thin primary melanomas (≤1 mm), the utility of SLNB in this population is controversial (49, 50, 52, 54, 55, 59-62).

When sentinel lymph node biopsy results positive for melanoma metastasis it is necessary observe some factors to decide performed or not lymph node dissection, as the likelihood for non-sentinel lymph node metastasis is around 20%. These factors are: size of sentinel lymph node metastasis, number of sentinel lymph nodes involved, distribution of metastasis inside de sentinel lymph node and primary tumor characteristics (thickness and ulceration). The prognosis evaluation obtained after lymph node dissection and non-sentinel lymph node metastasis demonstrate an important independent predictor of disease specific survival. This population is more likely to have distant metastasis than negative non sentinel lymph node population (46, 56, 63-66).

In a prespecified retrospective subset analysis of patients who developed nodal metastases from intermediate-thickness (1.2–3.5 mm) melanoma, MSLT-I confirmed a survival advantage to those with microscopic versus macroscopic disease at the time of detection and removal (10-year DSS for those detected by SLNB versus nodal basin observation: 62% vs. 41.5%, $p = 0.006$). A similar survival advantage was not seen in patients with thick (>3.5 mm) melanomas and positive nodes (67).

Two recent randomized clinical trials failed to demonstrate improved overall survival for complete lymph node dissection over observation with ultrasound after positive sentinel lymph node evaluation, but both demonstrated improved local control after complete lymph node dissection. Immediate completion lymph node dissection increased the rate of regional disease control and provided prognostic information but did not increase melanoma-specific survival among patients with melanoma and sentinel node metastases (45, 68).

Clinically positive lymph node

If there is a clinically positive lymph node but no distant metastasis, the best treatment is still complete lymph node dissection. The survival rates are between 30-50% after five years (69).

Pelvic lymph node dissection

In patients with clinical positive inguinal-femoral nodes, three or more positive inguinal-femoral nodes, or Cloquet's positive lymph node the risk of pelvic nodes metastasis is increased. The overall survival benefit of pelvic dissection is unknown in this population (70).

Morbility after lymph node dissection

Several studies report high rates of complications after lymph node dissection as 40-60%. Wound dehiscence, infection, neuropathy and lymphedema are the most important complications after this procedure (69-71).

RADIOTHERAPY

The major role of radiotherapy (RT) in melanoma treatment is in the adjuvant postoperative setting, mainly in patients who are at high risk of nodal recurrence. The aggressive desmoplastic subtype may require local irradiation after wide excision. For definitive treatment of initial disease, RT may be used for selected patients who have contraindications to have a radical resection, impossible to achieve negative margins or in the lentigo forms, which frequently involves critical anatomical areas.

Adjuvant postoperative

Adjuvant RT to regional nodes

The most common indication of radiation therapy in melanoma is to prevent nodal recurrence at high-risk non metastatic patients with palpable disease who had undergone lymphadenectomy. The ANZMTG 01.02/TROG 02.01 randomised controlled trial enrolled patients estimating the risk according to areas of lymph-node field (parotid and cervical, axilla, or groin), number of involved nodes (≤3 vs >3), maximum involved node diameter (≤4 cm vs >4 cm), and extent of extracapsular extension (none, limited, or extensive) to adjuvant RT 48Gy in 20 fractions (n = 123, 109 eligible for efficacy assessments) or observation (n=127,108 eligible). Inclusion criterias where to have LDH < 1.5 times the upper limit, ≥ 1 parotid, ≥ 2 cervical or axillary or ≥ 3 groin positive nodes, diameter ≥ 3cm in neck, ≥ 4 cm in the axilla or groin, or nodal extracapsular extension. After a median follow-up of 73 months (IQR 61–91) 23 (21%) relapses occurred in the adjuvant radiotherapy group compared with 39 (36%) in the observation group (adjusted hazard ratio (HR) 0·52 (95% CI 0·31–0·88), p=0·023). Minor, long-term toxic effects from radiotherapy (predominantly pain, and fibrosis of the skin or subcutaneous tissue) were common, and 20 (22%) of 90 patients receiving adjuvant radiotherapy developed grade 3–4 toxic effects. Eighteen (20%) of 90 patients had grade 3 toxic effects, mainly affecting skin (nine (10%) patients) and subcutaneous tissue (six (7%) patients). Over 5 years, a significant increase in lower limb volumes was noted after adjuvant radiotherapy (mean volume ratio 15·0%) compared with observation (7·7%; difference 7·3% (95% CI 1·5–13·1), p=0·014). No significant differences in upper limb volume were noted between groups. Despite these findings, the indication of adjuvant RT to nodal regions is already a matter of debate, based in the survival. The overall survival (HR 1·27 (95% CI 0·89–1·79), p=0·21) and relapse-free survival (0·89 (0·65–1·22), p=0·51) did not differ between groups (72).

Adjuvant RT to primary site

Retrospectives studies have shown that adjuvant RT may be beneficial in the aggressive desmoplastic neurotropic melanoma (DNM). The major serie of literature reviewed 277 patients from 1989 through 2010 who were treated for nonmetastatic desmoplastic melanoma by surgery with or without adjuvant RT. A total of 113 patients (40.8%) received adjuvant RT. After a median follow-up of 43.1 months, adjuvant RT was found to be independently associated with improved local control on multivariable analysis (hazards ratio, 0.15; 95% confidence interval, 0.06-0.39 ($p < 0.001$)). Among 35 patients with positive resection margins, 14% who received RT developed a local recurrence versus 54% who did not ($p = 0.004$). In patients with negative resection margins, there was a trend ($p = 0.09$) toward improved local control with RT. In patients with negative resection margins and traditionally high-risk features, including a head and neck tumor location, a Breslow depth > 4 mm, or a Clark level V tumor, RT was found to significantly improve local control ($p < 0.05$) (73). This and other studies raised the hypothesis that RT may be used as adjuvant treatment in order to improves local control in DNM. An ongoing phase III trial is trying to clarify this matter, where patients are randomised to receive adjuvant curative post-operative radiation therapy aiming to reduce the rate of local recurrence. The recommended dose prescribed is 48 Gy in 20 fractions over four weeks (74).

Definitive RT

For the superficial lentigo maligna (LM), confined to the epidermis, and lentigo maligna melanoma, invasive into the dermis, RT may be an effective treatment to achieve local control. It should be considered in lesions not amenable for exicions, due to cosmesis, functional and/or medical conditions (75). Management of LM may be challenging, as frequently involves head and neck region. Sometimes, wide excision requires extensive reconstruction. Although lacking of evidence-based treatment, radiotherapy and nonsurgical therapies have beam increasingly used. A systematic review of retrospectives studies, revealed outcomes of 349 patients treated with RT, and found 18 (5%) recurrences after a median follow-up of three years. There were five marginal recurrences documented out of 123 assessable patients (4%). There were eight in-field recurrences documented with either LM (five) or LMM (three) out of 171 assessable patients (5%). The majority relapses as LM was salvage using further RT, surgery or other therapies. Progression as LM melanoma occurred in five patients (76). As the primary treatment, RT has a limited role for invasive melanomas at initial stages. There is limited evidence analysing its effectiveness in more deeply invasive disease and must be reserved only for carefully selected cases.

Radiotherapy and immunotherapy

The systemic effects of RT have long been observed, when tumoral response are seen outside treatment fields, known as abscopal effect. Molecular evidence support a immune response that may become systemic, when cancer antigens are exposed to defence cells by radiation and reverses some immunosuppressive barriers, driven an inflammatory cascade (77). Since the advent of immunotherapy, this phenomenon have gained considerable interest. There are plenty preclinical data supporting a synergistic response when this treatment is associated with RT, enhancing response rates in and outside fields (78). Although in the clinical setting, there is only a low level of evidence to support such findings. Further prospective data are needed to establish the efficacy and safety on the combination of targeted therapy and RT. With the widespread use of immunotherapy, there is a concern about how they interact in terms of toxicities.

Radiotherapy and BRAF inhibitors

Up to 50% of melanomas cases caries *BRAF* mutations. Their inhibitors (BRAFi) have been found to significantly improve survival. The prospective trial testing BRAFi and MEKi excluded RT, resulting in a lack of data when used combined. But there is reports regarding dermatologic and visceral toxicity in patients treated with RT prior to, during, or subsequent to treatment with vemurafenib or dobrafenib. The Eastern Cooperative Oncology Group (ECOG) reviewed literature and outlined a guideline, with the main recommendations summarized below (79).

- BRAFi and MEKi recommendations (eg, vemurafenib/dabrafenib and trametinib/cobimetinib)
- Hold ≥3 days before and after fractionated RT.
- Hold ≥1 day before and after SRS.
- RT recommendations
- Consider dose per fraction <4 Gy unless using a stereotactic approach or the patient has very poor prognosis/performance status.
- For adjuvant nodal basin RT, consider a dose ≤48 to 50 Gy in 20 fractions.
- For spine metastases, consider posterior oblique RT fields when feasible and safe to minimize exit dose through visceral organs.

Radiotherapy and checkpoint immunotherapy

Although several studies have reported improvement in some outcomes such as response rates and survival by combining RT with checkpoint inhibitors (ipilimumab or nivolumab), other retrospective data fail to demonstrate a benefit. Abscopal responses were also observed. In brain metastases, analyzes of these data have hypothesized that there may be an optimal sequence, crucial for the success of the combined modality treatment (80). In terms of toxicities, the evidence suggest the safety on the combination of checkpoint inhibitors (ipilimumab or nivolumab) both for brain and visceral metastasis (81, 82). There are ongoing prospective trials to further explore these findings. Until a solid platform of data is expected to be released, treatment choices must be carefully performed by a multidisciplinary team (83).

SYSTEMIC TREATMENT

Adjuvant treatment

Prior to approval of target therapies and checkpoint inhibitors, the only therapy that showed benefit in overall survival, although small (3% in five years), was interferon-alpha (84, 85). With significant toxicity, high doses of interferon-alpha result in frequent constitutional, hematological and neurological adverse events, and in most cases grade 3 cases (85). In the setting of the public health system, the use of adjuvant interferon can be considered in patients with good performance, ulcerated primary lesion and more than 2 mm thick Breslow (IIC-III) (84, 85).

Based on the RFS and OS results of the EORTC-18071 trial that evaluated the adjuvant use of cytotoxic T-lymphocyte-associated protein-4 (CTLA-4) blocking antibody ipilimumab, the FDA licensed its use for patients with stage-3 melanoma after lymphadenectomy, but its use in this scenario of adjuvancy was not approved in Brazil by the Brazilian Health Regulatory Agency (ANVISA) (85, 86).

For stage III patients in the private healthcare system, there are the options of targeted therapies (for patients with $BRAF^{V600E/K}$ mutation) and, more recently, the anti-PD-1 antibodies (for all comers) (87-89). Brazil was one of the first countries to approve the use of the combination of dabrafenib and trametinib in adjuvant, based on the results of COMBI-AD trial which showed benefits of RFS (HR 0.47 vs placebo) and OS (HR 0.57 vs placebo), with a reduction in risk of relapse or death of 53% (87).

At the beginning of this year the use of pembrolizumab in adjuvancy was approved in Brazil, based on the results of the Phase III study Keynote 054. This study showed, after a 15-month follow-up, a 43% reduction in the relative risk of relapse or death when compared to placebo (HR = 0.57; IC 98.4%: 0.43-0.74; $p < 0.001$) (88).

This year we also had the approval in Brazil of the use of nivolumab for adjuvant treatment. The Chekmate-238 study revealed superior RFS with nivolumab compared to ipilimumab (HR 0.65). With excellent tolerability, only 4% of patients discontinued nivolumabe compared to a 30% discontinuation for iplimumab (89).

Management of stage IV disease

Patients with stage IV distant metastatic disease are subjected to confirm the suspicion of metastatic disease with FNA or core, incisional, or excisional biopsy of the metastases. In private facilities, genetic analyses (eg, *BRAF* or *KIT* mutation status) are available for patients being considered for treatment with targed therapy, or to participation in a clinical trial. Brain metastases are often treated without histologic confirmation.

Initial studies showed that *BRAF* inhibitors have an objective response rates of approximately 50% and, subsequently, these rates increased to 70% with the combination with MEK inhibitors (90-94). With disease control rates exceeding 90% (complete response, partial response, or stable disease), and with increasing progression-free survival (7-9 months with BRAF inhibitor monotherapy to 11-14.9 months with BRAF and MEK inhibitors), the combined treatment has become an estabilished standard regimen in various parts of the world, including Brazil. Complete responses were reported in 16% of patients with metastatic melanoma treated with this combination, and 3-5 year overall survival has reached 40% (90, 95).

Three BRAF-MEK inhibitor combination are presently on the market: vemurafenibe and cobimetinib, dabrafenib and trametinib, and encorafenib and binimetinib. These treatment combinations have similar efficacy, whereas their toxicity profiles differ in some regards, for instance, dabrafenib-trametinib is more commonly associated with pyrexia, whereas the vemurafenib-cobimetinib combination is more associated with increased photosensitivity. On the other hand, the adding of MEK inhibitor reduced cutaneous toxicity and the development of non-melanoma skin cancer lesion by BRAF inhibitor monotherapy. These combinations are an excellent choice for patients with symptomatic melanoma with rapidly progression tumours who require rapid response regardless of localization of metastasis (including intracranial reponse rates of up to 55%) and of tumour burden (96). Special care must be taken when applying concurrent radiation therapy due to the risk of increased toxicity, including cases of radionecrosis and severe dermatitis (79).

Regarding new immunotherapies for melanoma, the use of monotherapy with checkpoint inhibitors against CTLA4 (ipilimumab) and PD-1 (pembrolizumab and nivolumab) is approved in Brazil, although not provided by SUS. In supplementary health, patients may receive monotherapy with ipilimumab, pembrolizumab or nivolumab. First to be approved in the market, ipilimumab presents an increase in the percentage of long-term survival to around 20% in patients with metastatic melanoma. On the other hand, nivolumab and pembrolizumab, present superior efficacy when compared to ipilimumab or chemotherapy, and with less toxicity (97-112). Therefore, PD-1 inhibitors are preferably used, where available, over ipilimumab (113). The latter is used as a rescue, after the use of PD-1 inhibitors, as suggested by the Checkmate-64 study (114). Immune Related Adverse Events (IrAEs), such as pneumonitis, hypothyroidism and hyperthyroidism, are monitored and managed according to guidelines developed and established by interdisciplinary groups around the world (115, 116). Combinations of immunotherapy, such as nivolumab and ipilimumab, are expected to be approved in Brazil, especially for those patients with worse prognostic factors (expression of PD-L1 in less than 1% of melanoma cells, elevated serum lactate dehydrogenase, mucosal melanoma, and cerebral metastasis) (117). Resistance to PD-1 checkpoint inhibition is predicted to occur around 20-30% of initial responders. In these cases, treatments to which the patient has not been exposed previously, such as ipilimumab, targeted therapy according to mutational status, or chemotherapy, are chosen (8, 114).

Although widely used in private facilities, neither immunotherapies nor target therapies are offered for patients treated in public healthcare in Brazil. Only treatment with chemotherapy, mostly with monotherapy with dacarbazine. Polichemotherapy therapy regimens such as CVD (cisplatin, vinblastine and DTIC) and Dartmouth regimen (cisplatin, DTIC and carmustine) are also used (118).

According to a study recently published by Melo et al., which evaluated the epidemiology of melanoma in Brazil between 2000 and 2014, the patients attended by the SUS represented 77.1% of the patients included and around 76% of the entire population of Brazil (12). Due to the recognized lower response of chemotherapy in metastatic melanoma, many isolated cases are judicialized to receive treatment with immunotherapy or target therapies.

CONCLUSION

Latin America has an extensive territorial area, with a wide range of exposure to solar UV radiation as well as a diversity of ethnic patterns. In addition, with an aging population trend, it is expected that the incidence of melanoma will continue to increase over the coming decades. In Brazil, efforts are being made with government health agencies, with the aim of reducing the disparity between the treatment offered to patients who depend on SUS and those privileged with access to supplementary health care.

REFERENCES

[1] Siegel R. L., Miller K. D., Jemal A. *Cancer Statistics, 2017*. CA Cancer J Clin 2017;67(1):7-30.

[2] Whiteman DC, Green AC, Olsen CM. *The growing burden of invasive melanoma: projections of incidence rates and numbers of new cases in six susceptible populations through 2031*. J Invest Dermatol 2016;136(6):1161-71.

[3] Siegel RL, Miller KD, Jemal A. *Cancer statistics, 2018*. CA Cancer J Clin 2018;68(1):7-30.

[4] *Cancer survival and prevalence in Australia: period estimates from 1982 to 2010.* Asia Pac J Clin Oncol 2013;9(1):29-39.

[5] INCA. Estimativa 2018: *Incidência de câncer no Brasil.* Rio de Janeiro: INCA, 2017.

[6] Schmerling RA, Loria D, Cinat G, Ramos WE, Cardona AF, Sanchez JL, et al. *Cutaneous melanoma in Latin America: the need for more data.* Rev Panam Salud Publica 2011;30(5):431-8.

[7] Miller AJ, Mihm MC Jr. *Melanoma.* N Engl J Med 2006;355(1):51-65.

[8] Schadendorf D, van Akkooi ACJ, Berking C, Griewank KG, Gutzmer R, Hauschild A, et al. *Melanoma.* Lancet 2018;392(10151):971-84.

[9] Bakos L, Masiero NC, Bakos RM, Burttet RM, Wagner MB, Benzano D. *European ancestry and cutaneous melanoma in Southern Brazil.* J Eur Acad Dermatol Venereol 2009;23(3):304-7.

[10] Eide MJ, Weinstock MA. *Association of UV index, latitude, and melanoma incidence in nonwhite populations--US Surveillance, Epidemiology, and End Results (SEER) Program*, 1992 to 2001. Arch Dermatol. 2005;141(4):477-81.

[11] Hu S, Ma F, Collado-Mesa F, Kirsner RS. *UV radiation, latitude, and melanoma in US Hispanics and blacks.* Arch Dermatol 2004;140(7):819-24.

[12] de Melo AC, Wainstein AJA, Buzaid AC, Thuler LCS. *Melanoma signature in Brazil: epidemiology, incidence, mortality, and trend lessons from a continental mixed population country in the past 15 years.* Melanoma Res 2018;28(6):629-36.

[13] Baxter AJ, Hughes MC, Kvaskoff M, Siskind V, Shekar S, Aitken JF, et al. *The Queensland Study of Melanoma: environmental and genetic associations (Q-MEGA); study design, baseline characteristics, and repeatability of phenotype and sun exposure measures.* Twin Res Hum Genet 2008;11(2):183-96.

[14] Davies H, Bignell GR, Cox C, Stephens P, Edkins S, Clegg S, et al. *Mutations of the BRAF gene in human cancer.* Nature 2002;417(6892):949-54.

[15] Pollock PM, Harper UL, Hansen KS, Yudt LM, Stark M, Robbins CM, et al. *High frequency of BRAF mutations in nevi.* Nat Genet 2003;33(1):19-20.

[16] Platz A, Egyhazi S, Ringborg U, Hansson J. *Human cutaneous melanoma; a review of NRAS and BRAF mutation frequencies in relation to histogenetic subclass and body site.* Mol Oncol 2008;1(4):395-405.

[17] Bauer J, Buttner P, Murali R, Okamoto I, Kolaitis NA, Landi MT, et al. *BRAF mutations in cutaneous melanoma are independently associated with age, anatomic site of the primary tumor, and the degree of solar elastosis at the primary tumor site.* Pigment Cell Melanoma Res 2011;24(2):345-51.

[18] Goel VK, Lazar AJ, Warneke CL, Redston MS, Haluska FG. *Examination of mutations in BRAF, NRAS, and PTEN in primary cutaneous melanoma.* J Invest Dermatol 2006;126(1):154-60.

[19] Curtin JA, Busam K, Pinkel D, Bastian BC. *Somatic activation of KIT in distinct subtypes of melanoma.* J Clin Oncol 2006;24(26):4340-6.

[20] Van Raamsdonk CD, Bezrookove V, Green G, Bauer J, Gaugler L, O'Brien JM, et al. *Frequent somatic mutations of GNAQ in uveal melanoma and blue naevi. Nature 2009*;457(7229):599-602.

[21] Mirmohammadsadegh A, Marini A, Nambiar S, Hassan M, Tannapfel A, Ruzicka T, et al. *Epigenetic silencing of the PTEN gene in melanoma.* Cancer Res 2006;66(13):6546-52.

[22] Ibrahim N, Haluska FG. *Molecular pathogenesis of cutaneous melanocytic neoplasms.* Annu Rev Pathol 2009;4:551-79.

[23] Levy C, Khaled M, Fisher DE. *MITF: master regulator of melanocyte development and melanoma oncogene.* Trends Mol Med 2006;12(9):406-14.

[24] Yajima I, Kumasaka MY, Thang ND, Goto Y, Takeda K, Iida M, et al. *Molecular Network Associated with MITF in Skin Melanoma Development and Progression.* J Skin Cancer 2011:730170.

[25] Ghosh P, Chin L. *Genetics and genomics of melanoma.* Expert Rev Dermatol 2009;4(2):131.

[26] Potrony M, Badenas C, Aguilera P, Puig-Butille JA, Carrera C, Malvehy J, et al. *Update in genetic susceptibility in melanoma.* Ann Transl Med 2015;3(15):210.

[27] Puig S, Potrony M, Cuellar F, Puig-Butille JA, Carrera C, Aguilera P, et al. *Characterization of individuals at high risk of developing melanoma in Latin America: bases for genetic counseling in melanoma*. Genet Med 2016;18(7):727-36.

[28] Bakos RM, Besch R, Zoratto GG, Godinho JM, Mazzotti NG, Ruzicka T, et al. *The CDKN2A p.A148T variant is associated with cutaneous melanoma in Southern Brazil*. Exp Dermatol 2011;20(11):890-3.

[29] Mangana J, Cheng PF, Schindler K, Weide B, Held U, Frauchiger AL, et al. *Analysis of BRAF and NRAS Mutation Status in Advanced Melanoma Patients Treated with Anti-CTLA-4 Antibodies: Association with Overall Survival?* PLoS One 2015;10(10):e0139438.

[30] Welsh CF, Roovers K, Villanueva J, Liu Y, Schwartz MA, Assoian RK. *Timing of cyclin D1 expression within G1 phase is controlled by Rho*. Nat Cell Biol 2001;3(11):950-7.

[31] Brunet A, Roux D, Lenormand P, Dowd S, Keyse S, Pouyssegur J. *Nuclear translocation of p42/p44 mitogen-activated protein kinase is required for growth factor-induced gene expression and cell cycle entry*. EMBO J 1999;18(3):664-74.

[32] Lin AW, Barradas M, Stone JC, van Aelst L, Serrano M, Lowe SW. *Premature senescence involving p53 and p16 is activated in response to constitutive MEK/MAPK mitogenic signaling*. Genes Dev 1998;12(19):3008-19.

[33] Albino AP, Nanus DM, Mentle IR, Cordon-Cardo C, McNutt NS, Bressler J, et al. *Analysis of ras oncogenes in malignant melanoma and precursor lesions: correlation of point mutations with differentiation phenotype*. Oncogene 1989;4(11):1363-74.

[34] Omholt K, Platz A, Kanter L, Ringborg U, Hansson J. *NRAS and BRAF mutations arise early during melanoma pathogenesis and are preserved throughout tumor progression*. Clin Cancer Res 2003;9(17):6483-8.

[35] Gajewski TF. *Molecular profiling of melanoma and the evolution of patient-specific therapy*. Semin Oncol 2011;38(2):236-42.

[36] Flaherty KT. *Narrative review: BRAF opens the door for therapeutic advances in melanoma*. Ann Intern Med 2010;153(9):587-91.

[37] Woodman SE, Davies MA. *Targeting KIT in melanoma: a paradigm of molecular medicine and targeted therapeutics*. Biochem Pharmacol 2010;80(5):568-74.

[38] Posch C, Moslehi H, Feeney L, Green GA, Ebaee A, Feichtenschlager V, et al. *Combined targeting of MEK and PI3K/mTOR effector pathways is necessary to effectively inhibit NRAS mutant melanoma in vitro and in vivo*. Proc Natl Acad Sci USA 2013;110(10):4015-20.

[39] Schalka S, Steiner D, Ravelli FN, Steiner T, Terena AC, Marcon CR, et al. *Brazilian consensus on photoprotection*. An Bras Dermatol 2014;89(6 Suppl 1):1-74.

[40] Smyth EC, Hsu M, Panageas KS, Chapman PB. *Histology and outcomes of newly detected lung lesions in melanoma patients*. Ann Oncol 2012;23(3):577-82.

[41] SBMN. Acesso à tecnologia é deficitário e assimétrico no País. 2016.. URL: http://sbmn.org.br/pet-ct-acesso-a-tecnologia-deficitario-e-assimetrico-no-pais-prejudica-assistencia-a-populacao-brasileira/.

[42] Balch CM, Gershenwald JE, Soong SJ, Thompson JF, Atkins MB, Byrd DR, et al. *Final version of 2009 AJCC melanoma staging and classification*. J Clin Oncol 2009;27(36):6199-206.

[43] Tadiparthi S, Panchani S, Iqbal A. *Biopsy for malignant melanoma--are we following the guidelines*? Ann R Coll Surg Engl 2008;90(4):322-5.

[44] Johnson TM, Sondak VK, Bichakjian CK, Sabel MS. *The role of sentinel lymph node biopsy for melanoma: evidence assessment*. J Am Acad Dermatol 2006;54(1):19-27.

[45] Faries MB, Thompson JF, Cochran AJ, Andtbacka RH, Mozzillo N, Zager JS, et al. *Completion Dissection or Observation for Sentinel-Node Metastasis in Melanoma*. N Engl J Med 2017;376(23):2211-22.

[46] Statius Muller MG, van Leeuwen PA, de Lange-De Klerk ES, van Diest PJ, Pijpers R, Ferwerda CC, et al. *The sentinel lymph node status is an important factor for predicting clinical outcome in patients with Stage I or II cutaneous melanoma.* Cancer 2001;91(12):2401-8.

[47] Bedrosian I, Faries MB, Guerry Dt, Elenitsas R, Schuchter L, Mick R, et al. *Incidence of sentinel node metastasis in patients with thin primary melanoma*(< or = 1 mm) with vertical growth phase. Ann Surg Oncol 2000;7(4):262-7.

[48] Statius Muller MG, van Leeuwen PA, van Diest PJ, Vuylsteke RJ, Pijpers R, Meijer S. *No indication for performing sentinel node biopsy in melanoma patients with a Breslow thickness of less than 0.9 mm.* Melanoma Res 2001;11(3):303-7.

[49] Rousseau DL, Jr., Ross MI, Johnson MM, Prieto VG, Lee JE, Mansfield PF, et al. *Revised American Joint Committee on Cancer staging criteria accurately predict sentinel lymph node positivity in clinically node-negative melanoma patients.* Ann Surg Oncol 2003;10(5):569-74.

[50] Olah J, Gyulai R, Korom I, Varga E, Dobozy A. *Tumour regression predicts higher risk of sentinel node involvement in thin cutaneous melanomas.* Br J Dermatol 2003;149(3):662-3.

[51] Kesmodel SB, Karakousis GC, Botbyl JD, Canter RJ, Lewis RT, Wahl PM, et al. *Mitotic rate as a predictor of sentinel lymph node positivity in patients with thin melanomas.* Ann Surg Oncol 2005;12(6):449-58.

[52] Sondak VK, Taylor JM, Sabel MS, Wang Y, Lowe L, Grover AC, et al. *Mitotic rate and younger age are predictors of sentinel lymph node positivity: lessons learned from the generation of a probabilistic model.* Ann Surg Oncol 2004;11(3):247-58.

[53] Fontaine D, Parkhill W, Greer W, Walsh N. *Partial regression of primary cutaneous melanoma: is there an association with sub-clinical sentinel lymph node metastasis*? Am J Dermatopathol 2003;25(5):371-6.

[54] Borgognoni L, Urso C, Vaggelli L, Brandani P, Gerlini G, Reali UM. *Sentinel node biopsy procedures with an analysis of recurrence patterns and prognosis in melanoma patients: technical advantages using computer-assisted gamma probe with adjustable collimation.* Melanoma Res 2004;14(4):311-9.

[55] Kruper LL, Spitz FR, Czerniecki BJ, Fraker DL, Blackwood-Chirchir A, Ming ME, et al. *Predicting sentinel node status in AJCC stage I/II primary cutaneous melanoma.* Cancer 2006;107(10):2436-45.

[56] Cascinelli N, Bombardieri E, Bufalino R, Camerini T, Carbone A, Clemente C, et al. *Sentinel and nonsentinel node status in stage IB and II melanoma patients: two-step prognostic indicators of survival.* J Clin Oncol 2006;24(27):4464-71.

[57] Morton DL, Thompson JF, Cochran AJ, Mozzillo N, Nieweg OE, Roses DF, et al. *Final trial report of sentinel-node biopsy versus nodal observation in melanoma.* N Engl J Med 2014;370(7):599-609.

[58] Nowecki ZI, Rutkowski P, Nasierowska-Guttmejer A, Ruka W. *Survival analysis and clinicopathological factors associated with false-negative sentinel lymph node biopsy findings in patients with cutaneous melanoma.* Ann Surg Oncol 2006;13(12):1655-63.

[59] Taylor RC, Patel A, Panageas KS, Busam KJ, Brady MS. *Tumor-infiltrating lymphocytes predict sentinel lymph node positivity in patients with cutaneous melanoma.* J Clin Oncol 2007;25(7):869-75.

[60] Azimi F, Scolyer RA, Rumcheva P, Moncrieff M, Murali R, McCarthy SW, et al. *Tumor-infiltrating lymphocyte grade is an independent predictor of sentinel lymph node status and survival in patients with cutaneous melanoma.* J Clin Oncol 2012;30(21):2678-83.

[61] Speijers MJ, Bastiaannet E, Sloot S, Suurmeijer AJ, Hoekstra HJ. *Tumor mitotic rate added to the equation: melanoma prognostic factors changed*? A single-institution database study on the prognostic value of tumor mitotic rate for sentinel lymph node status and survival of cutaneous melanoma patients. Ann Surg Oncol 2015;22(9):2978-87.

[62] Munsch C, Lauwers-Cances V, Lamant L, Gentil C, Rochaix P, Garrido I, et al. *Breslow thickness, clark index and ulceration are associated with sentinel lymph node metastasis in melanoma patients: a cohort analysis of 612 patients.* Dermatology 2014;229(3):183-9.

[63] Balch CM, Soong SJ, Gershenwald JE, Thompson JF, Reintgen DS, Cascinelli N, et al. *Prognostic factors analysis of 17,600 melanoma patients: validation of the American Joint Committee on Cancer melanoma staging system*. J Clin Oncol 2001;19(16):3622-34.

[64] Lima Sanchez J, Sanchez Medina M, Garcia Duque O, Fiuza Perez M, Carreteri Hernandez G, Fernandez Palacios J. *Sentinel lymph node biopsy for cutaneous melanoma: a 6 years study*. Indian J Plast Surg 2013;46(1):92-7.

[65] Yamamoto M, Fisher KJ, Wong JY, Koscso JM, Konstantinovic MA, Govsyeyev N, et al. *Sentinel lymph node biopsy is indicated for patients with thick clinically lymph node-negative melanoma*. Cancer 2015;121(10):1628-36.

[66] Wright BE, Scheri RP, Ye X, Faries MB, Turner RR, Essner R, et al. *Importance of sentinel lymph node biopsy in patients with thin melanoma*. Arch Surg 2008;143(9):892-9; discussion 9-900.

[67] Morton DL, Cochran AJ, Thompson JF, Elashoff R, Essner R, Glass EC, et al. *Sentinel node biopsy for early-stage melanoma: accuracy and morbidity in MSLT-I, an international multicenter trial*. Ann Surg 2005;242(3):302-13.

[68] Leiter U, Stadler R, Mauch C, Hohenberger W, Brockmeyer N, Berking C, et al. *Complete lymph node dissection versus no dissection in patients with sentinel lymph node biopsy positive melanoma (DeCOG-SLT): a multicentre, randomised, phase 3 trial*. Lancet Oncol 2016;17(6):757-67.

[69] Balch CM. *The role of elective lymph node dissection in melanoma: rationale, results, and controversies*. J Clin Oncol 1988;6(1):163-72.

[70] Chu CK, Delman KA, Carlson GW, Hestley AC, Murray DR. *Inguinopelvic lymphadenectomy following positive inguinal sentinel lymph node biopsy in melanoma: true frequency of synchronous pelvic metastases*. Ann Surg Oncol 2011;18(12):3309-15.

[71] Glarner CE, Greenblatt DY, Rettammel RJ, Neuman HB, Weber SM. *Wound complications after inguinal lymph node dissection for melanoma: is ACS NSQIP adequate?* Ann Surg Oncol 2013;20(6):2049-55.

[72] Henderson MA, Burmeister BH, Ainslie J, Fisher R, Di Iulio J, Smithers BM, et al. *Adjuvant lymph-node field radiotherapy versus observation only in patients with melanoma at high risk of further lymph-node field relapse after lymphadenectomy (ANZMTG 01.02/TROG 02.01): 6-year follow-up of a phase 3, randomised controlled trial*. Lancet Oncol 2015;16(9):1049-60.

[73] Strom T., Caudell J. J., Han D., Zager J. S., Yu D., Cruse C. W., et al. *Radiotherapy influences local control in patients with desmoplastic melanoma.* Cancer 2014;120(9):1369-78.

[74] NIH. *A randomised trial of post-operative radiation therapy following wide excision of neurotropic melanoma of the head and neck (RTN2)*. URL: https://clin icaltrials.gov/ct2/show/NCT00975520.

[75] Read T, Noonan C, David M, Wagels M, Foote M, Schaider H, et al. *A systematic review of non-surgical treatments for lentigo maligna*. J Eur Acad Dermatol Venereol 2016;30(5):748-53.

[76] Fogarty GB, Hong A, Scolyer RA, Lin E, Haydu L, Guitera P, et al. *Radiotherapy for lentigo maligna: a literature review and recommendations for treatment*. Br J Dermatol 2014;170(1):52-8.

[77] Formenti SC, Demaria S. *Systemic effects of local radiotherapy*. Lancet Oncol 2009;10(7):718-26.

[78] Formenti SC, Demaria S. *Combining radiotherapy and cancer immunotherapy: a paradigm shift*. J Natl Cancer Inst 2013;105(4):256-65.

[79] Anker CJ, Grossmann KF, Atkins MB, Suneja G, Tarhini AA, Kirkwood JM. *Avoiding Severe Toxicity From Combined BRAF Inhibitor and Radiation Treatment: Consensus Guidelines from the Eastern Cooperative Oncology Group (ECOG)*. Int J Radiat Oncol Biol Phys 2016;95(2):632-46.

[80] Schmidberger H, Rapp M, Ebersberger A, Hey-Koch S, Loquai C, Grabbe S, et al. *Long-term survival of patients after ipilimumab and hypofractionated brain radiotherapy for brain metastases of malignant melanoma: sequence matters.* Strahlenther Onkol 2018;194(12):1144-51.

[81] Patel KR, Shoukat S, Oliver DE, Chowdhary M, Rizzo M, Lawson DH, et al. *Ipilimumab and stereotactic radiosurgery versus stereotactic radiosurgery alone for newly diagnosed melanoma brain metastases.* Am J Clin Oncol 2017;40(5): 444-50.

[82] Barker CA, Postow MA, Khan SA, Beal K, Parhar PK, Yamada Y, et al. *Concurrent radiotherapy and ipilimumab immunotherapy for patients with melanoma.* Cancer Immunol Res 2013;1(2):92-8.

[83] Crittenden M, Kohrt H, Levy R, Jones J, Camphausen K, Dicker A, et al. *Current clinical trials testing combinations of immunotherapy and radiation.* Semin Radiat Oncol 2015;25(1):54-64.

[84] Ives NJ, Suciu S, Eggermont AMM, Kirkwood J, Lorigan P, Markovic SN, et al. *Adjuvant interferon-alpha for the treatment of high-risk melanoma: An individual patient data meta-analysis.* Eur J Cancer 2017;82:171-83.

[85] Napolitano S, Brancaccio G, Argenziano G, Martinelli E, Morgillo F, Ciardiello F, et al. *It is finally time for adjuvant therapy in melanoma.* Cancer Treat Rev 2018;69:101-11.

[86] Eggermont AM, Chiarion-Sileni V, Grob JJ, Dummer R, Wolchok JD, Schmidt H, et al. *Adjuvant ipilimumab versus placebo after complete resection of high-risk stage III melanoma (EORTC 18071): a randomised, double-blind, phase 3 trial.* Lancet Oncol 2015;16(5):522-30.

[87] Long GV, Hauschild A, Santinami M, Atkinson V, Mandala M, Chiarion-Sileni V, et al. *Adjuvant Dabrafenib plus Trametinib in Stage III BRAF-Mutated Melanoma.* N Engl J Med 2017;377(19):1813-23.

[88] Eggermont AMM, Blank CU, Mandala M, Long GV, Atkinson V, Dalle S, et al. *Adjuvant pembrolizumab versus placebo in resected stage III Melanoma.* N Engl J Med. 2018 May 10;378(19):1789-801.

[89] Weber J, Mandala M, Del Vecchio M, Gogas HJ, Arance AM, Cowey CL, et al. *Adjuvant Nivolumab versus Ipilimumab in Resected Stage III or IV melanoma.* N Engl J Med 2017;377(19):1824-35.

[90] Ascierto PA, McArthur GA, Dreno B, Atkinson V, Liszkay G, Di Giacomo AM, et al. *Cobimetinib combined with vemurafenib in advanced BRAF(V600)-mutant melanoma (coBRIM): updated efficacy results from a randomised, double-blind, phase 3 trial.* Lancet Oncol 2016;17(9):1248-60.

[91] Larkin J, Ascierto PA, Dreno B, Atkinson V, Liszkay G, Maio M, et al. *Combined vemurafenib and cobimetinib in BRAF-mutated melanoma.* N Engl J Med 2014 13;371(20):1867-76.

[92] Long GV, Stroyakovskiy D, Gogas H, Levchenko E, de Braud F, Larkin J, et al. *Dabrafenib and trametinib versus dabrafenib and placebo for Val600 BRAF-mutant melanoma: a multicentre, double-blind, phase 3 randomised controlled trial.* Lancet 2015;386(9992):444-51.

[93] Robert C, Karaszewska B, Schachter J, Rutkowski P, Mackiewicz A, Stroiakovski D, et al. *Improved overall survival in melanoma with combined dabrafenib and trametinib.* N Engl J Med 2015;372(1):30-9.

[94] Dummer R, Ascierto PA, Gogas HJ, Arance A, Mandala M, Liszkay G, et al. *Encorafenib plus binimetinib versus vemurafenib or encorafenib in patients with BRAF-mutant melanoma (Columbus): a multicentre, open-label, randomised phase 3 trial.* Lancet Oncol 2018;19(5):603-15.

[95] Long GV, Flaherty KT, Stroyakovskiy D, Gogas H, Levchenko E, de Braud F, et al. *Dabrafenib plus trametinib versus dabrafenib monotherapy in patients with metastatic BRAF V600E/K-mutant melanoma: long-term survival and safety analysis of a phase 3 study.* Ann Oncol 2017;28(7):1631-9.

[96] Davies MA, Saiag P, Robert C, Grob JJ, Flaherty KT, Arance A, et al. *Dabrafenib plus trametinib in patients with BRAF(V600)-mutant melanoma brain metastases (COMBI-MB): a multicentre, multicohort, open-label, phase 2 trial.* Lancet Oncol 2017;18(7):863-73.

[97] Hodi FS, O'Day SJ, McDermott DF, Weber RW, Sosman JA, Haanen JB, et al. *Improved survival with ipilimumab in patients with metastatic melanoma.* N Engl J Med 2010;363(8):711-23.

[98] Robert C, Thomas L, Bondarenko I, O'Day S, Weber J, Garbe C, et al. *Ipilimumab plus dacarbazine for previously untreated metastatic melanoma.* N Engl J Med 2011;364(26):2517-26.

[99] Ascierto PA, Del Vecchio M, Robert C, Mackiewicz A, Chiarion-Sileni V, Arance A, et al. *Ipilimumab 10 mg/kg versus ipilimumab 3 mg/kg in patients with unresectable or metastatic melanoma: a randomised, double-blind, multicentre, phase 3 trial.* Lancet Oncol 2017;18(5):611-22.

[100] Robert C, Long GV, Brady B, Dutriaux C, Maio M, Mortier L, et al. *Nivolumab in previously untreated melanoma without BRAF mutation.* N Engl J Med 2015;372(4):320-30.

[101] Weber JS, D'Angelo SP, Minor D, Hodi FS, Gutzmer R, Neyns B, et al. *Nivolumab versus chemotherapy in patients with advanced melanoma who progressed after anti-CTLA-4 treatment (CheckMate 037): a randomised, controlled, open-label, phase 3 trial.* Lancet Oncol 2015;16(4):375-84.

[102] Larkin J, Minor D, D'Angelo S, Neyns B, Smylie M, Miller WH, Jr., et al. *Overall survival in patients with advanced melanoma who received nivolumab versus investigator's choice chemotherapy in CheckMate 037: a randomized, controlled, open-label phase III trial.* J Clin Oncol 2018;36(4):383-90.

[103] Larkin J, Hodi FS, Wolchok JD. *Combined nivolumab and ipilimumab or monotherapy in untreated melanoma.* N Engl J Med 2015;373(13):1270-1.

[104] Wolchok JD, Chiarion-Sileni V, Gonzalez R, Rutkowski P, Grob JJ, Cowey CL, et al. *Overall survival with combined nivolumab and ipilimumab in advanced melanoma.* N Engl J Med 2017;377(14):1345-56.

[105] Postow MA, Chesney J, Pavlick AC, Robert C, Grossmann K, McDermott D, et al. *Nivolumab and ipilimumab versus ipilimumab in untreated melanoma.* N Engl J Med 2015;372(21):2006-17.

[106] Hodi FS, Chesney J, Pavlick AC, Robert C, Grossmann KF, McDermott DF, et al. *Combined nivolumab and ipilimumab versus ipilimumab alone in patients with advanced melanoma: 2-year overall survival outcomes in a multicentre, randomised, controlled, phase 2 trial.* Lancet Oncol 2016;17(11):1558-68.

[107] Ribas A, Puzanov I, Dummer R, Schadendorf D, Hamid O, Robert C, et al. *Pembrolizumab versus investigator-choice chemotherapy for ipilimumab-refractory melanoma (KEYNOTE-002): a randomised, controlled, phase 2 trial.* Lancet Oncol 2015;16(8):908-18.

[108] Robert C, Schachter J, Long GV, Arance A, Grob JJ, Mortier L, et al. *Pembrolizumab versus ipilimumab in advanced melanoma.* N Engl J Med 2015;372(26):2521-32.

[109] Schadendorf D, Hodi FS, Robert C, Weber JS, Margolin K, Hamid O, et al. *Pooled analysis of long-term survival data from phase ii and phase iii trials of ipilimumab in unresectable or metastatic melanoma.* J Clin Oncol 2015;33(17):1889-94.

[110] Hamid O, Puzanov I, Dummer R, Schachter J, Daud A, Schadendorf D, et al. *Final analysis of a randomised trial comparing pembrolizumab versus investigator-choice chemotherapy for ipilimumab-refractory advanced melanoma.* Eur J Cancer 2017;86:37-45.

[111] Schachter J, Ribas A, Long GV, Arance A, Grob JJ, Mortier L, et al. *Pembrolizumab versus ipilimumab for advanced melanoma: final overall survival results of a multicentre, randomised, open-label phase 3 study (KEYNOTE-006).* Lancet 2017;390(10105):1853-62.

[112] Robert C, Ribas A, Hamid O, Daud A, Wolchok JD, Joshua AM, et al. *Durable complete response after discontinuation of pembrolizumab in patients with metastatic melanoma.* J Clin Oncol 2018;36(17):1668-74.

[113] National Comprehensive Cancer Network. NCCN guidelines. URL: https://www.nccn.org/professionals/physician_gls/default.aspx.

[114] Weber JS, Gibney G, Sullivan RJ, Sosman JA, Slingluff CL, Jr., Lawrence DP, et al. *Sequential administration of nivolumab and ipilimumab with a planned switch in patients with advanced melanoma (CheckMate 064): an open-label, randomised, phase 2 trial.* Lancet Oncol 2016;17(7):943-55.

[115] Eigentler TK, Hassel JC, Berking C, Aberle J, Bachmann O, Grunwald V, et al. *Diagnosis, monitoring and management of immune-related adverse drug reactions of anti-PD-1 antibody therapy.* Cancer Treat Rev 2016;45:7-18.

[116] Haanen J, Carbonnel F, Robert C, Kerr KM, Peters S, Larkin J, et al. *Management of toxicities from immunotherapy: ESMO Clinical Practice Guidelines for diagnosis, treatment and follow-up.* Ann Oncol 2017;28(Suppl 4):iv119-iv42.

[117] Schadendorf D, Wolchok JD, Hodi FS, Chiarion-Sileni V, Gonzalez R, Rutkowski P, et al. *Efficacy and safety outcomes in patients with advanced melanoma who discontinued treatment with nivolumab and ipilimumab because of adverse events: a pooled analysis of randomized phase II and III trials*. J Clin Oncol 2017;35(34):3807-14.

[118] Chapman PB, Einhorn LH, Meyers ML, Saxman S, Destro AN, Panageas KS, et al. *Phase III multicenter randomized trial of the Dartmouth regimen versus dacarbazine in patients with metastatic melanoma*. J Clin Oncol 1999;17(9):2745-51.

In: Cancer Management in Latin America II
Editors: Maurício F Silva et al.
ISBN: 978-1-53616-735-1

Chapter 3

MANAGEMENT OF SOFT TISSUE SARCOMA OF THE EXTREMITIES IN ADULTS

Célia Regina Soares[1,2,*], MD, Marineide Prudêncio de Carvalho[3], MD(C), PhD, Pedro Péricles Ribeiro Baptista[4], MD, PhD, Fiona Lim[5], MBBS, Bo Angela Wan[6], MD(C) and Maurício F Silva[7,8,9], MD, PhD

[1]Radiation Oncology Unit, Hospital Santa Marcelina, Brazil
[2]Radiation Oncology, Instituto do Cancer Arnaldo Vieira de Carvalho, São Paulo, Brazil
[3]Clinical Oncology Unit, Santa Casa de Misericordia de SãoPaulo, São Paulo, Brazil
[4]Orthopedic Surgery Unit, Institutodo Cancer Arnaldo Vieira de Carvalho, São Paulo, Brazil
[5]Department of Oncology, Princess Margaret Hospital, Hong Kong, P R China
[6]Odette Cancer Centre, Sunnybrook Health Sciences Centre, University of Toronto, Toronto, Ontario, Canada
[7]Radiation Oncology Unit, Santa Maria Federal University, Santa Maria, Brazil,
[8]Hospital de Caridade Astrogildo de Azevedo, Santa Maria, Brazil
[9]Latin America Cooperative Oncology Group, Porto Alegre, Brazil

ABSTRACT

Soft tissue sarcomas (STS) comprise a heterogeneous and rare group of tumors derived from mesenchymal cells that can rise in any anatomic site and present with diverse

* Corresponding Author's Email: cecersoares@gmail.com.

biological behaviors. Radical surgery was a common procedure for STS and used to be the standard treatment for many years. However, despite good results regarding local control (LC), it had poor functional outcomes. Nowadays amputations are rarely needed, and the treatment is always multidisciplinary. Many papers have been published on the use of conservative surgery (CS) associated with adjuvant treatments using radiotherapy (RT) and chemotherapy (CT), reporting the possibility of avoiding radical surgeries, maintaining the same results of LC and better quality of life than amputations. Exclusive resection is indicated in low-grade superficial tumors or in small intramuscular tumors. There are benefits of using neoadjuvant and adjuvant RT; however neoadjuvant RT is associated with a higher incidence of healing difficulties, while adjuvant RT is associated with a higher incidence of fibrosis. RT is indicated for almost all cases of STS. Advanced technology RT is associated with greater LC and lower morbidity than conventional RT and brachytherapy (BRT). CT is not routinely used adjuvancy but may be employed in high-grade tumors, or tumors greater than 5 cm. Neoadjuvant CT may have benefits through early treatment of micrometastases and increased resectability rates. New drugs such as targeted therapy, monoclonal antibodies and immunotherapy are under investigation.

INTRODUCTION

Soft tissue sarcomas (STS) comprise a heterogeneous and rare group of tumors derived from mesenchymal cells of muscle, adipose, nerve, blood vessel, tendon and synovial tissues, with more than 50 histological subtypes. They can arise in any anatomic site but are more frequent in the limbs, especially the thigh (1). They represent only about 1% of all malignant tumors in adults and 12% of pediatric neoplasias. In the United States, it is estimated that 12,000 new cases of soft tissue sarcomas occur per year, which leads to about 4,700 deaths (2).

The great majority of STS has an unknown etiology. However, some cases are attributed to environmental factors or genetic factors, such as exposure to radiation, immunosuppression, lymphedema, viruses (ex. type 8 herpes virus), Li-Fraumeni Syndrome, Gardner's Syndrome and Neurofibromatosis type 1, among others (1).

Up to the 1970's, amputation was a common procedure for STS of the extremities. Local excision, that is, resection of the tumor and its false capsule as is the standard for benign tumors, was the first type of resection used, but was accompanied by high rates of local recurrence (LR). Resection with histological confirmation of free margins is essential to reduce the risk of LR and is the standard potentially curative treatment for adult-type, localized STS. Wide excision followed by radiotherapy (RT) is the gold standard treatment for high-grade (G2-G3) and extensive lesions (> 5 cm) (2, 3). The use of adjuvant RT promotes the destruction of tumor cells around the main lesion and, when associated with surgical resection of the limb, it promotes an increase in local control (LC), minimizing recurrence to 10-15% (4).

Pre- and postoperative RT have equivalence in LC and survival, but preoperative RT is associated with more complications of the surgical wound while postoperative RT is associated with more irreversible late morbidity (5). An individualized and careful evaluation should be performed to determine the best adjuvant timing. The use of advanced technology can improve the results regarding LC and toxicity of RT.

Adjuvant chemotherapy (CT) is not the standard treatment for adult-type STS, but neoadjuvant CT has the advantage of treating micrometastases early, improving the resection index in responsive tumors. Doxorubicin remains standard of care as the first-line treatment for locally advanced or metastatic STS (6, 7).

There is strong evidence that multidisciplinary treatment involving healthcare professionals who prescribe CS, RT, and CT allows the preservation of the limb, decreased morbidity, and better quality of life c compared to radical surgery. Nowadays, wide resection/CS combined with pre- or postoperative RT is the current standard of care for most high-grade STS (8).

This chapter is a review of the modern approach of STS of the extremities in adults, with evidence that conservative treatment can offer good LC and OS with acceptable adverse effects and better quality of life than radical surgery.

Table 1. Studies comparing surgery and adjuvant RT

Study	Randomization	Local failure	OS or DFS
Rosenberg et al. NCI 1982 N = 43 (extremities)	Amputacion vs. Surg + EBRT (60-70 Gy) both arms received CT	0% (0/16) 15% (4/27) p = 0.06	88% 83% p = 0.99 (5 years OS)
Pisters et al. MSKCC 1996 N = 164 (extremities and trunk)	High-grade (n = 19) Surg. vs Surg. + BRT (42-45 Gy) Low-grade (n = 45) Surg. vs Surg. + BRT (42-45 Gy)	30% (19/63) 9% (5/56) p = 0.0025 26% (6/23) 36% (8/22) p = 0.49	All patients 81% 84% p = 0.65 (5 years OS)
Yang et al. NCI 1998 N = 141 (extremities)	High-grade (n = 91) Surg. vs Surg. + EBRT (63 Gy) both arms received CT Low-grade (n = 50) Surg. vs Surg. + EBRT (63 Gy)	19% (9/47) 0% (0/44) p = 0.003 33% (8/24) 4% (1/26) p = 0.016	74% 75% p = 0.71 (10 years OS) 92% (2/24) 92% (24/26)

LITERATURE SEARCH

We performed a literature review through a Medline search of using the PubMed and Medscape databases. Selected articles were in the English-language and included manuscripts published on randomized studies and guidelines.

The most important prognostic factor is Tumour-Nodes-Metastases (TNM) staging. Five-year disease-free survival (DFS), based on the 7th Edition of the American Joint Committee on Cancer (AJCC), is 86% in stage I, 72% in stage II and 52% in stage III (8). The degree of cell differentiation is the most important independent prognostic factor. High-grade-tumor 5-year DFS ranges from 44 to 67% while a low-grade-tumor ranges from 90 to 100% (9). The second isolated prognostic factor is the size of the lesion. An M.D. Anderson Hospital study found that 5-year overall survival (OS) was 85% for tumors smaller than 5 cm, 68% for tumors between 5 and 15 cm and 52% for tumors larger than 15 cm (10).

Surgical resection

Wide resection is the most commonly used type of resection, also described as CS, limb-sparing surgery, or function-sparing surgery. It involves *en bloc* removal of the tumor with a margin of normal tissue in longitudinal, transverse and deep directions. This procedure preserves good function (limb salvage) without adjuvant treatment but is usually associated with moderately high LR rates, ranging from 25% to 60% (11, 12).

Radiotherapy

Combining CS and adjuvant RT decreased the rate of limb amputation from 50% in the 1970s to 1% currently, without compromising LC or survival (13).

Rosenberg et al. (4) showed that OS and DFS results are similar when performing amputation or CS followed by RT. Two other prospective and randomized studies demonstrated significant improvement in LC by the addition of adjuvant RT to limb sparing surgery. One study used external beam radiotherapy (EBRT) and randomized 141 patients (91 with high-grade tumors, 50 with low-grade tumors) to receive or not receive postoperative RT (12). Patients with high-grade tumors also received CT. The 10-year LR rate in high-grade tumors was 0% for the RT group and 22% for the non-RT group ($p = 0.0001$). This benefit was also observed in low-grade tumors ($p = 0.003$). The other study evaluated postoperative brachytherapy (BRT), randomizing 164 patients to BRT or without additional treatment (14). The 60-month LR-free survival rate was 82% and 69% for the BRT and non-BRT groups, respectively ($p = 0.04$). Table 1 shows the results of these 3 studies.

Strander et al. (15) observed that adjuvant RT improves LC when combined with CS in the treatment of STS of the extremities or trunk in patients with negative margins or microscopically positive surgical margins. In addition, an analysis of 6,960 patients from the Surveillance, Epidemiology, and End Results (SEER) database demonstrated a survival benefit for the addition of RT to surgery in STS, especially for large and high-grade tumors (73% vs 63% reduced risk) (16).

Table 2. Trial NCIC SR2 – Results - Wound complications

Wound complications*	Preoperative	Post-operative
Any complication	31 (35%)	16 (17%)
Wound surgical reparir	14 (45%)	5 (31%)
Invasive procedure for wound management	5 (16%)	4 (25%)
Hospital readjustment for wound care	1 (3%)	0
No complications	57 (65%)	78 (83%)

*p = 0.001 for any complication vs. no complication.

Table 3. SR-2 results – Local failure, OS/DFS

Trial	Randomization	Local failure	OS or DFS
O'Sullivan	Pre-op RT (50 Gy) + Surgery	7%	73%
CSG 2004	Surgery + post-op RT (60 Gy)	8%	67%
N = 190 (extremities)		p = NS; 5 years LC	p = 0.48; 5 years OS

The National Cancer Institute of Canada (NCIC SR2) (6) evaluated 182 eligible patients and compared preoperative and postoperative RT in patients with STS. The primary endpoint was the presence or absence of operative wound complications. The study compared 50 Gy in 25 preoperative fractions and 66 Gy in 33 postoperative fractions. Among patients receiving preoperative RT, 35 had complications of the surgical wound compared with 17% in the postoperative RT group (p = 0.01) (see Table 2). This difference was predominantly seen in the lower limb, particularly the thigh. Six weeks after surgery, patients treated with postoperative RT had better functional results than the preoperative RT group, although this effect was subsequently lost, probably because the wound complications had resolved. No difference was found between the 2 groups in relation to LC, progression-free survival or OS (5) (see Table 3).

Davis et al. evaluated the results after 2 years of follow-up of patients treated in the NCIC SR2 study, observing worse results in patients who received postoperative RT (19, 20). Of the 129 patients eligible for late toxicity assessment, 48.2% in the postoperative group and 31.5% in the preoperative group had grade 2 or higher fibrosis (p = 0.07). Although no statistical significance was observed, edema was more frequently observed in the postoperative RT group (23.2% vs 15.5%), as well as joint stiffness (23.2% vs 17.8%). The size of the field was predictive of higher fibrosis rates (p = 0.002) and joint stiffness (p = 0.006) and marginally predictive of edema (p = 0.06) (17) (see Table 4).

Table 4. Late toxicity

Toxicity	Grade	Preoperative N = 73 (%)	Post-operative N = 56 (%)	p-value*
Subcutaneous fibrosis	< 2	50 (68.5)	29 (51.8)	0.07
	> 2	23 (31.5)	27 (48.2)	
Joint stiffness	< 2	60 (82.2)	43 (76.8)	0.51
	> 2	13 (17.8)	13 (23.2)	
Edema	< 2	62 (84.9)	43 (76.8)	0.26
	> 2	11 (15.1)	13 (23.2)	

*p-value calculated by Fisher's test.

Table 5. Toxicity grade 2 or more in conventional RT and IMRT

Toxicity	All	Conventional RT	IMRT	p-value
Wound complications	18.2%	17.5%	18.8%	1.0
Radiodermatitis	39.8%	48.7%	31.5%	0.002
Fracture	6.9%	9.1%	4.8%	0.18
Joint stiffness	12.9%	11%	14.5%	0.40
Edema	11.3%	14.9%	7.9%	0.05

Two papers were recently published in order to demonstrate the benefits of IMRT in reducing morbidity compared to conventional RT. Folkert et al. compared 319 patients with non-metastatic STS treated between 1996 and 2010, randomizing them between surgery followed by conventional RT vs CS followed by IMRT (follow-up of 58 months). There was less LR in 5 years in those patients treated with IMRT compared to those treated with conventional RT (7.6% and 15.1%, respectively, p = 0.05) (18) (see Table 5). The factors associated with local failure were lesion size (>10 cm) and age (>50 years). There was also less acute radiodermatitis in the arm treated with IMRT (31.5% vs 48.7%, p = 0.002) and less chronic edema in favor of IMRT over conventional RT (7.9% vs 14.9%, p = 0.05). The RTOG 0630 study evaluated 79 patients with STS treated in a neoadjuvant regimen using a daily Image Guided Radiation Therapy (IGRT) technique in order to reduce the treatment margins. The primary endpoint of this work was toxicity after two years of treatment. The results were compared to those obtained in the Canadian study NCIC-SR2 and found that despite the decrease in RT margin, LC remained satisfactory. The complication index of the surgical wound remained high despite the most modern techniques, but there were fewer grade 2 or higher late toxicities, in favor of those who used IGRT daily (10.5% vs 37%, p = 0.001) (19).

Another clinically important late effect of RT to consider is bone fracture. Dickie et al. (20) investigated the incidence of bone fractures in 691 patients with lower limb STS. After a mean follow-up of seven years, 31 fractures (4.5%) were observed in an average interval of three years. For 21 of the 31 fractures, dose-volume parameters could be revised. This group was compared to 53 patients without fractures. Patients who developed bone fractures received a maximum bone dose of 64 Gy and a mean dose of 45 Gy, compared to a maximum dose of 59 Gy and a mean dose of 37 Gy for patients without fractures. The risk of fractures was reduced when the bone volume receiving 40 Gy was maintained <64%. Thus, the risk of fracture seems to be related to the dose and volume of bone treated (20).

No bolus is used during preoperative RT and its use during RT after surgery is debatable. It is indispensable when no biopsy scar excision is performed (21).

Brachytherapy can be used as an adjuvant treatment (monotherapy). If it is exclusive and used at a low-dose-rate (LDR), the recommended dose is 45 Gy; with a high-dose-rate (HDR) it ranges from 30 to 50 Gy, using 2.0 Gy to 4.0 Gy per fraction, twice a day. If used as a boost associated with external RT, the dose is 15 to 20 Gy for LDR and 12 to 20 Gy for HDR, using 2.0 Gy to 4.0 Gy per fraction, twice daily. The advantages of BRT are the use of a high dose administered in a limited volume, in a shorter treatment duration. Its disadvantages are dose heterogeneity, with an increase in the risk of fibrosis, in addition to the possibility of marginal failure. The treatment technique consists of placing parallel catheters equidistant about 1 cm from each other, in order to allow the more homogenous dose contribution (22). Contact or proximity of catheters with large vessels, nerves, or bone structures should be avoided. To allow better healing of the surgical wound, treatment should be performed from the sixth postoperative day. It is a complex technique, although an effective form of dose delivery, with a considerably shorter treatment time and with potentially less volume of treatment (14).

Oertel et al. presented the treatment of 153 patients with diagnoses of primary or recurrent sarcoma, in which CS and intraoperative radiotherapy (IORT) were performed at a dose of 10 Gy at 20 Gy, followed by postoperative RT at a dose of 36 to 50 Gy. Five-year OS was 77% and 78% for LC. Better LC was observed when the IORT dose was greater than 15 Gy, which had an 17% acute wound-related toxicity (23).

Stereotactic body radiation therapy (SBRT) is a safe and effective local treatment option for oligomestastatic pulmonary metastases in patients with contraindications to surgery or for palliation of symptomatic pulmonary metastases and spine metastases. LC ranging from 73% to 96% have been reported for treatment of metastases to the lung as well as other sites for a mix of tumors including sarcoma (24). There are fewer data regarding the role of SBRT for definitive treatment of primary sarcomas. A study of SBRT for 14 patients with primary sarcoma of the spine reported LC for 5 of 7 patients treated with SBRT alone and for 5 of 7 patients treated with SBRT and surgery (25).

Unresectable tumors can be initially treated with RT or RT plus CT. When they remain unresectable, RT may be used exclusively with doses between 70-80 Gy in selected cases. Lesion size and dose administered influence the results, with 51% LC at 5-years for tumors smaller than 5 cm and 9% for tumors larger than 10 cm. Doses above 63 Gy also show higher LC rates (26).

Chemotherapy

Adjuvant CT is not a standard treatment for adult-type STS, but it may be an option for high-risk patients (high-grade, deep lesions >5 cm, regional lymph node metastasis). Adjuvant CT should never be intended to rescue inadequate surgery and should never be used in CT-insensive histological subtypes (7).

Neoadjuvant CT has the advantage of treating micrometastasis early, improving the resection index in responsive tumors, treating a more vascularized tumor, and assessing the tumor response to the drug regimen used. It should be reserved for localized, clinically unresectable tumours, large numbers of tumor-positive lymph nodes and/or extranodal spread, or high-risk patients.

Histotype-tailored neoadjuvant CT vs standard CT in patients with high-risk STS (ISG-STS 1001) is being studied in an international, open-label, phase III, multicentre trial. In the standard CT group, treatment had to be repeated every 21 days, consisting of epirubicin 60 mg/m² per day plus ifosfamide 3 g/m² per day. All patients in the standard CT group, irrespective of histotype, were given the same scheme. In the histotype-tailored CT group, CT was tailored to histological subtypes. For high-grade myxoid liposarcoma, CT had to be repeated every 21 days and consisted of trabectedin 1.3 mg/m², given as a 24-h continuous infusion. Notably, at the start of the study, trabectedin was not yet available and three patients with high-grade myxoid liposarcoma received a tailored regimen of doxorubicin 75 mg/m² per day, every three weeks. Trabectedin was then introduced with the first amendment (Jan 25, 2012).

For leiomyosarcomas, CT had to be repeated every 14 days and consisted of gemcitabine 1800 mg/m² and dacarbazine 500 mg/m². For synovial sarcomas, CT consisted of high-dose ifosfamide 14 g/m², given over 14 days, every 28 days. For malignant peripheral nerve sheath tumours, CT had to be repeated every 21 days with etoposide 150 mg/m² per day and ifosfamide 3 g/m² per day. For undifferentiated pleomorphic sarcomas, CT had to be repeated every 21 days and consisted of gemcitabine 900 mg/m² and docetaxel 75 mg/m².

In high-grade myxoid liposarcomas, undifferentiated pleomorphic sarcoma, and leiomyosarcomas, RT was delivered postoperatively when indicated to a total dose of 60–66 Gy. In malignant peripheral nerve sheath tumours and synovial sarcomas, RT could be either delivered in the preoperative or postoperative setting according to the standard practice.

The results did not show any benefit of a neoadjuvant histotype-tailored CT regimen over the standard CT regimen. These findings provide support to the notion that the use of neoadjuvant CT with a full-dose anthracycline plus ifosfamide regimen is associated with a prognostic advantage, in terms of both OS and DFS. The benefit seen with the standard CT regimen suggests that this benefit might be the added value of neoadjuvant CT itself in patients with high-risk STS (7).

The combination of dacarbazine (DTIC) and doxorubicin is one of the oldest drugs to demonstrate efficacy in advanced STS. DTIC was primarily used as a monotherapy in advanced STS, and had a rate response (RR) of 18% but a short time to progression with a median duration of 8 weeks (range 5-19) (27).

A study compared doxorubicin alone with the combination of doxorubicin and DTIC and showed an increase in RR in advanced STS. The regimens using doxorubicin as a single agent resulted in an equivalent response frequency (18%) and survival (median, 8.0 months). DTIC significantly increased the overall response frequency of doxorubicn to 30%. However, DTIC did not influence survival (median, 8.0 months) or increase the number of complete responses (28).

Since 1986, there have been reports about the association of doxorubicin plus ifosfamide in the treatment of locally advanced and/or metastatic adult STS. The randomized phase III EORTC 62012 trial was conducted, which analyzed 455 locally advanced or metastatic, grade 2 or 3 STS patients randomly assigned to receive either single-agent doxorubicin (75 mg/m^2) or doxorubicin (75 mg/m^2) with ifosfamide (10 g/m^2 over 4 days) with mesna and growth factor support. Patients were treated every three weeks for a maximum of sex cycles or until progression. At a median follow-up of 56 months, the difference of OS did not achieve statistical significance. Median OS was 14.3 months with the combination and 12.8 months with doxorubicin alone (HR = 0.83; p = 0.076). Median progression free survival (PFS), however, was 7.4 months with the combination and 4.6 months with doxorubicin alone, for a 26% reduction in risk that was statistically significant (HR = 0.74; p = 0.003) (29).

The GeDDiS trial was a phase III, randomized, multicenter study to compare the combination of gemcitabine and docetaxel with doxorubicin in patients with previously untreated advanced unresectable or metastatic STS. Patients were randomly assigned to the control arm (75 mg/m^2 of doxorubicin) or the investigational arm (675 mg/m^2 of gemcitabine plus 75 mg/m^2 of docetaxel, every 21 days. A total of 257 patients were enrolled with a median follow-up of 19 months. The primary endpoint of 24-week PFS was identical between arms at 46%. However, patients in the investigational arm had lower dose intensity (83.3% *vs.* 94.6% for doxorubicin), more dose delays (55.5% *vs.* 45.7% for doxorubicin), and more withdrawals because of unacceptable toxicity (10.2% *vs.* 0.8% for doxorubicin). Moreover, no differences in efficacy were found between histology subtype groups, such as leiomyosarcoma or non-leiomyosarcoma (30).

Targeted therapy

Pazopanib is a potent and selective multi-targeted receptor tyrosine kinase (RTK) inhibitor that blocks tumour growth and inhibits angiogenesis that has demonstrated single-agent activity in patients with advanced STS subtypes except lipogenic sarcoma

(LPS). In the phase III study PALETTE (EORTC 62072), 367 patients with metastatic non-lipogenic STS that had failed at least one anthracycline-based chemotherapy regimen were randomized to either pazopanib or placebo. Pazopanib significantly prolonged median PFS (4.6 months vs 1.6 months for placebo, $p < 0.001$). The results of the PALETTE study led pazopanib to be approved by the Food and Drug Administration (FDA) in 2012 (31).

Palbociclib, an inhibitor of cyclin-dependent kinases (CDKs) 4 and 6, induced objective tumor responses and an increase in PFS from 56% to 66% in patients with CDK-4-amplified, well-differentiated or de-differentiated liposarcoma (32).

Olaratumab is a recombinant monoclonal antibody that targets PDGFRα, blocking PDGF-AA, PDGF-BB and PDGF-CC. Previous studies revealed that olaratumab may exert anti-tumour activity in human sarcoma xenograft models (33). The results of the phase Ib/II study that randomized 133 patients to receive olaratumab plus doxorubicin or doxorubicin alone showed a median PFS of 6.6 months (95% CI: 4.1–8.3 months) and 4.1 months (95% CI: 2.8–5.4 months), respectively. The addition of olaratumab to doxorubicin produced a greater improvement in OS, with a 11.8-month difference between these two arms. The median OS was 26.5 months (95% confidence interval (CI): 20.9–31.7 months) and 14.7 months (95% CI: 9.2–17.1 months), respectively ($p = 0.0003$) (34). Due to its improvement to OS, olaratumab was approved by both the FDA and the European Medicines Agency for its use in the first-line setting in combination with doxorubicin.

Tumor PD-L1 expression has been reported in up to 65% of different subtypes of sarcomas and the degree of PD-1 positivity in tumor-infiltrating lymphocytes (TILs) and PD-L1 expression in tumor specimens from 105 cases of STS, has been correlated with a poorer prognosis and more aggressive disease (35).

Discussion

Pathophysiology

STS are a rare and heterogeneous group of tumors that can rise in any anatomic site, with different biological behaviours. The World Health Organization (WHO) classifies STS according to its histology (2). There are more than 50 subtypes, but the following represent approximately 75% of all STS: undifferentiated pleomorphic sarcoma, liposarcoma, leiomyissarcoma, mixofibrosarcoma and synovial sarcoma (1). Immuno-histochemical examination assists in refinement of diagnosis.

There are several histological grade assay systems. The NCI-US National Cancer Institute and the French National Federation both define low, intermediate or high-grade lesions based on mitotic index, degree of necrosis, and differentiation (36).

The distribution of STS is approximately 45% in upper limb and 15% in lower limb. The most frequent histologies for these sites are liposarcoma, malignant fibrous histiocytoma/undifferentiated pleomorphic sarcoma, synovial sarcoma, fibrosarcoma, and myxoid liposarcoma, the latter being more frequent in the medial and proximal region of the thigh.

Fibrosarcomas have an infiltrative behavior, with a high incidence of compromised margins and local recurrence; epithelioid sarcomas may present as skip metastases in the limbs. Synoviossarcoma is usually of a high degree and presents itself close to the joints and is most frequent in young adults. Rhabdomyosarcomas are more frequent in children (37).

Desmoid tumor, or aggressive fibromatosis, is a low grade, locally aggressive but no metastasizing tumor, usually with a long natural history. It is often associated with patients with fibromatosis (6).

STS usually presents as a painless mass, and can reach large dimensions, especially in the lower limb. Some patients may report pain or paresthesia as a result of compression. They tend to invade longitudinally along the musculoaponeurotic planes, rarely invading fascia or bone, growing and compressing the surrounding tissues. STS form a pseudo capsule, which is the result of an inflammatory process produced by aggressive tumors and is not a barrier to neoplastic cells, as they can infiltrate and extend beyond 5 to 10 cm from it (38).

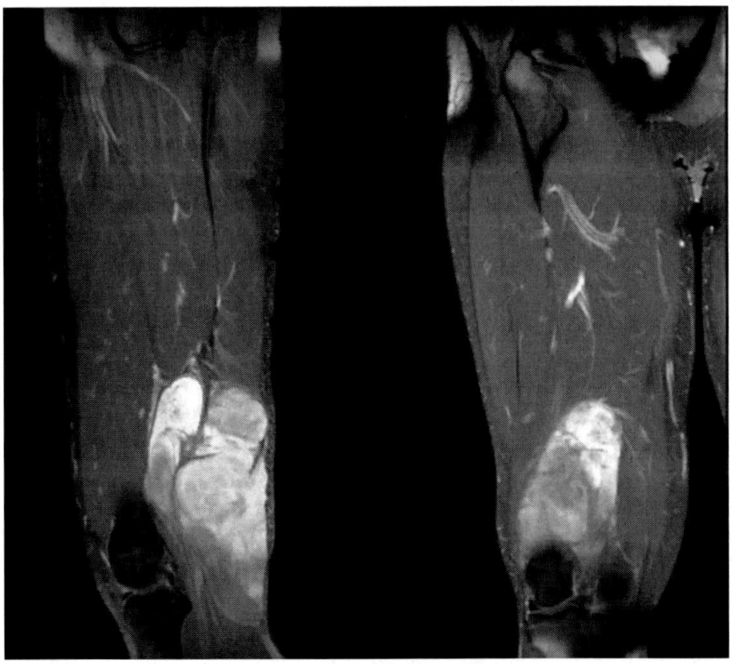

Figure 1. MRI of leg - Magnetic Resonance shows a popliteal cavity with a large, deep and heterogeneous tumor with intense contrast.

At diagnosis, approximately 23% of STS present with metastatic disease to the viscera, usually lung (34%), bone, liver, and brain (39). Lymph node metastasis is an adverse prognostic factor although they are rarely observed at diagnosis (1.8 to 3.7%) (12). Some histological subtypes show increased likelihood of lymph node involvement, such as synovial sarcomas (14%), clear cell sarcomas (10% to 18%), angiosarcomas (10% to 15%), rhabdomyosarcomas (20% to 35%), and epithelioid sarcomas (20% to 35%); collectively, these are known as "SCARE" (40).

Imaging

In addition to physical examination and assessment of tumor characteristics such as mobility, suprajacent skin infiltration, size, location and associated symptoms, imaging tests will assist in the investigation of the primary lesion and possible areas of dissemination.

In the evaluation of the primary lesion, the use of Magnetic Resonance (MR) (see Figure 1) imaging is preferential to Computed Tomography (CT) because it elucidates local boundaries of the tumor and the surrounding affected structures (41, 42). However, it is important to do both exams. CT is specifically used to search for pulmonary metastases. MR is still the ideal imaging test to evaluate local recurrence after STS resection if there are no metal elements such as orthopedic prostheses.

The positron emission tomography with fluorine deoxyglucose (FDG-PET/CT) allows, with high sensitivity, differentiation of high-grade STS from benign soft tissue tumors. However, it loses value when trying to differentiate low- or intermediate-grade STS from benign disease. Although FDG-PET/CT should not be used when first assessing patients with tissue tumors, its use is indicated for prognosis and for evaluating the response to the chemotherapy (43).

Biopsy

Biopsy is indicated for the histological diagnosis of STS. Biopsies should be limited to the compromised compartment to reduce the risk of contamination to other areas and the necessity for more extensive surgeries (44). The incisional biopsy (i.e., those performed through a surgical incision) exposing part of the tumor is the most used biopsy for STS. It should be performed along the resection axis.

Currently, percutaneous biopsies have gained popularity with the development of appropriate needles (e.g., trucut®) and imaging methods, which include the use of ultrasound and tomography to guide them.

In some cases, biopsies can be substituted by excisional resection, also called excisional biopsy. This needs to be performed by the same surgeon who will be responsible for the definitive treatment. The biopsy wound should be in-line with the incision that will be used during the resection and the path of the biopsy should be removed in block with the tumor.

The pathologist should be in the room to obtain a frozen section, which helps guarantee that the collected material is representative of the lesion, which avoids redoing the procedure later. The definitive histologic result should be concluded only after the histology is obtained in paraffin and, eventually, with immunohistochemistry.

Staging and prognosis

The current staging is based on the 8th Edition of the AJCC, published in 2017 (45) (see Table 6). Predictive factors of worse prognosis for OS and DFS are vascular invasion, leiomyosarcoma, synovial sarcoma, nerve sheath infiltration and early lymph node involvement (9). Older age at presentation, positive margins, bone or neurovascular invasion, gender and race are predictive for worse DFS (46). Important predictors for LR include positive margins, recurrent disease and older age. LR with positive margins range 28% to 56%, while for negative margins ranges from 0% to 20% (14, 47, 48). Among the main risk factors for LR include compromised margin of resection, older patients, deeper location (compared to superficial) and tumors with previous LR.

Table 6. American Joint Committtee on Cancer TNM Stage Grouping - 8th Ed (2017)

Stage	Grade tumor	T	N	M
IA	G1, GX	T1	N0	M0
IB	G1, GX	T2, T3, T4	N0	M0
II	G2, G3	T1	N0	M0
IIIA	G2, G3	T2	N0	M0
IIIB	G2, G3	T3, T4	N0	M0
IV	Any G	Any T	N0	M1
IV	Any G	Any T	N1	M0

Definitions: Primary Tumor (T) T1: Tumor ≤ 5 cm; T2: Tumor 5 to ≤ 10 cm.

T3: Tumor of 10 and ≤ 15 cm; T4: Tumor > 15 cm; Regional Lymph Nodes (N).

N0: No regional lymph node metastases or unknown lymph node status; N1: Regional lymph node metastasis; Distant Metastasis (M) M0: Not distant metastasis; M1: Distant metastasis.

Principles of management

The goal of STS treatment is to preserve the patient's life, avoid local recurrence, maximize the function of the affected limb, and minimize functional deficits (see Figure 2). STS management can be very complex and should be treated at a specialized sarcoma Center. Surgeons who specializes in treating these tumors should be thoroughly familiar with the biological behavior of the disease and be trained in cancer procedures. They will need to be able to assess the indication and timing of the association with other therapies, as well the technical ability to perform the act within the principles of modern oncologic surgery.

It is important to have a team consisting of different specialists who interact to manage cases of STS. Such professionals include an orthopedic oncologist, oncologist surgeon, plastic surgeon, pathologist, radiologist, radiation oncologist, clinical oncologist, physiotherapist, social worker and a psychologist.

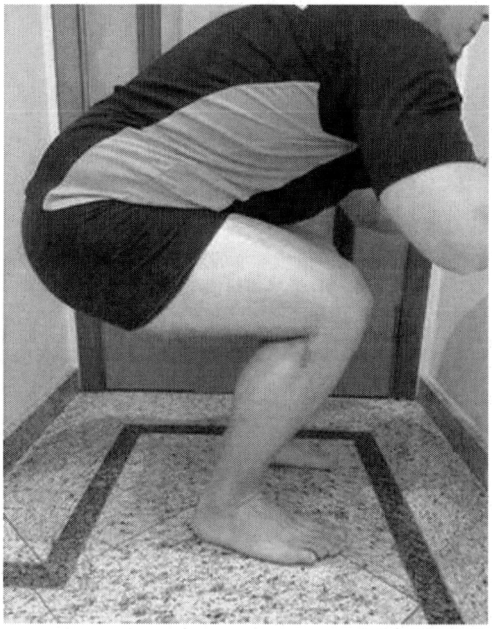

Figure 2. Squatting with support - Total lower limb function after conservative surgery and adjuvant radiotherapy.

Surgery

Tumor resection through a pseudo capsule leaves microscopic neoplastic tissue and is a risk factor for LF and worse prognosis. The dissection should be through grossly normal tissue planes uncontaminated by order, in order to reduce surgical field contamination (Figure 3).

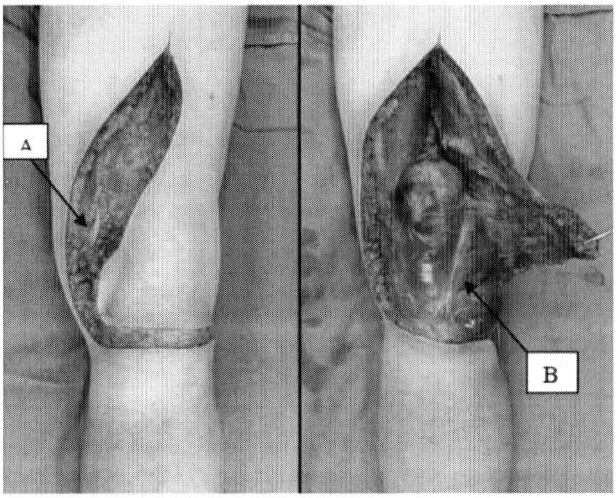

Figure 3. Large posterior medial incision curving over the popliteal fold, with excision of the biopsy site (A), exposing the external sciatic nerve (B).

Recommended thickness of the broad margins around the tumor is questionable. Traditionally, it is recommended to have 1 cm to several centimeters depending on anatomic constraints. At least one cm is considered adequate (6). Intralesional or marginal resections are inadmissible. To preserve fine tissues such as large nerves or vessels, the surgeon can this margin to avoid resection of such structures. On the other hand, anatomical tissues represent different barriers to the tumor. Whereas 1 to 2 mm of margin may be suitable for a safe resection in the muscle fascia, much wider margins are needed for other tissues such as abdominal fat and muscle. In the presence of resection with positive surgical margins, the recommendation is to enlarge it surgically (47). However, which anatomical structure should be resected for this enlargement needs to be evaluated in order to avoid impairment of limb function.

R0 resection are those with no residual microscopic disease, R1 are those with microscopic residual disease, and R2 resection those ones with gross residual disease. Large nerves can be preserved by dissecting and withdrawing the outer nerve sheath as a margin since STS do not infiltrate nerves. However, when the tumor surrounds the nerve, the nerve may need to be removed along with the tumor (6).

Surgical clips should be placed to mark the surgical field and other relevant structures to help RT planning. If suction drainage is used, the drains should exit the skin close to the edge of the surgical incision, in case RT or new resection is indicated (6).

Therefore, the indication of amputation in the presence of STS may be necessary for excessively extensive tumors (e.g., residual limb has no function), when resecting a main nerve (e.g., brachial plexus) or when it is impossible to obtain sufficiently large margins. The damage of large vessels by a tumor used to be a reason for amputation, but with vascular reconstruction techniques it became possible to resect the tumor in block with the vessels and reconstruct them with vascular grafts, allowing for a viable limb. Lymph nodes should be resected only if compromised by disease.

Surgery also plays an important role in the treatment of oligometastatic lesions, whether for lung or bone, with lesion excision, followed or not by adjuvant CT.

The New York Memorial Sloan-Kattering Cancer Center suggests the use of a nomogram to evaluate the outcome 5 or 12 years after resection of the lesion, considering histological type, age, sex, location of presentation, size of the lesion, degree of differentiation, conditions and thickness of the surgical margin, applicable for initial or recurrent disease, characterizing the importance of all these factors in the tumor control after only surgical procedure (49).

Radiotherapy

As discussed above, the gold standard of treating patients with STS of the extremities is surgery. Larger local excision decreases the likelihood of local failure and amputations are rarely needed. Adjuvant RT is offered in conjunction with limb-conserving surgery to optimize LC.

The initial studies about conservative treatment were with patients with STS submitted to CS and postoperative RT. In this approach, the RT planning is performed using information about the resected sample, including histological type and margin status after resection, adjusting the radiation dose to the high-risk areas in the surgical bed, including all wound areas within the field of irradiation. However, the optimal RT time in STS is still debated and several studies on preoperative RT have been performed. This approach has the advantage of irradiating a very well-defined target, a better oxygenated tumor, using smaller doses and smaller fields since there is no surgical scar to be included, and having greater potential for sterilization of margins and increased resectability.

Comfortable patient position is important issue to ensure reproducibility. IMRT allows more possibilities of positioning, besides offering the advantage of reducing the morbidity on the normal tissue, maintaining good rates of LC. The 94% LC rate at 5 years in STS patients treated with IMRT has recently been reported, with lower potential morbidities compared to conventional RT (50).

The most frequent acute toxicities of RT are fatigue and skin changes, such as hyperemia, desquamation, alopecia, moist desquamation and healing changes. RT of the abdominal and thoracic regions can lead to nausea, vomiting, intestinal changes and esophagitis. RT should be initiated after four weeks of surgery to reduce the chance of healing issues. When CT using doxorubicin is associated to concomitant RT, the daily dose should be reduced in order to reduce the intensity of radiodermatitis.

With the use of any RT technique, some details are important to keep in mind to reduce late toxicity, such as: protecting a range of circumference of the limb in order to avoid lymphedema and pain, protecting genitalia when treating lesions near the perineum, and avoiding treating all thickness of the bone to avoid fractures. The entire joint should receive less than 40-45 Gy because when higher doses are required, at least part of the joint should be protected to avoid joint stiffness (51).

A trend in the use of preoperative RT is currently observed, since it apparently produces better functional results in the long term. However, an individualized and careful evaluation should be performed in order to determine the adequate adjuvant timing. Both postoperative RT and preoperative RT have advantages and disadvantages. Preoperative RT uses smaller fields and doses, avoids surgical implants during surgery, and evidences lower rates of edema and fibrosis, but is associated with greater complications in operative wound-healing. Postoperative RT uses larger fields and doses, presents higher rates of fibrosis and edema, but with lower rates of wound complications.

Brachytherapy can be used as an adjuvant treatment, either exclusively (monotherapy) in high-grade tumors with free surgical margins or combined with external RT. The treatment technique consists of placing parallel catheters equidistant (about 1 cm) from one another in order to allow a more homogenous dose contribution (22). Important care should be made to avoid contact or proximity of catheters with large vessels, nerves, or bone structures. The treatment should be performed from the sixth postoperative day to allow better healing of the surgical wound. Although an effective form of dose delivery with a considerably shorter treatment time and with potentially less volume of treatment, it is a complex technique (14).

Intraoperative RT allows evaluation of the volume of risk at the moment of its resection, under direct vision, allowing the protection of the adjacent structures and reducing the potential morbidity of the treatment. It can be performed using electron beams or high-dose rate (HDR) BRT.

SBRT is a technique that delivers highly focused photon radiation doses to extracranial lesions. The dose schedules are hypofractionated, with large ablative fraction sizes rarely used to treat primary tumors.

Another technique that has been studied is the use of proton beam therapy, especially in sarcomas located in proximity to risk organs, where the use of protons may decrease the dose in these organs. There is still no randomized study to prove that this type of radiation would be more effective than the traditional use of photons in LC.

Local recurrences should be treated with the same principles as patients with initial tumor. New resection and RT are suggested if this was not previously employed (52).

Chemotherapy

CT can be administered with single agents (dacarbazine, doxorubicin, epirubicin or ifosfamide) or antracycline-based combination regimes (doxorubicin or epirubicin with ifosfamide and/or dacarbazine) for patients with advanced, unresectable, or metastatic disease.

The overall clinical conclusion should be that doxorubicin remains the standard of care as the first-line treatment for locally advanced or metastatic STS. Dose exceeding 75 mg/m^2 are associated with cardiotoxicities, myelosuppression and mucositis.

Standard first line CT comprises of anthracycline, with addition of ifosfamide, particularly in subtypes sensitive to ifosfamide, when a tumor response is felt to be likely.

Gemcitabine in combination with docetaxel, vinorelbine or dacarbazine has been shown to be beneficial in patients with unresctable or metastatic STS of various histologic subtypes.

Use of the doxorubicin and ifosfamide combination is for selected patients who need to optimize their chances of tumour shrinkage; use of gemcitabine and docetaxel combination is for patients with cardiac dysfunction which is a contraindication for doxorubicin.

For most patients, existing studies hopefully provide sufficient guidance for clinicians to consider in the selection of the first-line treatment for advanced STS (see Table 7).

Table 7. Chemotherapy by sarcoma histology

Histology	Drug
Leiomyosarcoma	Gemcitabine – Docetaxel Gemcitabine – Dacarbazine Doxorubicin Doxorubin – Ifosfamide – Mesna Pazopanib
Liposarcoma	Doxorubicin Epirubicin Liposomal Doxorubicin Doxorubin – Ifosfamide – Mesna
Synovial Sarcoma	Ifosfamida Epirubicin – Ifosfamide – Mesna
Angiosarcoma	Paclitaxel Liposomal Doxorubicin Doxorubicin
Pleomorphic Sarcoma	Epirubicin – Ifosfamide – Mesna Gemcitabine – Docetaxel Epirubicin

There is no standard regimen in second-line treatment for STS. Beside anthracyclines and ifosfamide, there are other drugs with moderate activity in this disease. As different subtypes may have different sensitivity to different cytotoxic agents, beyond the first line, the treatment for STS is being increasingly driven by histology.

Rhabdomyosarcoma is treated with neoadjuvant and adjuvant chemotherapeutic protocols. In the rare cases of this neoplasm occurring in adults, the pediatric CT protocol is adopted.

The investigations of sarcoma genomics and mutations of signaling pathway have revealed several candidates for targeted therapy, and the angiogenetic pathway was found to be one of the promising targets (see Table 8). Small molecular TKI targeting angiogenesis including pazopanib, sunitinib, sorafenib, regorafenib, cediranib and apatinib have shown activity in leiomyosarcoma, synovial sarcoma, alveolar soft part sarcomas, solitary fibrous tumours and angiosarcomas. The selection should be based on histologic subtype, patient characteristics, toxicity profile and accessibility of the drug.

Imatinib is specific for the *TK* domain in *able* (the Abelson proto-oncogene), *c-kit* and *PDGF-R* and sunitinib inhibits cellular signaling by targeting multiple receptor tyrosine kinases (RTKs), these include all receptors for platelet-derived growth factor (PDGF-Rs) and vascular endothelial growth factor receptors (VEGFRs), have also shown efficacy in patients with advanced and/or metastatic STS other than GIST(gastrointestinal stromal tumor) (53).

Sorafenib is a small inhibitor of several tyrosine protein kinases, such as VEGFR, PDGFR and Raf family kinases (more avidly C-Raf than B-Raf) appeared to be active in patients with solitary fibrous tumor, leiomyosarcoma, and desmoid tumors (54).

Olaratumab is also being studied in other combinations. ANNOUNCE-2 is an open-label phase 1b and randomized, double-blind phase II study evaluating gemcitabine and docetaxel with or without olaratumab for the treatment of advanced STS. This trial is expected to enroll 211 patients, with the primary endpoint for phase Ib being identification of an olaratumab dose for phase II, and the phase II primary endpoint being OS (55).

Table 8. Sarcoma biomarkers with pharmacological inhibition

Soft Tissue Sarcoma (VEGFR)	**Pazopanib**
Inflamatory myofibroblastic tumor (ALK)	Crizotinib
Liposarcoma (CDK4 amplification)	Palbociclib
Angiosarcoma (KDR, VEGF)	Sorafenib, Bevacizumab
Perivascular epithelioid cell tumor (PECOMA)	Everolimus

CONCLUSION

In conclusion, because of the variety of histological subtypes and different biological behavior the treatment of STS is multidisciplinary, although the most important is the surgical approach. Amputations are rarely needed. Wide excision followed by RT is the gold standard treatment for high-grade (G2-G3) and extensive lesions (>5 cm). Initial stages of extremities STS show 80% of LC rates and 85% and 5-year survival rates of 90%. It is important to reduce treatment-related morbidity and improve quality of life using more conformal adjuvant RT, define which patients should receive only surgery and which ones need more aggressive treatment. Patient stage III have a high rate of distant metastasis and death. For these patients CT should be consider and novel therapy are needed.

REFERENCES

[1] *World Health Organization classification of tumours of soft tissue and bone*. In: Fletcher CDM, Bridge JA, Hogendoorn PC, et al. eds. Lyon, France: IARC Press, 2013.

[2] Siegel R, Ma J, Zou Z, Jemal A. *Cancer statistics*, 2014. CA Cancer J Clin 2014;64(1):9-29.

[3] Casali PG, Abecassis N, Aro HT, Bauer S, Biagini R, et al. *Soft tissue and visceral sarcomas: ESMO–EURACAN Clinical Practice Guidelines for diagnosis, treatment and follow-up.* Ann Oncol 2018;29(Suppl 4):iv268-9.

[4] Rosenberg SA, Tepper J, Glatstein E, Costa J, Baker A, Brennan M, et al. *The treatment of soft-tissue sarcomas of the extremities: prospective randomized evaluations of (1) limb-sparing surgery plus radiation therapy compared with amputation and (2) the role of adjuvant chemotherapy*. Ann Surg 1982;196(3):305-15.

[5] O'Sullivan B, Davis AM, Turcotte R, Bell R, Catton C, Chabot P, et al. *Preoperative versus postoperative radiotherapy in soft-tissue sarcoma of the limbs: A randomized trial.* Lancet 2002;359(9325):2235-41.

[6] *National Comprehensive Network* (NCCN Clinical Practice Guidelines in Oncology). 2018.

[7] Gronchi A, Ferrari S, Quagliuolo V, Broto JM, Pousa AL, Grignani G, et al. *Histotype-tailored neoadjuvant chemotherapy versus standard chemotherapy in patients with high-risk soft-tissue sarcomas (ISG-STS 1001): an international, open-label, randomized, controlled, phase 3, multicentre trial.* Lancet Oncol 2017;18(6):812-22.

[8] *AJCC cancer staging manual.* In: Edge SB, Byrd DR, Compton CC, et al, eds. New York: Springer, 2010.

[9] Callegaro D, Miceli R, Bonvalot S, Ferguson P, Strauss DC, Levy A, et al. *Development and external validation of two nomograms to predict overall survival and occurrence of distant metastases in adults after surgical resection of localized soft-tissue sarcomas of the extremities: a retrospective analysis*. Lancet Oncol 2016;17(5):671-80.

[10] Lahat G, Tuvin D, Wei C, Anaya DA, Bekele BN, Lazar AJ, et al. *New perspectives for staging and prognosis in soft tissue sarcoma.* Ann Surg Oncol 2008;15:2739-48.

[11] Riad S, Griffin AM, Liberman B, Blackstein ME, Catton CN, Kandel RA, et al. *Lymph node metastasis in soft tissue sarcoma in an extremity*. Clin Orthop Relat Res 2004;(426):129-34.

[12] Yang JC, Chang AE, Baker AR, Sindelar WF, Danforth DN, Topalian SL, et al. *Randomized prospective study of the benefit of adjuvant radiation therapy in the treatment of soft tissue sarcomas of the extremity*. J Clin Oncol 1998;16(1):197-203.

[13] Canter RJ, Beal S, Borys D, Martinez SR, Bold RJ, Robbins AS. *Interaction of histologic subtype and histologic grade in predicting survival for soft-tissue sarcomas*. J Am Coll Surg 2010;210(2):191-8.

[14] Pisters PW, Harrison LB, Leung DH, Woodruff JM, Casper ES, Brennan MF. *Long-term results of a prospective randomized trial of adjuvant brachytherapy in soft tissue sarcoma*. J Clin Oncol 1996;14(3):859-8.

[15] Strander H, Turesson I, Cavallin-Stahl E. *A systematic overview of radiation therapy effects in soft tissue sarcomas*. Acta Oncol 2003;42(5-6):516-31.

[16] Koshy M, Rich SE, Mohiuddin MM. *Improved survival with radiation therapy in high-grade soft tissue sarcomas of the extremities: A SEER analysis*. Int J Radiat Oncol Biol Phys 2010;77(1):203-9.

[17] Davis AM, O'Sullivan B, Turcotte R, Bell R, Catton C, Chabot P, et al. *Late radiation morbidity following randomization to preoperative versus postoperative radiotherapy in extremity soft tissue sarcoma*. Radiother Oncol 2005;75(1):48-53.

[18] Folkert MR, Singer S, Brennan MF, Kuk D, Qin LX, Kobayashi WK, et al. *Comparison of local recurrence with conventional and intensity-modulated radiation therapy for primary soft-tissue sarcomas of the extremity*. J Clin Oncol 2014;32(29):3236-41.

[19] Wang D, Zhang Q, Eisenberg BL, Kane JM, Li XA, Lucas D, et al. *Significant reduction of late toxicities in patients with extremity sarcoma treated with image-guided radiation therapy to a reduced target volume: results of Radiation Therapy Oncology Group RTOG-0630 Trial*. J Clin Oncol 2015;33(20):2231-8.

[20] Dickie CI, Parent AL, Griffin AM, Fung S, Chung PW, Catton CN, et al. *Bone fractures following external beam radiotherapy and limb-preservation surgery for lower extremity soft tissue sarcoma: Relationship to irradiated bone length, volume, tumor location and dose*. Int J Radiat Oncol Biol Phys 2009;75(4):1119-24.

[21] Baldini EH, Lapidus MR, Wang Q, Manola J, Orgill DP, Pomahac B, et al. *Predictors for major wound complications following preoperative radiotherapy and surgery for softtissue sarcoma of the extremities and trunk: importance of tumor proximity to skin surface*. Ann Surg Oncol 2013;20(5):1494-9.

[22] Naghavi AO, Fernandez DC, Mesko N, Juloori A, Martinez A, Scott JG, et al. *American Brachytherapy Society consensus statement for soft tissue sarcoma brachytherapy*. Brachytherapy 2017;16(3):466-89.

[23] Oertel S, Treiber M, Zahlten-Hinguranage A, Eichin S, Roeder F, Funk A, et al. *Intraoperative electron boost radiation followed by moderate doses of external beam radiotherapy in limb-sparing treatment of patients with extremity soft tissue sarcoma*. Int J Radiat Oncol Biol phys 2006;64(5):1416-23.

[24] Hof H, Hoess A, Oetzel D, Debus J, Herfarth K. *Stereotactic single-dose radiotherapy of lung metastases*. Strahlenther Onkol 2007;183(12):673-8.

[25] Levine AM, Coleman C, Horasek S. *Stereotactic radiosurgery for the treatment of primary sarcomas and sarcoma metastases of the spine*. Neurosurgery 2009;64(2 Suppl):A54-9.

[26] Kepka L, DeLaney TF, Suit HD, Goldberg SI. *Results of radiation therapy for unresected soft-tissue sarcomas*. Int J Radio Oncol Biol Phys 2005;63(3):852-9.

[27] Buesa JM, Mouridsen HT, van Oosterom AT, Verweij J, Wagener T, Steward W, et al. *High-dose DTIC in advanced soft-tissue sarcomas in the adult*. A phase II study of the E.O.R.T.C. Soft Tissue and Bone Sarcoma Group. Ann Oncol 1991;2(4):307-9.

[28] Borden EC, Amato DA, Rosenbaum C, Enterline HT, Shiraki MJ, Creech RH, et al. *Randomized comparison of three adriamycin regimens for metastatic soft tissue sarcomas*. J Clin Oncol 1987;5(6):840-50.

[29] Judson I, Verweij J, Gelderblom H, Hartmann JT, Schöffski P, Blay JY, et al. *Doxorubicin alone versus intensified doxorubicin plus ifosfamide for first-line treatment of advanced or metastatic soft-tissue sarcoma: a randomized controlled phase 3 trial.* Lancet Oncol 2014;15(4):415-23.

[30] Seddon B, Strauss SJ, Whelan J, Leahy M, Woll PJ, Cowie F, et al. *Gemcitabine and docetaxel versus doxorubicin as first-line treatment in previously untreated advanced unresectable or metastatic soft-tissue sarcomas (GeDDiS): a randomized controlled phase 3 trial.* Lancet Oncol 2017;18(10):1397-410.

[31] Kollár A, Jones RL, Stacchiotti S, Gelderblom H, Guida M, Grignani G, et al. *Pazopanib in advanced vascular sarcomas: an EORTC Soft Tissue and Bone Sarcoma Group (STBSG) retrospective analysis.* Acta Oncol 2017;56(1):88-92.

[32] Dickson MA, Tap WD, Keohan ML, D'Angelo SP, Gounder MM, Antonescue CR, et al. *Phase II trial of the CDK4 inhibitor PD0332991 in patients with advanced CDK4-amplified well-differentiated or dedifferentiated liposarcoma.* J Clin Oncol 2013;31(16):2024-8.

[33] Loizos N, Xu Y, Huber J, Liu M, Lu D, Finnerty B, et al. *Targeting the platelet-derived growth factor receptor alpha with a neutralizing human monoclonal antibody inhibits the growth of tumor xenografts: implications as a potential therapeutic target.* Mol Cancer Ther 2005;4(3):369-79.

[34] Tap WD, Jones RL, Van Tine BA, *Chmielowski B, Elias AD, Adkins D, et al. Olaratumab and doxorubicin versus doxorubicin alone for treatment of soft-tissue sarcoma: an open-label phase 1b and randomized phase 2 trial.* Lancet 2016;388(10043):488-97

[35] Toulmonde M, Penel N, Adam J, Chevreau C, Blay JY, Le Cesne A, et al. *Use of PD-1 Targeting, Macrophage Infiltration, and IDO Pathway Activation in Sarcomas: A Phase 2 Clinical Trial.* JAMA Oncol 2018;4(1):93-7.

[36] Guillou L, Coindre JM, Bonichon F, Nguyen BB, Terrier P, Collin F, et al. *Comparative study of the National Cancer Institute and French Federation of Cancer Centers Sarcoma Group grading systems in a population of 410 adult patients with soft tissue sarcoma.* J Clin Oncol 1997;15(1):350-62.

[37] Siegel RL, Miller KD, Jemal A. *Cancer statistics*, 2017. CA Cancer J Clin 2017;67(1):7-30.

[38] Enneking WF, Spanier SS, Malawer MM. *The effect of the anatomic setting on the results of surgical procedures for soft parts sarcoma of the thigh.* Cancer 1981;47(5):1005-22.

[39] Lawrence W Jr, Donegan WL, Natarajan N, Mettlin C, Beart R, Winchester D, et al. *Adult soft tissue sarcomas.* A pattern of care survey of the American College of Surgeons. Ann Surg 1987;205(4):349-59.

[40] Daigeler A, Kuhnen C, Moritz R, Stricker I, Goertz O, Tilkorn D, et al. *Lymph node metastases in soft tissue sarcomas: a single Center analysis of 1,597 patients.* Langenbecks Arch Surg 2009;394(2):321-29.

[41] Demas BE, Heelan RT, Lane J, Marcove R, Hajdu S, Brennan MF. *Soft-tissue sarcomas of the extremities: comparison of MR and CT in determining the extent of disease.* AJR Am J Roentgenol 1988;150(3):615-20.

[42] Aisen AM, Martel W, Braunstein EM, McMillin KI, Phillips WA, Kling TF. *MRI and CT evaluation of primary bone and soft-tissue tumors.* AJR Am J Roentgenol 1986;146(4):749-56.

[43] Folpe AL, Lyles RH, Sprouse JT, Conrad EU 3rd, *Eary JF. (F-18) fluorodeoxyglucose positron emission tomography as a predictor of pathologic grade and other prognostic variables in bone and soft tissue sarcoma.* Clin Cancer Res 2000;6(4):1279-87.

[44] Mankin HJ, Mankin CJ, Simon MA. *The hazards of the biopsy, revisited. Members of the Musculoskeletal Tumor Society.* J Bone Joint Surg Am 1996;78(5):656-63.

[45] AJCC cancer staging manual. 8th ed. In: Amin MB, Edge SB, Greene FL, et al., eds. Chicago, IL: Springer International Publishing, 2017.

[46] Gutierrez JC, Perez EA, Franceschi D, Moffat FL Jr, Livingstone AS, Koniaris LG. *Outcomes for soft-tissue sarcoma in 8249 cases from a large state cancer registry.* J Surg Res 2007;141(1):105-14.

[47] Gundle KR, Gupta S, Kafchinski L, Griffin AM, Kandel RA, Dickson BC, et al. *An analysis of tumor- and surgeryrelated factors that contribute to inadvertent positive margins following soft tissue sarcoma resection*. Ann Surg Oncol 2017;24(8):2137-44.

[48] Zagars GK, Ballo MT, Pisters PW, Pollock RE, Patel SR, Benjamin RS, et al. *Prognostic factors for patients with localized soft-tissue sarcoma treated with conservation surgery and radiation therapy: an analysis of 1,225 patients*. Cancer 2003;97(10):2530-43.

[49] Sarcoma Nomogram: Disclaimer. URL: http://normograms.mskcc.org/Sarc om/Post Surgery.aspx.

[50] Alektiar KM, Brennan MF, Healey JH, Singer S. *Impact of intensity-modulated radiation therapy on local control in primary soft-tissue sarcoma of the extremity*. J Clin Oncol 2008;26(20):3440-4.

[51] Catton C, Davis A, Bell R, O'Sullivan B, Fornasier V, Wunder J, et al. *Soft tissue sarcoma of the extremity*. Limb salvage after failure of combined conservative therapy. Radiother Oncol 1996;41(3):209-14.

[52] Cassier PA, Gelderblom H, Stacchiotti S, Thomas D, Maki RG, Kroep JR, et al. *Efficacy of imatinib mesylate for the treatment of locally advanced and/or metastatic tenosynovial giant cell tumor/pigmented villonodular synovitis*. Cancer 2012;118(6):1649-55.

[53] Gounder MM, Lefkowitz RA, Keohan ML, D'Adamo DR, Hameed M, Antonescu CR, et al. *Activity of sorafenib against desmoid tumor/deep fibromatosis*. Clin Cancer Res 2011;17(12):4082-90.

[54] *A study of olaratumab (LY3012207) in participants with advanced soft tissue sarcoma.* Identifier NCT02659020. URL: https://clinicaltrials.gov/ct2/show/NCT0 2659020

[55] Canter RJ, Beal S, Borys D, Martinez SR, Bold RJ, Robbins AS. *Interaction of histologic subtype and histologic grade in predicting survival for soft-tissue sarcomas*. J Am Coll Surg 2010;210(2):191-8.

In: Cancer Management in Latin America II
Editors: Maurício F Silva et al.
ISBN: 978-1-53616-735-1

Chapter 4

MANAGEMENT OF PEDIATRIC CANCER

Maria Luísa Sucharski Figueiredo[1,2,*], MD, Cristiane de Lacerda Gonçalves Chaves[1,2], MD, Michael Jenwei Chen[1,3], MD, Gustavo Nader Marta[2], MD, PhD, Fiona Lim[4], MBBS, Bo Angela Wan[5], MD(C) and Mauricio F Silva[6,7,8], MD, PhD

[1]Department of Radiation Oncology, Grupo de Apoio ao Adolescente e a Criança com Câncer (GRAACC), São Paulo, Brazil
[2]Department of Radiation Oncology, Instituto do Câncer do Estado de São Paulo (ICESP), São Paulo, Brazil
[3]Department of Radiation Oncology, A. C. Camargo Cancer Center (ACCCC), São Paulo, Brazil
[4]Department of Oncology, Princess Margaret Hospital, Hong Kong, PR China
[5]Odette Cancer Centre, Sunnybrook Health Sciences Centre, Toronto, Ontario, Canada
[6]Radiation Oncology Unit, Santa Maria Federal University, Santa Maria, Brazil
[7]Radiation Oncology Unit, Hospital de Caridade Astrogildo de Azevedo, Santa Maria, Brazil
[8]Latin America Cooperative Oncology Group, Porto Alegre, Brazil

ABSTRACT

Despite its low incidence, pediatric cancer comprises a significant percentage of malignant neoplasms. Radiation therapy represents an integral component in the treatment of many pediatric tumors, notwithstanding a certain aversion to it due to its

[*] Corresponding Author's Email: mariafigueiredo@graacc.org.br.

possible detrimental effects. Technological improvements have emerged within radiation oncology with the purpose of enhancing disease control while limiting treatment related toxicity and optimizing the therapeutic ratio. These, however, are often not within reach of Latin American countries due to its high cost, making it difficult to radiation oncologists to apply them in daily practice. This chapter describes some of the aspects of pediatric radiation therapy, highlighting and discussing some of the pitfalls radiation oncologists might face when dealing with pediatric patients beyond the technological improvements that radiation oncology is undergoing.

INTRODUCTION

When driven to elaborate about the childhood cancer treatment in Latin America, the first thought that comes up is the fragmentation of population-based registries. Data, when it exists, do not necessarily represent the national population as a whole, or fall short from any detailed description sought. That is the case of local registries in Brazil, Colombia, Ecuador, Honduras and Peru. Only Argentina and Chile have national pediatric cancer-specific registries: Argentina's national pediatric cancer registry, the Registro Oncopediátrico Hospitalario Argentino (ROHA) and Chile's national pediatric cancer registry, the Registro Nacional de Cáncer Infantil (RENCI) (1). In Brazil, since 1995, the National Institute of Cancer (Instituto Nacional do Câncer, INCA) calculates and publishes cancer estimates. In order to render these estimates to be viable, the information produced mostly originates from the population-based cancer registries and the Mortality Information System (Sistema de Informação sobre Mortalidade - SIM), supervised by INCA and by the Ministry of Health (Secretaria de Vigilância à Saúde - SVS) (2).

Despite their own unique characteristics, Latin American countries have similarities in terms of historical, political and social conformation. In general, they are characterized by high income concentrations, social inequalities and political and economic instability (3). Scarce resources can be only partly responsible for the lack of consistent information. The countries of this region have several parallel health systems, where generally, even individuals who are able to pay for a particular health insurance and can achieve good health outcomes can still be missed from data collection. The lack of easily accessible organized information could be improved through legal mechanisms. Instead, public health and official health is used as a bandage-solution for emergencies. Thus, discontinuity is a recurring factor in the history of Latin American health. This pattern is defined as a culture of survival. This culture in adversity not only damages the evaluation of initiatives that are already in progress, preventing regional and international comparisons, but mainly limits the elaboration and materialization of therapeutic protocols in the long-term (4). Overcoming these difficulties, pediatric oncologists and radiation oncologists tend to follow rigorous international protocols, keeping daily practice dilemmas and doubts nearly identical with those observed worldwide. This chapter aims to present and briefly discuss some of these pitfalls in dealing with pediatric patients.

Clinical features of malignant neoplasms that affect both adults and children

The treatment of pediatric cancer requires not only the expansion of knowledge to embryonic and other histological types that more rarely present in adults, but also the re-interpretation of several others that although may exist in common cancers, can behave in a totally different way in the pediatric population. A common example of this is the glioma. Children with gliomas show different disease evolution when compared to adults (5). Their prognosis, when tumors with identical pathological grade or similar brain site involvement are analyzed, are significantly better compared to adults, highlighting the possibility that they are truly distinct biological entities.

Low-grade gliomas, such as juvenile pilocytic astrocytomas, are the most common brain tumors of childhood. In pathological analysis, they tend to represent multiple tumor subtypes (6), yet in most cases, they pursue a common genomic mutation of the *BRAF* oncogene related to the mitogen-activated protein kinase (MAPK) pathway (7-9). Unlike low-grade tumours among older adolescents or adults, childhood tumors almost never express *IDH1* or *IDH2* mutations and rarely undergo malignant transformation into higher-grade neoplasms (10). Neither do they fit on the 1p/19q co-deletion prognostic subtype classification (11, 12). Instead, their levels of IL1RAP (soluble interleukin 1 receptor accessory protein) are high and may be the reason for their better prognosis as it IL1RAP is linked to apoptosis and inhibition of proliferation through blocking IL-6 secretion and IL-1β on glioma cells (see Table 1) (5).

Table 1. Gene expression differences among childhood and adult glioma tumors

High expression in tissue from children		**High expression in tissue from adults**	
Gene symbol	Fold change (children/adults)	Gene symbol	Fold change (children/adults)
IL1RAP	8.1	*EZR*	6.7
APOD	5.4	*MMP9*	3.2
TIMP4	5.0	*MST1*	4.1
OPCML	3.2		

Pediatric treatment decisions also diverge as it is largely based on the tumor's location in the brain and age at diagnosis, rather than histologic subtype or tumor biology. When required, interventions are mostly surgical resection followed by observation only, whereas carboplatin-containing chemotherapy and/or localized radiation is reserved for recurrent or progressive evolutions (13-16) (see Figure 1). This strategy is associated with pediatric 10- to 20-year overall survival of around 83% to 94% (17-19). The long survival requires judicious use of radiotherapy in children. Unfortunately, radiotherapy is associated with cognitive deficits, especially when used in children under five years and in the presence of other correlated factors including neurofibromatosis type 1, tumor volume and location, extent of resection and total radiation dose (20). On the other hand, in the adult population, age, good neurologic status, oligodendroglia histology and low proliferation indexes are associated with improved outcomes while Ki-67 (MIB-I) index of >3% is associated with to poorer outcomes (21). Although adult patients receive substantially more chemotherapy and radiation, the expected 5-year survival rates are 37% for adults with astrocytoma, 56% for mixed oligoastrocytoma, and 70% for oligodendroglioma, with malignant transformations associated with poor outcomes (22).

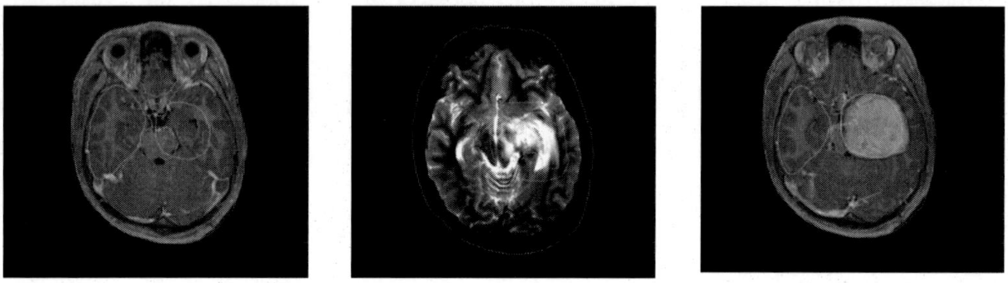

A B C

A. Image fusion with MRI-T1Gd allowing residual disease volume high quality definition. B. The same MRI with T2-FLAIR showing hipersinal. C. Final prescription dose selected in colorwash distribution dose.

Figure 1. Radiation treatment planning of a capsule nuclear astrocytoma, WHO grade II, partially resected.

High-grade gliomas represent >50% of all primary malignant brain tumors in adults whereas similar neoplasms arising outside the brainstem constitute only 10% of all primary brain tumors in children (23). Pediatric high-grade gliomas are also heterogeneous and diffusely infiltrative and carry a dismal prognosis (24, 25), but present very different characteristics with regards to their specific location in the brain (superficial cerebral or diencephalic masses), and specific molecular and genetic profile (26) (*BRAF* V600E mutation in place of *IDH1* or *IDH2* mutations) (27). Current studies are looking at how progenitor and mature cell types as well as the microenvironment within the developing brain may influence the disease process. Until recently, it was thought that pediatric high-grade gliomas resembled adult "secondary" tumors, which arise from a preceding lower-grade lesion. However, recent genomic studies found related numerous genes within the p53, PI3K/RTK and RB pathways, targeted by focal gain or loss mutations (with the exception of *PDGFRA* and *CDKN2A*, other alterations are found only at low frequency) (26). Despite a better understanding of their molecular or genetic profile, these high-grade tumors remain particularly difficult to treat because they do not usually respond to most aggressive therapies. Surgery and radiation are the usual modes of therapy, with the efficacy of chemotherapy being uncertain (28). Combination of radiation and temozolomide showed superior outcome in the treatment of adults with grade IV gliomas (25) but results in children have been disappointing (29), with *MGMT* overexpression inversely associated with survival.

Table 2. Different outcomes among children and adult with sarcomas

Type	**No.**	**Study years**	**Results**	**Reference**
Rhabdomyosarcoma				
Children	1,529	1973-2005	Adults had significantly worse outcome than children, tumors were more likely to be at unfavorable site; 5-year survival rate 27% vs. 61%	Sultan et al., 2009
Adults	1,071			
Adults	171	1975-2001	Overall rate of response to chemotherapy was 85%; 5-year event-free survival was 28% and 5-year overall survival was 61%	Ferrari et al., 2003
Adults	113		5-year survival rate 26%	Ariel and Briceno, 1975
Ewing's sarcoma/PNET				
Age $\leq$ 14	190	1972-1992	Rate of relapse $\leq$14 years vs. >14 years: 15.9 vs. 13.8 ($p < 0.94$)	Bacci et al., 2004
Age > 14	212			
Adults	19	1995-2003	Median OS of patients $\leq$ 20 years vs. > 20 years did not differ ($p = 0.27$)	Yamada et al., 2006
Children	353			
Adults	24	1990-2005	Localized disease: 3-year survival 59%	Gupta et al., 2010
Desmoplastic small round cell tumor				
Adults	18	1998-2006	5-Year survival rate 27.9%	Liping et al., 2008
Adults	84	1995-2009	Median OS 33.1 months	Ahn et al., 2011

PNET: Primitive neuroectodermal tumor.

Sarcomas can also be matched between children and adults for purposes of comparison. Soft tissue sarcomas originate from mesenchymal cells. They are rare adult malignancies, comprising 1% of all cancers, but represent 12% of pediatric solid tumors (30), being responsible for a mortality burden of around 13% of cancer related deaths in patients 0-19 years of age (31). Some sarcomas, including rhabdomyosarcomas, Ewing's sarcomas, primary neuroectodermal tumors and desmoplastic small round cell tumors rarely occur in adults. When they do, unfavorable histology and distant metastasis are more common, resulting in a higher mortality (see Table 2). In pediatric trials, older age is also associated with worse outcomes (32). Despite the biology of individual sarcomas subtypes being vastly different, historically the treatment has been very similar between children and adults, including a combination of conventional chemotherapeutics, surgery and radiation (33), where the complete surgical excision remains the mainstay of therapy (see Figure 2).

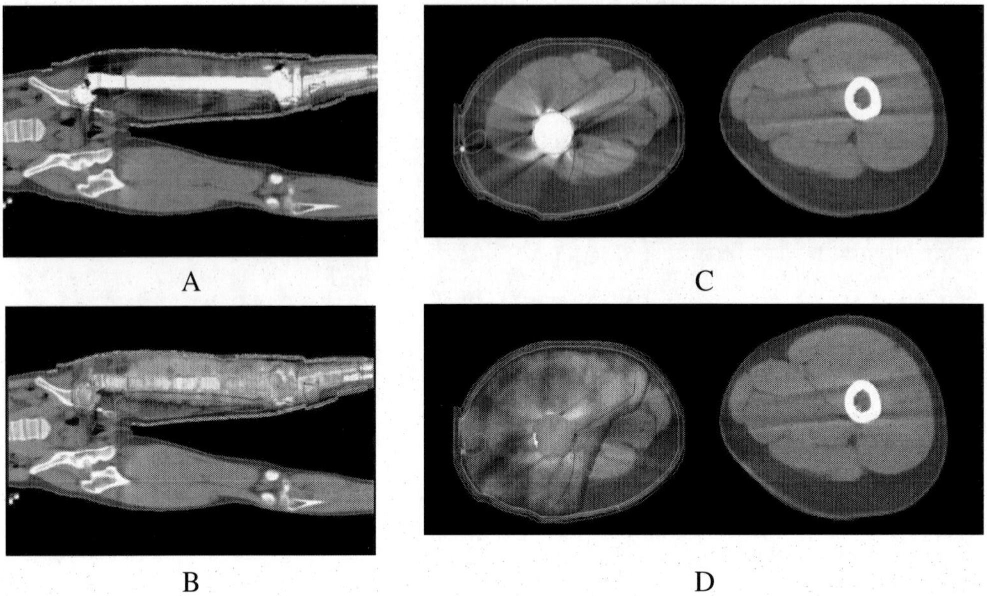

A. Coronal perspective of an adjuvant treatment volume for ressected sarcoma. B. Coronal perspective of the delivered dose with modulated technique. C. Axial perspective of the same adjuvant treatment volume for ressected sarcoma. D. Axial perspective of the same delivered dose with modulated technique.

Figure 2. Radiation adjuvant treatment for ressected sarcoma.

International trends in radiotherapy approach for different pediatric malignancies

A remarkable characteristic of radiotherapy's role in the multimodal management of pediatric malignant neoplasms is how radiation prescriptions (regarding treatment doses, volumes and moment to initiate) may vary amongst diverse therapeutic schemes. Although differences in combinations of chemotherapeutic agents and even in their dose intensity are observed between regional, national, and transnational protocols, they result in reasonably homogeneous outcomes in terms of cure.

Hodgkin's lymphoma

Hodgkin's lymphoma is a clear example of the absence of an international single "gold standard" protocol, with numerous choices of therapeutic schemes, including ones with lower or higher usage of chemotherapeutic agents or radiation doses. Variation not only occurs geographically, but also based on the age of the patient: children *vs.* adolescents and young adults *vs.* adults (34-38). Due to the success of these diverse treatment protocols in offering high local control, event-free and overall survival rates, the focus of researchers has progressively concentrated on the development of risk-adapted protocols aiming at improvements on late side effects. For example, the use of radiotherapy, due to the deleterious effects of ionizing radiation (34, 35), or even the intensity of all treatment, might be modulated in accordance to the presence or absence of clinical factors to which greater risks of therapeutic failure are attributed, or in accordance with the initial treatment response (36, 37).

Table 3. Wilms' tumor staging (NWST vs. SIOP)

Stage	NWTS	SIOP
I	Tumor limited to the kidney and completely resected. Renal surface intact, without tumor rupture.	Tumor limited to the kidney and completely resected. Renal surface intact, without tumor rupture.
II	Extra-renal extension, but completely resected. Tumor biopsy or rupture confined to flank. Macroscopic invasion or thrombus in peri-renal vessels (e.g., inferior vena cava and renal vein), but totally resected.	Extra-renal extension, but completely resected. Invasion of adjacent organs or vessels, but completelly resected. Peri-hilar lymph nodes may be involved, but completely resected.
II	Residual tumor after surgery, confined to the abdomen. Invasion of adjacent organs without possibility of surgical resection, regional lymph node metastases, intraperitoneal rupture during surgical procedure, or peritoneal surface invasion.	Residual tumor after surgery, confined to the abdomen. Invasion of adjacent organs without possibility of surgical resection, metastases to abdominal lymph nodes, intraperitoneal rupture before or during surgery, or peritoneal surface invasion. Tumor biopsied prior to initial treatment.
IV	Hematogenous metastases to the lung, liver, bones, or brain, or metastases to extra-abdominal lymph nodes.	Hematogenous metastases to the lung, liver, bones, or brain, or metastases to extra-abdominal lymph nodes.
V	Bilateral synchronous tumor. Each side must be defined amongst stages I and III.	Bilateral synchronous tumor. Each side must be defined amongst stages I and III.

NWST: National Wilms' Tumor Study (NWTS). SIOP: Societe Internationale D'oncologie Pediatrique.

In addition to those from many American and European cooperative groups, a similar effort has been exerted Latin America to offer risk-adapted management for childhood Hodgkin's lymphoma, limiting the usage of radiotherapy usually for patients with more advanced disease (39) (see Figure 3). In general, radiation doses are around 15 to 20 Gy, with addition of a "boost" of 5 to 10 Gy. Daily-recommended doses vary from 1.5 to 2.0 Gy, 5 times a week. It is important to note the dissimilarities of the treatment volumes, i.e., fields ("involved-field," "involved-site" and "involved-node"), and the specific radiotherapy recommendations of each treatment protocol. Also, apart from target delineation issues, these protocols sometimes demand different staging and response evaluation imaging exams; for example: computed tomography (CT) or positron emission tomography (PET)/CT, that will affect the extension of the consolidative radiation (40, 41).

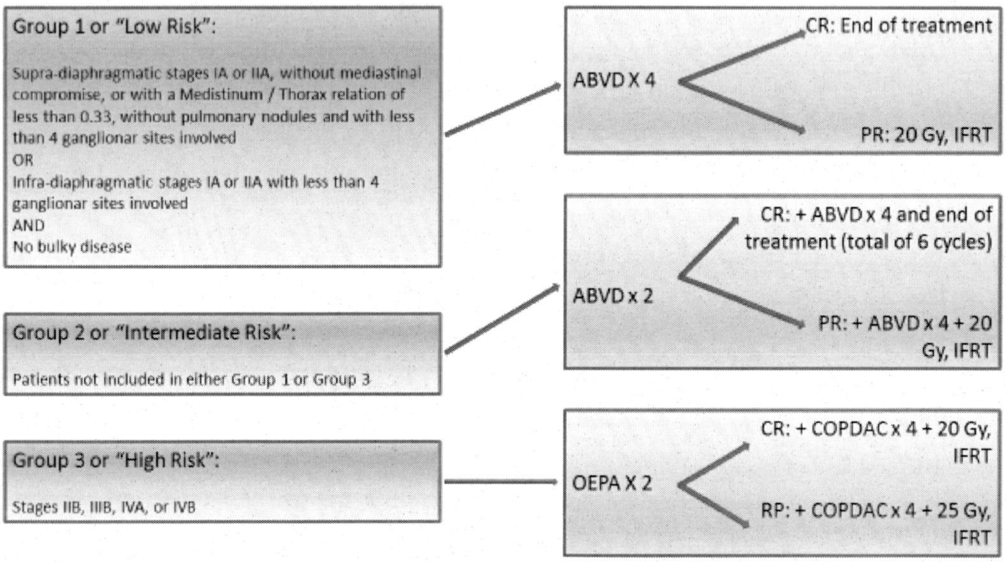

RC: complete response; RP: partial response; IFRT: "Involved-field" radiotherapy; Bulky: defined as tumor volume >6 cm in cross-section; ABVD: Adriamycin (25 mg/m²), Bleomycin (10 U/m²), Vinblastine (6 mg/m²), Dacarbazine (375 mg/m²); OEPA: Prednisone/prednisolone (60 mg/m²), Vincristine (1.5 mg/m²), Doxorubicin (40 mg/m²), Etoposide (125 mg/m²); COPDAC: Prednisone/prednisolone (40 mg/m²), Dacarbazine (250 mg/m²), Vincristine (1.5 mg/m²), Cyclophosphamide (500 mg/m²), Mesna (500 mg/m²).

Figure 3. Treatment algorithm of the LHBRA2015 Protocol of Brazilian Society of Pediatric Oncology (SOBOPE).

Wilms tumor

The greatest difference in terms of therapeutic approaches for pediatric verses adult malignancies occur with Wilms' Tumor protocols, as exemplified by the American National Wilms' Tumor Study (NWTS) and the European Société Internationale d'Oncologie Pédiatrique (SIOP). In NWTS, staging is performed after initial surgical treatment, while in SIOP, staging is performed after neoadjuvant chemotherapy and surgery, with the treatment recommendations directly related to therapeutic response (see Table 3). SIOP results demonstrate that preoperative therapy decreases the incidence of tumor rupture and seeding by the time nephrectomy is performed, and has a low toxicity profile (42, 43). Histological classifications defined by the NWTS and SIOP also differ. Anaplasia for example, is the pinnacle of the NWTS' classification, whereas SIOP classifications are based on cellular differentiation and chemotherapy-induced changes. In both protocols, the presence of diffuse anaplasia, morphologically defined, is considered a high-risk feature. However, the terminology "focal anaplasia" is not wholly equivalent in both protocols. The effect of neoadjuvant chemotherapy is grouped as an intermediate-risk feature by the SIOP's classification and recently categorized as a high-risk feature in the recent protocols from the "Cooperative Oncology Group" (COG), in continuity with NWTS protocols (44).

Table 4. Radiotherapy doses for Wilms' tumor treatment (NWST vs. SIOP)

Region	NWTS	SIOP
Flank	10.8 Gy (CS III, favorable histology, CS I - III, focal anaplasia, CS I - II, diffuse anaplasia) 19.8 Gy (CS III, diffuse anaplasia)	14,4 Gy (CS III, intermediate risk) 25,2 Gy (CS II and III, high risk, diffuse anaplasia, CS III, high risk and blastematous type)
Whole abdomen	10.5 Gy (CS III, tumor rupture or peritoneal metastasis)	15 Gy (CS III, intermediate risk, tumor rupture) 19.5 Gy (CS III, high risk, tumor rupture) 12 Gy (tumor rupture and age ≤ 24 months)
Dose "boost"	10.8 Gy (residual disease) 9 Gy (ES III, diffuse anaplasia and age >12 months)	10,8 Gy (residual disease)
Whole lung	10.5 Gy if age ≤ 12 months and 12 Gy if age > 12 months, (favorable histology and incomplete response at week 6, focal or diffuse anaplasia)	12 Gy (intermediate risk) * 15 Gy (high risk) * *dose "boost" of 10 to 13 Gy (intermediate risk) and 15 to 20 Gy (high risk) should be considered for residual disease after surgery
Metastasis	19.8 Gy to 30.6 Gy	14.4 to 36 Gy

NWST: National Wilms' Tumor Study (NWTS). SIOP: Societe Internationale D'oncologie Pediatrique. Adapted from Dome JS et al. (16) and the SIOP-RTSG-GCBTTW 2015 protocol.

Radiotherapy planning should be consistent with the proposed treatment scheme, with strict attention to the uniqueness of each approach, whether it is COG or SIOP. In general, treatment volumes for Wilms' Tumor remain very similar to the ones historically recommended at the conventional two-dimensional radiotherapy era, involving the tumor bed, (preferably determined by the imaging exams conducted at the initial diagnosis), with additional margins to include part of the affected hemi-abdomen ("flank") or all the abdominal cavity ("whole abdomen"). For the flank irradiation volume, cranium-caudal margins are limited to the initial disease extent and ought to include the total width of the vertebral bodies. In case of tumor rupture or intraperitoneal involvement, irradiation volume shall include the entire abdominal cavity, comprised between the diaphragm, pelvic floor, and abdominal walls. Caution is required to avoid radiation dose in excess to normal tissues, in example, the remaining kidney, heart, and lung.

Current recommendations from NWTS and COG studies suggest minimum treatment doses of 10.5 and 10.8 Gy for whole abdominal or flank irradiation, respectively, and reserve higher doses for residual or recurrent disease. In the SIOP studies, doses range from 14.4 to 15 Gy for flank or whole abdominal irradiation respectively, also reserving higher doses for residual or recurrent disease (45, 46) (see Table 4). Daily doses vary from 1.5 to 1.8 Gy, depending on the volume of irradiation, with smaller fractions indicated for larger volumes, (e.g., pulmonary or abdominal irradiation).

Despite these different approaches, the overall and event free survival observed by both groups are very similar (47, 48).

Childhood leukemia

Childhood leukemia has a wide variety of morphological and immunophenotypical presentations. Similar to Hodgkin's lymphoma, there is also a very large number of available therapeutic schemes, which can be used in the treatment of both lymphoid and myeloid variants (49, 50). In this setting, the role of radiotherapy over the last decade has been gradually restricted. Radiotherapy was a former agent of secondary prevention of recurrences in the central nervous system and spinal cord. Its use has since declined due to considerations of the potential risks of late side effects, such as cognitive alterations and induction of second primary neoplasms (51, 52).

Under a historical perspective, several of the international cooperative groups assessed the impact of radiotherapy de-intensification in some of their consecutive treatment protocols, especially for acute lymphoid leukemia and its replacement for intrathecal chemotherapy. Over the last five decades, the "total therapy" studies of St Jude Children's Research Hospital and the Berlin-Frankfurt-Munich group evaluated the impact of volume reduction (from craniospinal radiotherapy to whole cranial irradiation), dose reduction (24 Gy down to 12 Gy), and most importantly, the impact of a better selection of patients for whom prophylactic cranial irradiation (PCI) would then be indicated. PCI is now restricted to a minority of patients with higher recurrence risk (53, 54). In a recent meta-analysis published by Vora et al. (55) the use of PCI in patients from 1 to 18 years of age, diagnosed and treated between 1996 and 2007, has been reassessed with data from 10 cooperative groups from around the world. The proportion of patients eligible for PCI ranged from 0% to 33%, concluding that PCI was associated with a reduced risk of relapse in the subgroup of patients with CNS disease that manifested at the initial diagnosis (4% *vs.* 17%; $p = 0.02$) (55) (see Table 5).

Table 5. Indications of PCI in several studies for the treatment of childhood lymphocytic leukemia

Group and protocol	% of patients submitted to PCI	Indications
AIEOP ALL 2000	18	CNS3*, t(4;11) T cell with WBC > 100 x 10^9 / L, T cell and B cell with slow early response (prednisone poor response) or no CR at day 33 or high-risk MRD (≥ 5 x 10^{-4}) at week 12
BFM ALL 2000	18	CNS3*, t(4;11) T cell, B cell with slow early response (prednisone poor response) or no CR at day 33 or high risk MRD (≥ 5 x 10^{-4}) at week 12
COALL 06-97 and 07-03	12	CNS3 for both protocols. For 06-97: T cell and B cell with WBC > 100 x 10^9 / L. For 07-03: T cell with WBC > 50 x 10^9 / L, B cell with WBC > 200 x 10^9 / L and with WBC 100-200 x 10^9 / L and 1 x 10^9 / L blasts in the PB after prophase
DCOG ALL 09	0	Standard no PCI
JACLS ALL 02	10	CNS3, T cell with WBC > 100 x 10^9 / L
NOPHO ALL 2000	14	CNS3, T cell with mediastinal mass, T cell and B cell with WBC 100-200 x 10^9 / L; for all, only if age > 5 years at diagnosis
SJCRH Total Therapy Study XV	0	Standard no PCI
UK ALL 2003	2	CNS3
DFCI 00-01	22	T cell and B cell with CNS3 and / or WBC > 100 x 10^9 / L
GBTLI ALL 99	1,2	CNS3

Adapted from Vora A et al. (55) and Brandalise SR et al. (86).

AIEOP: Associazione Italiana Ematologia ed Oncologia Pediatrica; ALL: acute lymphoblastic leukemia; B-ALL: B cell acute lymphoblastic leukemia; BFM: Berlin-Frankfurt-Münster; BM: bone marrow; COALL: Cooperative Acute Lymphoblastic Leukemia Group; CNS3: overt CNS involvement; CR: complete remission; PCI: prophylactic cranial irradiation; DCOG: Dutch Children's Oncology Group; DFCI: Dana-Farber Cancer Institute; JACLS: Japanese Childhood Leukemia Study Group; MRD: minimal residual disease; NOPHO: Nordic Pediatric Hematology and Oncology Study Group; PB: peripheral blood; POG: Pediatric Oncology Group; SJCRH: St Jude Children's Research Hospital; T-ALL: T cell acute lymphoblastic leukemia; UK: United Kingdom and Ireland Group; GBTLI: Brazilian Childhood Cooperative Group for ALL Treatment.

*Includes patients with retinal infiltrates and cerebral/meningeal involvement on imaging in addition to those with blasts in CSF. Patients with normal CSF account for 52 of the 110 BFM patients included as having CNS3.

As with other pediatric malignant neoplasms such as those mentioned earlier, the radiation-oncologist ought to be alert to specific protocol details to correctly assign the therapeutic irradiation.

Technical aspects of childhood radiotherapy: choosing from conformal 3D to other more sophisticated modalities, and the cost-benefits and the risk of second primary malignancies

The current radiation oncologist faces an uncomfortable situation that may be the greatest of their challenges: to reconcile the scientific advances continuously presented in the medical literature with the resources available in the daily practice, often limited, and the real benefits expected from it. Proton therapy is probably the major contemporary focus of pediatric radiotherapy research, given its potential to reduce late complications from ionizing radiation, the Achilles' heel from this therapeutic modality. On the other hand, due to very high costs of proton therapy, much is discussed about its relevance in the current context of oncological care in developing countries, in which the amount of financial investment historically devoted to pediatric radiotherapy are usually very limited, not only for patient assistance but also for education and research (56, 57). On a lesser extent, questions regarding the cost-effectiveness of the proton therapy can be extended to other more mature technological advances, such as intensity modulated radiotherapy (IMRT), volumetric arc therapy (VMAT) and image-guided radiotherapy (IGRT). Currently there still are discussions regarding the possibility of an increased IMRT long-term carcinogenic potential due to larger volumes of tissues exposed to radiation low doses (58).

The standard procedure in treatment plan optimization is where the yes/no effect of tumor cure is a typical probabilistic (i.e., stochastic) endpoint achieved with the prescribed radiation dose and simultaneously, early and late normal tissues effects are yes/no avoided, or at least, the severity of effects are limited (i.e., deterministic) (59). For both early and late effects, the dose, amount of irradiated volumes, and even more relevant, the functional importance of the affected part of the organ must be considered and verified through dose-volume histograms treatment plans. For example, non-randomized clinical trials with patients submitted to adjuvant irradiation for medulloblastoma suggest lower incidences of ototoxicity in patients subjected to the posterior fossa "boost" with IMRT compared to RT3D (60). For rhabdomyosarcoma, subgroup analysis of a major clinical study suggests better coverage of the treatment target with IMRT (61).

Fortunately, the number of adult childhood-cancer survivors has increased over recent years (62). Sadly, their long-term survival also permits the long-latency radiation-associated secondary cancers to rise. In addition to two major studies, the US childhood survivor study (63) and the French-British Childhood survivor study (64), the recently published data from the German Childhood Hodgkin's Disease group provide the most convincing clinical data on the dependence of breast cancer risk on age and radiation dose (65, 66). High doses, which occur in or very close to the treatment volume, most often cause soft tissue sarcomas (which amount to 50% of all secondary cancers in the entire study population of childhood cancer survivors in the French/British cohort), whereas carcinomas, in particular adenocarcinomas of breast and thyroid, occur mostly in the penumbra of the radiation field.

The main reason for considering particle radiotherapy for childhood cancers is the possibility provided by the physical characteristics of protons to reduce the radiation exposure to organs and tissues close to the primary cancer. However, it doesn't without its own pitfalls: Hall's publication in 2006 stirred a lot of concern on the relative biological effectiveness of neutrons, which are inevitably produced, and the risk of secondary cancers induced from it (67). In order to investigate this, a comprehensive European project called ANDANTE is in progress (68).

Overall, there is no evidence based on randomized clinical trials to justify the use of routine proton therapy for the most prevalent malignant neoplasms in the pediatric age group. Clinical evidence is still lacking, where possibly future clinical studies reporting outcomes may reveal the real impact of the assumed theoretical dosimetric benefit from this technology (69, 70).

Anesthesia for radiotherapy

Radiotherapy is one of the main components of modern cancer treatment. Particularly for children, it requires substantial capital investment and trained professionals, where one of the very first obstacles found is the scarcity of centers with available anesthesia. It is part of a very sophisticated and complex care that has contributed to major disparities in cancer outcomes between high-income countries and low-and-middle income countries (71). Anesthesia is a crucial set-up to treat younger patients, as immobilization is a fundamental cornerstone for properly daily radiation dose delivery, keeping in mind that the irradiation applied is fixed in shape based on a previous CT image acquired for this purpose. Patient immobilization is especially important when modern planning techniques are used; when fields are created to be tight into the target volume, it allows for lower doses to normal surrounding structures.

Nearly all children aged 4 years or under require anesthesia, along with approximately 50% of children aged 4-6 years, and in some cases even children aged 10 years and over (72). In 2017 at Grupo de Apoio ao Adolescente e a Criança com Câncer (GRAACC), from a total of 223 children that started radiation sessions, 60 received daily anesthesia, of which 53 were less than 5 years old (see Figure 4). The remaining older children required it due to neurologic status (movement disorders or cognitive impairment) or psychological distress. There are some interventions that affect the proportion of children able to withstand the treatment without sedation. Unergoing treatment not only requires children to have the ability to keep still, but also to face the treatment room far away from their parents. In our experience, humanized interventions with psychologists resulted in reduction of anesthesia in 40% of designated cases for evaluation (73). In addition, a warm integration from all the radiotherapy team and available treatment room time large enough to permit a ludic experience are all utilised to help children feel safe enough to accept their treatment awake.

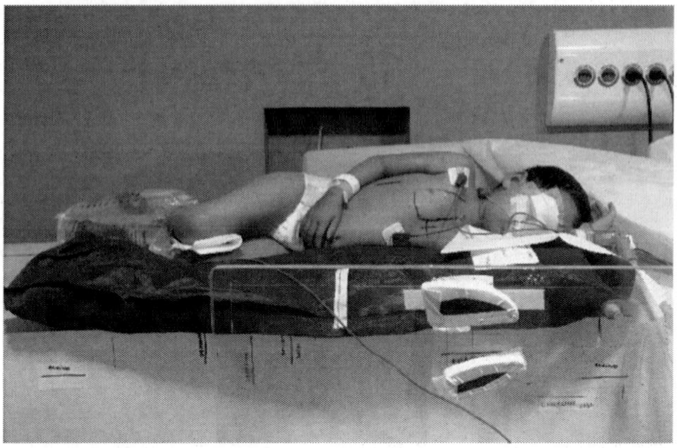

A

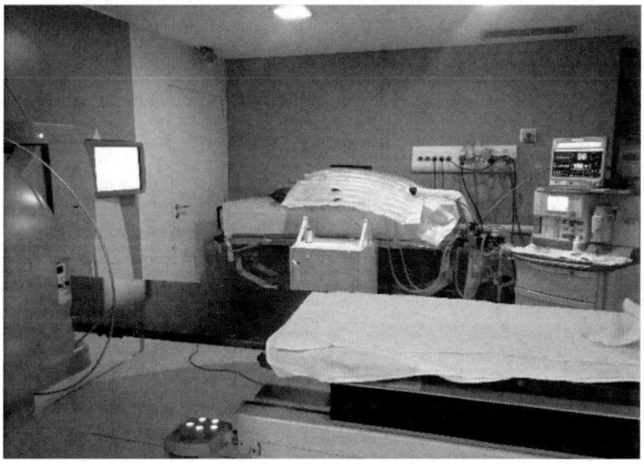

B

A. Child under anesthesia in the lateral decubitus position and alignment for the total-body irradiation with pulmonar partial blockage. B. Treatment room equipped with required instruments.

Figure 4. Anesthesia for total-body irradiation.

Not without reason, anesthesiologists need to be aware of the side effects and complications that are influenced by cancer type/location, the receipt of chemotherapy, and the dynamic of positioning each patient within specific accessories of immobilization. In the same way, radiation oncologists and pediatric oncologists have to be familiarized with anesthetic risk scales, types of anesthetic used, duration and degree of sedation, airway access and other salient medical conditions. In anticipation of each new treatment schedule, preferably soon after the first consultation with the radiation oncologist, the anesthesiologist will take the perioperative risk of the patient. The ASA-

PS (American Society of Anesthesiology Physical Status) classification system is one of several classification systems that estimate perioperative mortality for non-cardiac surgeries (74). The pertinence of this system is due to its property of translating the general medical condition of the patient and associating it with a risk. This may well correlate with our oncology patients who usually present with neoplasms or paraneoplastic syndromes or toxicities acquired through treatment, which cause systemic repercussions both for the cardiovascular system and for the respiratory system. These would correspond to category ASA 3 - severe systemic disease. The implications and cardiopulmonary complications of our patients cannot be explained by conventional cardiovascular risk factors such as coronary artery disease, heart failure or chronic obstructive pulmonary disease, for which there are other more targeted classification systems, such as Lee's Revised Cardiac Index, Goldman's Index, Detsky's Index, and the ACP (American College of Physicians) score. Instead, changes in the central regulation of the cardiovascular system and in the respiratory centers in the brainstem are found most often, as radiation treatment is often required for pediatric central nervous system tumors (75).

The clinical evaluation of patient risk should be revisited on a daily basis, considering the fluidity of the general health condition through the entire radiation course. There are some concomitant chemotherapeutic protocols, such as for medulloblastoma (76). Since it predicts that craniospinal irradiation and hematopoietic toxicity are expected, this demands a rigorous routine of checking laboratory values. Fever and mucous secretions impose session suspensions (77), unfortunately more often than the theoretical mechanism of radiobiology ideally permits, so every effort is applied to avoid infections, enact rapid screening of the infected individuals, apply contact insulation measures, and reinforcement of hygiene habits with the family.

The dose prescription of some radiotherapy regimens for sarcomas and CNS tumors can reach 30 to 35 sessions, imposing a long period of daily fasting. Associated with the nausea and hyporexia expected from radiation itself, there is a great negative impact on the weight of the patients. With this in mind, the Brazilian Society of Nutrition in line with the Society of Anesthesiology (78, 79), keeping up to date with the ERAS fasting protocol (Enhanced Recovery after Surgery) (80), is stimulating shorter periods of fasting through the use of specific glyco-solutions for oncologic patients. Patients are allowed to ingest clear liquids up to two hours before anesthetic induction. Also, aiming to avoid catabolic effects, a complex carbohydrate oral solution, such as malt dextrin in relatively high (12.5%) concentration is given up to two hours pre-procedure. Scheduling priority daily treatment, in order of youngest age and worst nutritional status, is another complementary action to combat the malnutrition of these children.

Until the end of 2017 at GRAACC, all craniospinal simulations were usually planned in the ventral decubitus position. Through 2016 and 2017, we counted 35 patients treated like this. In addition to rectifying the spine, this position allows direct visualization of the light field on the skin and so, the junction of the fields between the skull and the spine (81). However, anesthesia in the ventral decubitus requires the airway to be guaranteed by orotracheal intubation. Repeated intubation traumatizes the airway, making subsequent intubations increasingly difficult, and causing apophony and odynophagia, further decreasing oral intake and contributing to malnutrition. With the aid of an IGRT established algorithm (82), since 2017 our team reassigned all craniospinal simulations to a dorsal decubitus position, leaving the ventral position to very specific situations.

The treatment room time required for a procedure under anesthesia varies according to the expertise of each center. Disregarding delays, a single isocenter treatment takes about 40 minutes. There are routines for optimization, such as having an anteroom for the anesthetic induction, taking preferential use of fast-clearance anesthetic drugs and acquisition of the weekly IGRT images in different days rather than the beginning of the week (when patient's central lines are usually needled). Total intravenous anesthesia using propofol for maintenance sedation is not necessarily obligatory, as volatile agents such as sevoflurane are also an option. It is important to avoid anesthetic agents that stimulate nausea such as nitrous oxide, to provide a better and faster anesthetic recovery (83, 84). Externally published literature and data from our own survey report low complications rates on anesthesia for radiotherapy. The most prevalent complications being laryngospasm, bronchospasm, nausea and vomiting, with apnea and arrhythmias possible as well (77).

Besides specialized health care providers, including one anesthesiologist and two nurses (one can assist the anesthetic procedure while the other one takes care of the children treated earlier who are still recovering), specific material resources are required (85, 86). The room needs to be equipped with an anesthesia cart, monitors, emergency drugs and emergency equipment; medications should be stocked daily and include atropine, epinephrine, succinylcholine, lidocaine, salbutamol and ondansetron. The cart must also contain a box of controlled psychotropic medications. A capnograph is required to ensure visualization of the patient's tissue oxygenation profile, as well as the rate of anesthetic inhalation and exhalation. The capnograph information is transmitted to the anesthesiologist through a multiparameter monitor because during the irradiating beam, no one except the patient itself can remain inside the treatment room. A functioning vacuum suction is indispensable. The purchase of the accessories (laryngeal masks, Guedel airway) should be regular, as no session of treatment can be suspended because of a lack of material. An adequately staffed recovery room is in the same manner requisite to address emergencies properly.

REFERENCES

[1] Fedorovsky JM, Cuervo LG, Luciani S. *Pediatric cancer registries in Latin America: the case of Argentina's pediatric cancer registry*. Rev Panam Salud Pública 2017:41:e152.

[2] Brazilian Society of Pediatric Oncology. *Childhood and Adolescent Cancer in Brazil: Data from Mortality and Population-Based Registries*. Rio de Janeiro: National Cancer Institute, 2009.

[3] De Souza A. *América Latina, conceito e identidade: algumas reflexões da história*. Pr Rev Eletrônica Humanidades do Curso Ciências Sociais da UNIFAP [*Latin America, concept and identity: some reflections of history. Pr Eletr Eletrônica Humanities of the Social Sciences Course at UNIFAP*]. 2012;4(4): 29-39.

[4] Cueto M PS. Medicina E Saúde Pública Na América Latina: Uma História [*Medicine and Public Health in Latin America: A History*]. 1st ed. Rio de Janeiro: Editora Fiocruz, 2016.

[5] He J, Li X, Zhu W, Yu Y, Gong J. Research of differential expression of sIL1RAP in low-grade gliomas between children and adults [*Research on the differential expression of sIL1RAP in low-grade gliomas among children and adults*]. Brain Tumor Pathol 2018;35(1):19-28.

[6] Gajjar A, Bowers DC, Karajannis MA, Leary S, Witt H, Gottardo NG. *Pediatric brain tumors: Innovative genomic information is transforming the diagnostic and clinical landscape*. J Clin Oncol 2015;33(27):2986-98.

[7] Bar EE, Lin A, Tihan T, Burger PC, Eberhart CG. *Frequent gains at chromosome 7q34 involving BRAF in pilocytic astrocytoma*. J Neuropathol Exp Neurol 2008;67(9):878-7.

[8] Pfister S, Janzarik WG, Remke M, Ernst A, Werft W, Becker N, et al. *BRAF gene duplication constitutes a mechanism of MAPK pathway activation in low-grade astrocytomas*. J Clin Invest 2008;5(118):1739-49.

[9] Sievert AJ, Jackson EM, Gai X, Hakonarson H, Judkins AR, Resnick AC, et al. *Duplication of 7q34 in pediatric low-grade astrocytomas detected by high-density single-nucleotide polymorphism- based genotype arrays results in a novel BRAF fusion gene*. Brain Pathol 2009;3(19):449-58.

[10] Korshunov A, Meyer J, Capper D, Christians A, Remke M, Witt H, et al. *Combined molecular analysis of BRAF and IDH1 distinguishes pilocytic astrocytoma from diffuse astrocytoma.* Acta Neuropathol 2009;118(3):401-5.

[11] Cancer Genome Atlas Research Network, Brat DJ, Verhaak RG, Aldape KD, *Yung WK, Salama SR, et al. comprehensive, integrative genomic analysis of diffuse lower-grade gliomas*. N Engl J Med 2015;372(26):2481-98.

[12] Eckel-Passow JE, Lachance DH, Molinaro AM, Walsh KM, Decker PA, Sicotte H, et al. *Glioma groups based on 1p/19q, IDH, and TERT promoter mutations in tumors*. N Engl J Med 2015;372(26):2499-508.

[13] Wisoff JH, Sanford RA, Heier LA, Sposto R, Burger PC, Yates AJ, et al. *Primary neurosurgery for pediatric low-grade gliomas: A prospective multi-institutional study from the children's oncology group*. Neurosurgery 2011;68(6):1548-54.

[14] Merchant TE, Kun LE, Wu S, Xiong X, Sanford RA, Boop FA. Phase II trial of conformal radiation therapy for pediatric low-grade glioma. J Clin Oncol. 2009;27(22):3598-604.

[15] Müller K, Gnekow A, Falkenstein F, Scheiderbauer J, Zwiener I, Pietsch T, et al. *Radiotherapy in pediatric pilocytic astrocytomas: A subgroup analysis within the prospective multicenter study HIT-LGG 1996 by the German Society of Pediatric Oncology and Hematology (GPOH)*. Strahlentherapie und Onkol 2013;189(8):647-55.

[16] Packer RJ, Lange B, Ater J, Nicholson HS, Allen J, Walker R, et al. *Carboplatin and vincristine for recurrent and newly diagnosed low-grade gliomas of childhood*. J Clin Oncol 1993;(11):850-6.

[17] Bandopadhayay P, Bergthold G, London WB, Goumnerova LC, Morales La Madrid A, Marcus KJ, et al. *Long-term outcome of 4,040 children diagnosed with pediatric low-grade gliomas: an analysis of*

the surveillance epidemiology and end results (SEER) database. Pediatr Blood Cancer 2014;7(61): 1173-79.

[18] Fisher PG, Buerger PC. *Outcome Analysis of Childhood low-grade astrocytomas.* Pediatr Blood Cancer 2008;(51):245-50.

[19] Gnekow AK, Falkenstein F, von Hornstein S, Zwiener I, Berkefeld S, Bison B, et al. *Long-term follow-up of the multicenter, multidisciplinary treatment study HIT-LGG-1996 for low-grade glioma in children and adolescents of the German Speaking Society of Pediatric Oncology and Hematology*. Neuro Oncol 2012;10(14):1265-84.

[20] Merchant TE, Conklin HM, Wu S, Lustig RH, Xiong X. *Late effects of conformal radiation therapy for pediatric patients with low-grade glioma: Prospective evaluation of cognitive, endocrine, and hearing deficits.* J Clin Oncol 2009;27(22): 3691-7.

[21] Heegaard S, Brcendstrup O. *Proliferating Cell Nuclear Antigen and Ki-67 Immunohistochemistry of oligodendrogliomas with special reference to prognosis.* Cancer 1995;76(10):1809-13.

[22] Westphal M, Lamszus K, Hilt D. *Intracavitary chemotherapy for glioblastoma: present status and future directions.* Acta Neurochir Suppl 2003;88:61-7.

[23] Omuro AMP, Faivre S, Raymond E. *Lessons learned in the development of targeted therapy for malignant gliomas*. Mol Cancer Ther 2007;6(7):1909-19.

[24] MacDonald J, Aguillera D, Kramm C. *Treatment of high-grade glioma in children and adolescents*. Neuro Oncol 2011;13(10):1049-58.

[25] Stupp R, Mason WP, van den Bent MJ, Weller M, Fisher B, Taphoorn MJ, et al. *Radiotherapy plus concomitant and adjuvant temozolomide for glioblastoma*. N Engl J Med 2005;352(10):987-96.

[26] Paugh BS, Qu C, Jones C, Liu Z, Adamowicz-Brice M, Zhang J, et al. *Integrated molecular genetic profiling of pediatric high-grade gliomas reveals key differences with the adult disease*. J Clin Oncol 2010;28(18):3061-68.

[27] Louis DN, Perry A, Reifenberger G, von Deimling A, Figarella-Branger D, Cavenee WK, et al. *The 2016 World Health Organization classification of tumors of the central nervous system: a summary*. Acta Neuropathol 2016;131(6):803-20.

[28] Fangusaro J. *Pediatric high-grade gliomas and diffuse intrinsic pontine gliomas*. J Child Neurol 2009;24(11):1409-17.

[29] Cohen KJ, Pollack IF, Zhou T, Buxton A, Holmes EJ, Burger PC, et al. *Temozolomide in the treatment of high-grade gliomas in children: a report from the Children's Oncology Group*. Neuro Oncol 2011;13(3):317-23.

[30] Jo VY, Fletcher CD. *WHO classification of soft tissue tumours: An update based on the 2013 (4th) edition*. Pathology 2014;46(2):95-104.

[31] SEER Program. *Cancer incidence and survival among children and adolescents: United States SEER program 1975-1995*. Bethesda, MD: National Cancer Institute, 1999.

[32] Joshi D, Anderson JR, Paidas C, Breneman J, Parham DM, Crist W, et al. *Age is an independent prognostic factor in rhabdomyosarcoma: a report from the Soft Tissue Sarcoma Committee of the Children's Oncology Group*. Pediatr Blood Cancer 2004;42(1):64-73.

[33] Hingorani P, Janeway K, Crompton BD, Kadoch C, Mackall CL, Khan J, et al. *Current state of pediatric sarcoma biology and opportunities for future discovery: A report from the sarcoma translational research workshop*. Cancer Genet 2016;209(5):182-94.

[34] Donaldson SS, Link MP, Weinstein HJ, Rai SN, Brain S, Billett AL, et al. *Final results of a prospective clinical trial with VAMP and low-dose involved-field radiation for children with low-risk Hodgkin's disease.* J Clin Oncol 2007;3(25):332-7.

[35] Metzger ML, Weinstein HJ, Hudson MM, Billett AL, Larsen EC, Friedmann A, et al. *Association between radiotherapy vs no radiotherapy based on early response to VAMP chemotherapy and survival among children with favorable-risk Hodgkin lymphoma.* JAMA 2012;27(307):2609-16.

[36] Tebbi CK, Mendenhall NP, London WB, Williams JL, Hutchison RE, Fitzgerald TJ, et al. *Response-dependent and reduced treatment in lower risk Hodgkin lymphoma in children and adolescents, results of P9426: A report from the Children's Oncology Group*. Pediatr Blood Cancer 2012;7(59):1259-65.

[37] Dörffel W, Lüders H, Rühl U, Albrecht M, Marciniak H, et al. *Preliminary results of the multicenter trial GPOH-HD 95 for the treatment of Hodgkin's disease in children and adolescents: analysis and outlook*. Klin Padiatr 2003;3(215):139-45.

[38] Pieters RS, Wagner H, Baker S, Morano K, Ulin K, Cicchetti MG, et al. *The impact of protocol assignment for older adolescents with hodgkin lymphoma*. Front Oncol 2014;4(317).

[39] Pavlovsky S, Corrado C, Pavlovsky MA, Prates MV, Zoppegno L, Giunta M, et al. *Risk-adapted therapy with three or six cycles of doxorubicin/ bleomycin/ vinblastine/dacarbazine plus involved-field radiation therapy in Hodgkin lymphoma, based on prognosis at diagnosis and early response: results from the GATLA study*. Clin Lymphoma Myeloma Leuk 2010;3(10):181-5.

[40] Specht L, Yahalom J, Illidge T, Berthelsen AK, Constine LS, Eich HT, et al. ILROG. *Modern radiation therapy for Hodgkin lymphoma: field and dose guidelines from the international lymphoma radiation oncology group (ILROG)*. Int J Radiat Oncol Biol Phys 2014;4(89):854-62.

[41] Hodgson D, Dieckmann K, Terezakis S, Constine L, *International Lymphoma Radiation Oncology Group. Implementation of contemporary radiation therapy planning concepts for pediatric Hodgkin lymphoma: Guidelines from the International Lymphoma Radiation Oncology Group*. Pr Radiat Oncol 2015;2(5):85-92.

[42] Lemerle J, Voute PA, Tournade MF, Delemarre JF, Jereb B, Ahstrom L, et al. *Preoperative versus postoperative radiotherapy, single versus multiple courses of actinomycin D, in the treatment of Wilms' tumor. Preliminary results of a controlled clinical trial conducted by the International Society of Paediatric Oncology (S.I.O.P.)*. Cancer 1976;2(38):647-54.

[43] Lemerle J, Voute PA, Tournade MF, Rodary C, Delemarre JF, Sarrazin D, et al. *Effectiveness of preoperative chemotherapy in Wilms' tumor: results of an International Society of Paediatric Oncology (SIOP) clinical trial*. Clin Oncol 1983;10(1):604-9.

[44] Davidoff A. Wilms tumor. Adv Pediatr 2012;1(59):247-67.

[45] Tournade MF, Com-Nougué C, Voûte PA, Lemerle J, de Kraker J, Delemarre JF, et al. *Results of the Sixth International Society of Pediatric Oncology Wilms' Tumor Trial and Study: a risk-adapted therapeutic approach in Wilms' tumor*. J Clin Oncol 1993;6(11):1014-23.

[46] Nicolin G, Taylor R, Baughan C, Shannon R, Stevens S, Richardson D, et al. *Outcome after pulmonary radiotherapy in Wilms' tumor patients with pulmonary metastases at diagnosis: a UK Children's Cancer Study Group, Wilms' Tumour Working Group Study*. Int J Radiat Oncol Biol Phys 2008;1(70):175-80.

[47] Grundy PE, Breslow NE, Li S, Perlman E, Beckwith JB, Ritchey ML, et al. *Loss of heterozygosity for chromosomes 1p and 16q is an adverse prognostic factor in favorable-histology Wilms tumor: a report from the National Wilms Tumor Study Group*. J Clin Oncol 2005;29(23):7312-21.

[48] Pritchard-Jones K, Bergeron C, de Camargo B, van den Heuvel-Eibrink MM, Acha T, Godzinski J, et al. *Omission of doxorubicin from the treatment of stage II-III, intermediate-risk Wilms' tumour (SIOP WT 2001): an open-label, non-inferiority, randomised controlled trial*. Lancet 2015;9999(386):1156-64.

[49] Pui CH, Yang JJ, Hunger SP, Pieters R, Schrappe M, Biondi A, et al. *Childhood acute lymphoblastic leukemia: progress through collaboration*. J Clin Oncol 2015;27(33):2938-48.

[50] Zwaan CM, Kolb EA, Reinhardt D, Abrahamsson J, Adachi S, Aplenc R, et al. *Collaborative efforts driving progress in pediatric acute myeloid leukemia*. J Clin Oncol 2015;27(33):2949-62.

[51] Löning L, Zimmermann M, Reiter A, Kaatsch P, Henze G, Riehm H, et al. *Secondary neoplasms subsequent to Berlin-Frankfurt-Münster therapy of acute lymphoblastic leukemia in childhood: significantly lower risk without cranial radiotherapy*. Blood 2000;9(95):2770-5.

[52] Pui CH, Pei D, Campana D, Bowman WP, Sandlund JT, Kaste SC, et al. *Treating childhood acute lymphoblastic leukemia without cranial irradiation*. N Engl J Med 2009;26(360):2730-41.

[53] Schrappe M, Reiter A, Zimmermann M, Harbott J, Ludwig WD, Henze G, et al. *Long-term results of four consecutive trials in childhood ALL performed by the ALL-BFM study group from 1981 to 1995.* Leukemia 2000;12(14):2205-22.

[54] Pui C, Evans W. *A 50-year journey to cure childhood acute lymphoblastic leukemia*. Semin Hematol 2013;3(50):185-96.

[55] Vora A, Andreano A, Pui CH, Hunger SP, Schrappe M, Moericke A, et al. *Influence of cranial radiotherapy on outcome in children with acute lymphoblastic leukemia treated with contemporary therapy.* J Clin Oncol 2016;9(34):919-26.

[56] Rosenblatt E, Meghzifene A, Belyakov O, Abdel-Wahab M. Relevance of particle therapy to developing countries. Int J Radiat Oncol Biol Phys 2016;1(95):25-29.

[57] Kortmann RD, Freeman C, Marcus K, Claude L, Dieckmann K, Halperin E, et al. *Paediatric radiation oncology in the care of childhood cancer: A position paper by the International Paediatric Radiation Oncology Society (PROS)*. Radiother Oncol. 2016;2(119):357-60.

[58] Hall E. *The inaugural Frank Ellis Lecture-latrogenic cancer: the impact of intensity-modulated radiotherapy*. Clin Oncol 2006;4(18):277-82.

[59] Bentzen S. Dose-response relations in radiotherapy. In: Joiner M, van der Kogel A, eds. Basic clinical radiobiology. London: Edward Arnold, 2009:56-67.

[60] Huang E, Teh BS, Strother DR, Davis QG, Chiu JK, Lu HH, et al. *Intensity-modulated radiation therapy for pediatric medulloblastoma: early report on the reduction of ototoxicity*. Int J Radiat Oncol Biol Phys 2002;3(52):599-605.

[61] Lin C, Donaldson SS, Meza JL, Anderson JR, Lyden ER, Brown CK, al. *Effect of radiotherapy techniques (IMRT vs. 3D-CRT) on outcome in patients with intermediate-risk rhabdomyosarcoma enrolled in COG D9803--a report from the Children's Oncology Group*. Int J Radiat Oncol Biol Phys 2012;5(82):1764-70.

[62] Armstrong GT, Chen Y, Yasui Y, Leisenring W, Gibson TM, Mertens AC, et al. *Reduction in late mortality among 5-year survivors of childhood cancer*. N Engl J Med 2016; (374):833-42.

[63] Robison LL, Mertens AC, Boice JD, Breslow NE, Donaldson SS, Green DM. et al. *Study design and cohort characteristics of the childhood cancer survivor study: a multi-institutional collaborative project.* Med Pediatr Oncol 2002;(38):229-39.

[64] Tukenova M, Guibout C, Hawkins M, Quiniou E, Mousannif A, Pacquement H, et al. *Radiation therapy and late mortality from second sarcoma, carcinoma, and hematological malignancies after a solid cancer in childhood*. Int J Radiat Oncol Biol Phys 2011;(80):339-48.

[65] Dörffel W, Riepenhausen M, Lüders H, Brämswig J, Schellong G. Sekundäre maligne neoplasien nach therapie eines Hodgkin-Lymphoms im kindes-und jugendalter [*Secondary malignant neoplasia after therapy for Hodgkin's lymphoma in childhood and adolescence*]. Dtsch Arztebl 2015;(112):320-27.

[66] Schellong G, Riepenhausen M, Ehlert K, Brämswig J, Dörffel W, Schmutzler RK, et al. *Brustkrebs bei jungen Frauennach Therapie eines Hodgkin-Lymhoms im Kindes- und Jugendalter* [*Breast cancer in young women After therapy for Hodgkin's lymphoma in childhood and adolescence*]. Dtsch Arztebl 2015;(111):3-9.

[67] Hall E. *Intensity-modulated radiation therapy, protons, and the risk of second cancers*. Int J Radiat Oncol Biol Phys 2006;(65):12-22.

[68] The ANDANTE project. *Final Report Summary*. URL: https://cordis.europa.eu/result/rcn/182088_en.html.

[69] Leroy R, Benahmed N, Hulstaert F, Van Damme N, De ruysscher d. *proton therapy in children: a systematic review of clinical effectiveness in 15 pediatric cancers*. Int J Radiat Oncol Biol Phys 2016;1(95):267-78.

[70] Eaton BR, Esiashvili N, Kim S, Weyman EA, Thornton LT, Mazewski C, et al. *Clinical outcomes among children with standard-risk medulloblastoma treated with proton and photon radiation therapy: a comparison of disease control and overall survival.* Int J Radiat Oncol Biol Phys 2016;1(94):133-8.

[71] Magrath I, Epelman S. *Cancer in adolescents and young adults in countries with limited resources.* Curr Oncol Rep 2013;15(4):332-46.

[72] Owusu-Agyemang P, Popovich SM, Zavala AM, Grosshans DR, Van Meter A, Williams UU, et al. *A multi-institutional pilot survey of anesthesia practices during proton radiation therapy.* Pr Radiat Oncol 2016;(6):155-9.

[73] Viana LC, Cortez LS, Antunes NJ, Toledo TW, Garcia FB, Macedo TM, et al. *Psychologist intervention in radiotherapy treatment for patients with or without anesthesia/sedation: Report of a Brazilian experience in a radiotherapy unit in pediatric oncology.* XXIX Congress of SLAOP – Sociedad Latinoamericana de Oncología Pediátrica, Sao Paulo, 2018. [Portugese].

[74] Miller R, Cohen N, Eriksson L, Fleisher L, Wiener-Kronish J, Young W Miller's anesthesia, 8th ed. Philadelphia, PA: Elsevier, 2015.

[75] Bindra R, Wolden S. *Advances in radiation therapy in pediatric neuro-oncology.* J Child Neurol 2016;4(31):506-16.

[76] Jakacki RI, Burger PC, Zhou T, Holmes EJ, Kocak M, Onar A, et al. *Outcome of children with metastatic medulloblastoma treated with carboplatin during craniospinal radiotherapy: a Children's Oncology Group Phase I/II study.* J Clin Oncol 2012 20;30(21):2648-53.

[77] Verma V, Beethe A, LeRiger M, Kulkarni R, Zhang M, Lin C. *Anesthesia complications of pediatric radiation therapy.* Pr Radiat Oncol 2016;3(6):143-54.

[78] Nascimento JEA, Campos AC, Borges A, Correia MITD, Tavares GM. Sociedade Brasileira de Nutrição Parenteral e Enteral e Associação Brasileira de Nutrologia. Terapia Nutricional no Perioperatório. Projeto Diretrizes: Associação Médica Brasileira e Conselho Federal de Medicina, 2011. [Portugese].

[79] Aguilar-Nascimento J, Perrone F, Prado L. *Preoperative fasting of 8 hours or 2 hours: what does evidence reveal*? Rev Col Bras Cir 2009;(36):350-2.

[80] Feldheiser A, Aziz O, Baldini G, Cox B, KCH F, Feldman L et al. *Enhanced Recovery After Surgery (ERAS) for gastrointestinal surgery, part 2: Consensus statement for anaesthesia practice.* Acta Anaesthesiol Scand 2016;3(60):289-334.

[81] Verma J, Mazloom A1 Teh BS, South M, Butler EB, Paulino AC. *Comparison of supine and prone craniospinal irradiation in children with medulloblastoma.* Pr Radiat Oncol 2015;2(5):93-8.

[82] Figueiredo MLS, Chen MJ, Chaves CLG, Belletti F, Baptista L, Batista B, et al. *Apresentação de protocolo de image-guided radiotherapy (IGRT) na rotina do departamento de radioterapia do Grupo de Apoio ao Adolescente e Criança com Câncer (GRAACC) [Presentation of an image-guided radiotherapy (IGRT) protocol in the routine of the radiotherapy department of the Support Group for Adolescents and Children with Cancer (GRAACC)].* Braz J Oncol 2017;13(Supl): 1-402.

[83] George JA, Koka R, Gan TJ, Jelin E, Boss EF, Strockbine V, et al. *Review of the enhanced recovery pathway for children: perioperative anesthetic considerations.* Can J Anaesth 2017;65(5)569-77.

[84] Mazoit J. *Pharmacokinetic/pharmacodynamic modeling of anesthetics in children: therapeutic implications.* Paediatr Drugs 2006;3(8):139-50.

[85] Resolução CFM N 1.802/2006 (Publicado No D.O.U. de 01 Novembro 2006, Seção I, Pg. 102). *Retificação Publicada* No D.O.U. URL: https://sistemas.cfm.org.br/no rmas/visualizar/resolucoes/BR/2006/1802.

[86] Brandalise SR, Pinheiro VR, Aguiar SS, Matsuda EI, Otubo R, Yunes JA, et al. *Benefits of the intermittent use of 6-mercaptopurine and methotrexate in maintenance treatment for low-risk acute lymphoblastic leukemia in children: randomized trial from the Brazilian Childhood Cooperative Group-protocol ALL-99.* J Clin Oncol 2010;11(28):1911-8.

In: Cancer Management in Latin America II
Editors: Maurício F Silva et al.
ISBN: 978-1-53616-735-1

Chapter 5

MANAGEMENT OF LOW-GRADE GLIOMA

Eduardo Weltman*[1,2,*]*, MD PhD, Renato Ghelfond*[1]*, MD, Vinicius Calheiros*[1]*, MD, Fiona Lim*[3]*, MBBS, Bo Angela Wan*[4]*, MD(C) and Mauricio F Silva*[5,6,7]*, MD, PhD

[1]Radiation Oncology Discipline, Faculdade de Medicina da Universidade de São Paulo, São Paulo, Brazil
[2]Radiation Oncology Department at Hospital Israelita Albert Einstein, University of São Paulo, São Paulo, Brazil
[3]Department of Oncology, Princess Margaret Hospital, Hong Kong, PR China
[4]Odette Cancer Centre, Sunnybrook Health Sciences Centre, Toronto, Ontario, Canada
[5]Radiation Oncology Unit, Santa Maria Federal University, Santa Maria, Brazil
[6]Hospital de Caridade Astrogildo de Azevedo, Santa Maria, Brazil
[7]Latin America Cooperative Oncology Group, Porto Alegre, Brazil

ABSTRACT

Low grade gliomas are challenging tumors to manage. They are less aggressive than high grade gliomas but are frequently still fatal. Isocitrate dehydrogenase (IDH) mutation, Karnofsky performance score (KPS), age and pathological type are recognized prognostic factors. Surgery that aims at complete resection is the mainstay of treatment, but this may not always be feasible due to tumor extension to important functional areas of the brain. Radiotherapy has been proven to be useful in prolonging progression-free survival (PFS) following surgery, whether as adjuvant or salvage therapy. However, it has failed so far to confer overall survival (OS) benefit when employed as an isolated adjuvant treatment Adding chemotherapy to radiation is promising, with a possible better OS outcome. It is also a valuable option when postponement of radiotherapy is considered in order to avoid specific risks and side effects, especially in children.

* Corresponding Author's Email: eweltman@einstein.br.

INTRODUCTION

Gliomas are a group of neuroepithelial tumors originating from the supporting glial cells of the central nervous system (CNS). This group encompasses astrocytomas, oligodendrogliomas, glioblastomas and oligoastrocytomas (1). The World Health Organization (WHO) classification system categorizes gliomas from grade I (lowest grade) to grade IV (highest grade) based on histopathologic, genotypic and phenotypic characteristics, where a higher grade carries worse prognosis (2). Low grade gliomas include tumors that are classified as Grade I and Grade II. Treatment of these tumors usually require multimodal approaches.

Surgery is the mainstay of treatment in low grade glioma. There is growing evidence that early aggressive treatment improves overall survival and delays the time to malignant progression (4, 5). Multiple series had shown a better prognosis and an increase in overall survival when a complete resection is achieved (4-7). Similar outcomes were demonstrated in a recent meta-analysis published in 2018 (8). However, gross total resection is only feasible in the minority of cases. Most series reported no more than 38% of success due to the proximity between tumor and eloquent (functional) parts of the brain in which wide resections may lead to unacceptable risk of neurological deficit (5). Although the completeness of glioma resection independently correlates with patient survival (4-6), the final extent of surgery that can be achieved is often limited by the extent of tumor infiltration into critical structures and the expected permanent morbidities after surgery (9). Postoperative radiotherapy and chemotherapy are viable options for residual or unresectable tumors (10). Tailored treatments based on the identification of genetic markers with prognostic value, such as IDH-mutation and 1p/19q co-deletion, are also being vigorously studied (11). The RTOG-9802 study established a new landmark in 2016 by showing an increase in overall survival with adjuvant chemoradiation. This chapter aims to address the overall treatments of low-grade glioma, with focus on the role of radiotherapy in a multimodality approach.

OUR SEARCH

We performed a Medline search of the manuscripts published in the last 16 years (January 2002 to June 2018) using the following search terms in title and abstracts: 1- Low grade glioma, 2- Radiotherapy, 3-Adjuvant. We limited the search literature to published studies in human, English, Spanish and Portuguese which returned more than 1,000 publications. Studies were selected according to the interest of this paper, resulting in a total of 40 studies.

Table 1. Summary of most relevant included studies

Study	Primary Cancer	Intervention	Result	Notes
Louis DN et al. (2)	CNS tumors	Defines nomenclature for the different CNS tumors and their molecular signatures.	Restructured diffuse gliomas, medulloblastomas and other embryonal tumors. Incorporated entities that are defined by both histology and molecular features (glioblastoma, IDH-wildtype and glioblastoma, IDH-mutant; diffuse midline glioma, H3 K27M-mutant; RELA fusion-positive ependymoma; medulloblastoma, WNT-activated and medulloblastoma, SHH-activated; and embryonal tumor with multilayered rosettes, C19MC-altered). Added newly recognized neoplasms, and deleted some entities, variants and patterns that no longer have diagnostic and/or biological relevance. Addition of brain invasion as a criterion for atypical meningioma.	The 2016 WHO Classification of CNS Tumors.
Capelle L et al. (4)	WHO grade II gliomas	Retrospective study. Search of prognostic factors for survival in patients with grade II gliomas ($n = 1097$).	At the time of radiological diagnosis, independent spontaneous factors of a poor prognosis were age ≥ 55 years, impaired functional status, tumor location in nonfrontal area, and most significantly, a larger tumor size. When the study starting point was set at the time of first treatment, independent favorable prognostic factors were limited to a smaller tumor size, an epileptic symptomatology, and a greater extent of resection.	
McGirt MJ et al. (5)	Low grade gliomas (WHO grade II gliomas)	Retrospective study comparing outcomes for GTR (gross tumor resection), NTR (near total resection) or STR (subtotal resection). Outcomes were OS, PFS, and malignant degeneration-free survival (conversion to high-grade glioma) ($n = 170$).	132 primary and 38 revision resections were performed for low-grade astrocytomas ($n = 93$) or oligodendrogliomas ($n = 77$). GTR, NTR, and STR were achieved in 65 (38%), 39 (23%), and 66 (39%) cases, respectively. GTR versus STR was independently associated with increased OS (HR: 0.36; 95% CI: 0.16-0.84; $p < 0.017$) and PFS (HR:0.56; 95%CI:0.32-0.98; $p = 0.043$) and a trend of increased malignant degeneration-free survival (HR:0.46; 95% CI:0.20-1.03; $p < 0.060$). NTR versus STR was not independently associated with improved OS, PFS, or malignant degeneration-free survival. Five-year OS after GTR, NTR, and STR was 95, 80, 70%, respectively, and 10-year OS was 76, 57, and 49%, respectively. After GTR, NTR, and STR, median time to tumor progression was 7.0, 4.0, and 3.5 years, respectively. Median time to malignant degeneration after GTR, NTR, and STR was 12.5, 5.8, and 7 years, respectively.	

Table 1. (Continued)

Study	Primary Cancer	Intervention	Result	Notes
Duffau H. et al. (6)	Supratentorial low grade gliomas (WHO grade II gliomas)	Single-institution comparing survival, rate of severe neurological deficits and extent of resection following surgery with or without DES (direct electrical stimulation) ($n = 100$).	Comparison between the two series showed that 35% of LGGs were operated on in eloquent areas in S1 versus 62% in S2 ($p < 0.0001$), with 17% severe permanent deficits in S1 versus 6.5% in S2 ($p < 0.019$). On postoperative MRI, 37% of resections were subtotal and 6% total in S1 versus 50.8% and 25.4%, respectively, in S2 ($p < 0.001$). In both groups, survival was significantly related to the quality of resection.	
Xia L et al. (8)	Low grade gliomas	Meta-analysis comparing outcomes for GTR (gross total resection) or STR (subtotal resection) - 5-year OS and 10-year OS ($n = 20$ articles, 2128 patients).	5-year OS (OR:3.90, 95% CI:2.79-5.45, $p < 0.01$, $Z = 7.95$) and 10-year OS (OR:7.91, 95% CI:5.12-12.22, $p < 0.01$, $Z = 9.33$) associated with gross total resection (GTR) were higher than those associated with subtotal resection (STR). Similarly, as compared with biopsy, the 5-year and 10-year OS were higher after either GTR (5-year: OR:5.43, 95% CI: 3.57-8.26, $P < 0.01$, $Z = 7.9$; 10-year: OR:10.17, 95% CI: 4.02-25.71; $P < 0.00001$, $Z = 4.9$) or STR (5-year: OR: 2.59, 95% CI: 1.81-3.71, $p < 0.00001$, $Z = 5.19$; 10-year: OR:2.21, 95% CI:1.16-4.25, $P = 0.02$, $Z = 2.39$).	
Buckner JC et al. (10)	WHO grade II gliomas	Trial randomly assigning patients to receive RT alone or RT plus combination chemotherapy following biopsy or resection. Outcomes were PFS and OS ($n = 251$).	A total of 251 eligible patients were enrolled from 1998 through 2002. The median follow-up was 11.9 years; 55% of the patients died. Patients who received radiation therapy plus chemotherapy had longer median overall survival than did those who received radiation therapy alone (13.3 vs. 7.8 years, HR:0.59, $p = 0.003$). The rate of progression-free survival at 10 years was 51% in the group that received radiation therapy plus chemotherapy versus 21% in the group that received radiation therapy alone; the corresponding rates of overall survival at 10 years were 60% and 40%. A Cox model identified receipt of radiation therapy plus chemotherapy and histologic findings of oligodendroglioma as favorable prognostic variables for both progression-free and overall survival.	RTOG 9802 trial.

Study	Primary Cancer	Intervention	Result	Notes
Brat D, Verhaak et al. (11)	WHO grade II and III gliomas	Genome-wide analyses of lower-grade gliomas from adults, incorporating exome sequence, DNA copy number, DNA methylation, messenger RNA expression, microRNA expression, and targeted protein expression were performed. These data were integrated and tested for correlation with clinical outcomes (n = 293).	Unsupervised clustering of mutations and data from RNA, DNA-copy-number, and DNA-methylation platforms uncovered concordant classification of three robust, nonoverlapping, prognostically significant subtypes of lower-grade glioma that were captured more accurately by IDH, 1p/19q, and TP53 status than by histologic class. Patients who had lower-grade gliomas with an IDH mutation and 1p/19q codeletion had the most favorable clinical outcomes. Their gliomas harbored mutations in CIC, FUBP1, NOTCH1, and the TERT promoter. Nearly all lower-grade gliomas with IDH mutations and no 1p/19q codeletion had mutations in TP53 (94%) and ATRX inactivation (86%). The large majority of lower-grade gliomas without an IDH mutation had genomic aberrations and clinical behavior strikingly similar to those found in primary glioblastoma.	Part of Cancer Genome Atlas Network.
Baumert BG et al. (16)	WHO grade II gliomas	Randomized, open-label, phase 3 trial comparing PFS (intention-to-treat analysis), OS, adverse events, neurocognitive function, health-related quality of life and neurological function, and correlative analyses of progression-free survival by molecular markers, between 2 groups: conformal radiotherapy or dose-dense TMZ (n = 477).	Severe hematological toxicity occurred in 14% of TMZ-treated patients, infections in 3% of TMZ-treated patients, and 1% of RT-treated patients. Moderate to severe fatigue was recorded in 3% of patients in the RT group and 7% in the TMZ group. At a median follow-up of 48 months (IQR:31-56), median PFS was 39 months (IQR:16-46) in the TMZ arm and 46 months (IQR:19-48) in the RT group (HR:1.16, 95% CI:0.9-1.5, p = 0.22). Median OS has not been reached. Exploratory analyses identified treatment-dependent variation in outcome of molecular LGG subgroups (n = 318).	EORTC 22033-26033 trial.
Van den Bent MJ et al. (24)	Low-grade astrocytoma, oligodendroglioma, mixed oligoastrocytoma, and incompletely resected pilocytic astrocytoma	After surgery, patients were randomly assigned to early radiotherapy of 54 Gy in fractions of 1.8 Gy or deferred radiotherapy until the time of progression (control group). Analysis was by intention to treat, and primary endpoints were OS and PFS (n = 314).	157 patients were assigned early radiotherapy, and 157 control. Median progression-free survival was 5.3 years in the early radiotherapy group and 3.4 years in the control group (HR:0.59, 95% CI:0.45-0.77, p < 0.0001). However, overall survival was similar between groups: median survival in the radiotherapy group was 7.4 years compared with 7.2 years in the control group (HR:0.97, 95% CI:0.71-1.34; p = 0.872). In the control group, 65% of patients received radiotherapy at progression. At 1 year, seizures were better controlled in the early radiotherapy group.	EORTC 22845 trial.

Table 1. (Continued)

Study	Primary Cancer	Intervention	Result	Notes
Klein M et al. (26)	Low-grade gliomas (treated with early radiotherapy)	Prospective study evaluating neurocognitive deficits in 195 patients with low-grade glioma compared with 100 low-grade hematological patients and 195 healthy controls. Several neuropsychological tests were performed. Assessed effects of the tumor (e.g., disease duration, lateralization) and treatment (neurosurgery, radiotherapy, antiepileptic drugs) on cognitive function and on RR of cognitive disability (n = 295).	Low-grade glioma patients had lower ability in all cognitive domains than did low-grade haematological patients and did even less well by comparison with healthy controls. Use of radiotherapy was associated with poorer cognitive function; however, cognitive disability in the memory domain was found only in radiotherapy patients who received fraction doses exceeding 2 Gy. Antiepileptic drug use was strongly associated with disability in attentional and executive function.	
Gnekow AK et al. (30)	Low grade glioma (in children and adolescents)	Prospective study comparing observation, RT and chemotherapy (Vincristine-Carboplatin) in children (post-surgery when achievable), aiming to defer the start of irradiation in young children. Outcomes were OS, PFS and EFS (event-free survival) (n = 1031).	Ten-year progression-free survival was 0.62 following radiotherapy and 0.44 following chemotherapy. 61 out of 216 chemotherapy patients received radiotherapy 0.3-8.7 years after initial diagnosis. By multivariate analysis, diencephalic syndrome and incomplete resection were found to be unfavorable factors for OS and EFS, age ≥11 years for OS, and supratentorial midline location for EFS. Dissemination, age <1 year, and non-pilocytic histology were unfavorable factors for progression following radiotherapy (138 patients); and diencephalic syndrome, dissemination, and age ≥11 years were unfavorable factors following chemotherapy (210 patients). NF-1 patients and boys experienced prolonged tumor stabilization with chemotherapy.	HIT-LGG-1996 trial.
Fisher BJ et al. (36)	High-risk low-grade gliomas	Phase 2 prospective study comparing outcomes of patients receiving RT (54 Gy in 30 fractions) and concurrent and adjuvant TMZ with historical controls. Outcomes were 3-year OS, PFS and rate of grade 3 and 4 toxicities (n = 129).	Patients had median and minimum follow-up examinations of 4.1 years and 3 years, respectively. The 3-year OS rate was 73.1% (95% CI:65.3%-80.8%), which was significantly improved compared to that of prespecified historical control values ($p < .001$) and the study-hypothesized rate of 65%. Median survival time has not yet been reached. Three-year progression-free survival was 59.2%. Grades 3 and 4 adverse events occurred in 43% and 10% of patients, respectively. One patient died of herpes encephalitis.	RTOG 0424 trial.

OR: odds ratio; HR: hazard ratio; CI: confidence interval; RR: relative risk; OS: overall survival; PFS: progression-free survival.

FINDINGS

Low grade gliomas have been studied by various trials in the past years to define the most suitable treatments based on patient's performance, histology, location and stage of the tumor. Although most gliomas have an indolent course in comparison with other brain tumors, potential for malignant transformation is still present so that the choice of treatment must be very accurate to produce more benefit than harm.

Table 2. Molecular and genetic characteristics of low-grade gliomas differentiating astrocytoma to oligodendroglioma (18-20)

	Astrocytoma grade II	**Oligodendroglioma grade II**
Principal genetic markers	IDH mutation	IDH mutation + 1p/19q co-deletion
Associated genetic aberrations	TP53 mutation, ATRX loss	TERT mutation

Molecular and genetic characteristics of low-grade gliomas

Nowadays, it's clear that not only the histologic subtype or size of gliomas predict the aggressiveness of the tumor, but also molecular and genetic characteristics. The molecular and genetic characteristics of low-grade gliomas are summarized in Table 2, differentiating between astrocytomas and oligodendrogliomas.

Methylation of the *MGMT* (*O6-methylgaunine-DNA-methyltransferase*) promoter area (of DNA) causes loss of the corresponding protein which functions in DNA repair through inhibiting alkylation, and therefore leads to tumorigenesis. It is a predictive factor for better response to alkylating agents, namely temozolomide (TMZ) (12). It has also been found to predict a better overall survival in response not only to chemotherapy, but also to radiotherapy alone in glioblastomas (13). It can be assessed through methylation-specific polymerase chain reaction (MS-PCR or MSP).

Isocitrate dehydrogenase 1 and *2* (*IDH1* and *IDH2*) mutations, identifiable by immunohistochemistry (IHC), is emerging as another important prognostic factor for gliomas. Overall, tumors having it carry better outcomes than those with wildtype *IDH* (non-mutated) (11). Mutations in these genes occur in various types of malignancies, including over 80% of low-grade gliomas. The main driver of oncogenesis is the overproduction of R-2-hydroxyglutarate (R-2HG), which is involved in the Krebs cycle. The resulting R-2HG accumulation competitively inhibits α-ketoglutarate (αKG)-dependent enzymes, causing alterations in cellular metabolism, epigenetic regulation, redox states, and DNA repair, all of which may contribute to carcinogenesis (14). Most low-grade gliomas without IDH mutation are molecularly and clinically similar to glioblastomas, which are a much more aggressive type of glioma and frequently resistant to any kind of treatment. Alternatively, a glioblastoma with *IDH* mutation is probably a malignant progression from lower grade gliomas (11).

1p/19q co-deletion (loss of heterozygosity with the complete deletion of the short arm of chromosome 1 and the long arm of chromosome 19), a genetic biomarker of oligodendrogliomas of better overall prognosis (15), can be identified by fluorescent in situ hybridization (FISH). Array comparative genomic hybridization (aCGH) and single nucleotide polymorphism (SNP) array can identify these deletions with higher reliability and may be preferred over FISH when feasible. However, these techniques tend to be more labor demanding and require a higher proportion of neoplastic cells (16). 1p/19q co-deletion is usually mutually exclusive with TP53 and *ATRX* (*alpha-thalassemia/mental retardation syndrome X-linked*) mutations, and both characterize glial tumors of astrocytic lineage, while *TERT* (*telomerase reserve transcriptase*) mutations help assign the oligodendroglial subtype.

The EORTC 22033-26033 trial published their results in 2016 regarding treatment of low grade gliomas with either radiotherapy or temozolomide and showed a favorable prognosis for patients with *IDH* mutant tumors, with a median PFS (progression-free survival) of 62 months (95% CI (confidence interval): 41-upper limit not yet determined) for patients with *IDH* mutations with 1p/19q co-deletions; 48 months (95% CI: 41-55) for patients with non-*IDH* mutations and non-1p/19q co-deletions, and only 20 months (95% CI: 12–26) for *IDH* wild type patients. It's important to note that in the *IDH*-mutation, non-1p/19q co-deletion group, the majority (86%) had a methylated *MGMT* promoter; and in the *IDH*-mutation with 1p/19q co-deletion group, 100% them had a methylated *MGMT* promoter. The authors therefore concluded that *MGMT* testing failed to provide additional prognostic or predictive value in the *IDH*-mutated subgroup due to the nested dependency of these alterations (16). A study by Wick et al. (17) in 2013 came to a similar conclusion regarding grade III and IV gliomas. The genetic evaluation of *IDH* and 1p/19q co-deletion status has now become a standard of care in patients with low grade gliomas, with *MGMT* methylation status being reserved as a predictive marker for response to alkylating agents in the *IDH* wild type subpopulation (see Table 2).

Surgery

Surgery has been used for histopathological confirmation and for relieving mass-effect symptoms through debulking. The main goal of this treatment modality is to obtain histologic diagnosis, and when possible, to achieve complete tumor removal which has been shown to increase overall survival. Duffau et al. (6) published the outcomes of a series of 222 operated low-grade glioma cases in 2005. At a median follow-up of 4-years, 21% of those who underwent subtotal resection died compared with none after complete resection.

Most of the time, tumors either locate in eloquent parts of the brain, or show infiltrative growth with indistinct boundaries to adjacent functional areas, thus making complete resection very hard or even impossible without a high risk of neurological impairment (4). Historically under this situation, patients were set to have incomplete removal with the aim to relieve symptom or just to obtain biopsies (8).

With recent advances in neurosurgical techniques that allow bigger tissue removal under considerably lower risk of postoperative complications, the use of biopsy alone has been reduced. One reason is to avoid the risk of sampling errors on small pieces of tissue. An undergrading of actual WHO grade III gliomas has been reported in up to 28% of patients (18). The other reason is to have more comprehensive molecular tests when a large volume of tissue is available (19).

Newer neuroimaging techniques such as functional MRI (magnetic resonance imaging), DTI (diffusion tensor imaging), and intraoperative MRI (20) have now been employed pre-operatively to more accurately assess the tumor status. These together with the intraoperative use of electrostimulation mapping in an awake patient became the most reliable method to identify eloquent areas close to the tumor, thus allowing maximal tumor resection with reduced morbidity (approx. ≤ 2%) (20).

A supratotal resection (made beyond the MRI fluid-attenuated inversion recovery abnormalities (FLAIR)) for patients with diffuse low-grade glioma within non-eloquent areas of the brain has been recently suggested to further reduce the risk of anaplastic transformation (21).

If complete tumor removal is impossible, a multidisciplinary discussion involving a neurosurgeon, radio-oncologist and clinical oncologist is recommended to review the need of various non-surgical treatments, such as chemotherapy and/or radiotherapy. If not, the usual "watch-and-wait" approach can be adopted (8). However, patients put in this approach should be carefully followed with serial imaging to ensure a timely intervention can be provided at time of suspected tumor growth or anaplastic transformation before symptoms occur.

Finally, whether gliomas are incidentally found or symptomatic, surgery has been reported to reduce the incidence of seizures, which are usually the presenting symptom (6).

Table 3. Percentage of reported gross total resection from selected series

Studies	Rate of Complete Resection
Duffau H et al, 2005 (6)	37/222 (17%)
Smith JS et al. 2008 (7)	75/216 (35%)
McGirt MJ et al. 2008 (5)	65/170 (38%)
Capelle L et al. 2013 (4)	80/674 (12%)
Gnekow AK et al. 2012 (30)	359/1031 (35%)

Delivery of radiation therapy

Radiation treatment is delivered with conformal EBRT (external beam radiotherapy), at least two weeks after surgery to avoid interfering with healing process and to avoid transient edema changing the irradiated volumes. Treatment is given with immobilization through using a thermoplastic mask. Doses are around 45-54 Gy to the tumor over 5 to 6 weeks with a daily fraction size of 1.8-2.0 Gy. Contouring of the gross tumor volume (GTV) should contain the visible residual tumor at the MRI T1-enhanced images with use of contrast, and/or the signal abnormality area at T2/FLAIR images. A clinical target volume (CTV) margin of 1-2 cm around the GTV is used to account for possible microscopic spread, editing out natural expected barriers to tumor invasion (bone of skull, dura mater, intraventricular space). The planning target volumes (PTV), accounting for physical and positioning imprecision, must englobe the CTV and depends on the modality of treatment used (with or without image-guided radiotherapy (IGRT)) (see Figure 1). One should take into consideration the pre- and postoperative MRI images when available. A randomized trial has shown that dose escalation above 45-54 Gy failed to improve overall survival or progression-free survival (22). Intensity-modulated radiation therapy (IMRT) could be used to reduce volumes irradiated with full dose and protect organs at risk (like the cerebral stem, optic chiasm, optic nerves and lenses), with similar outcomes when compared to conformal radiotherapy.

Newer technologies in radiation delivery, such as proton beam therapy seem promising in dose escalation with better sparing of surrounding normal tissue, but evidence is still lacking (23). In addition, there is limited experience regarding reirradiation of recurrent disease, but toxicities seem to be mild and easily manageable.

Timing of radiation therapy

Historically, radiation therapy has been reserved for cases with disease progression or new symptoms caused by the residual tumor after surgery.

The EORTC 22845 phase III randomized trial (with mature results in 2005) showed that in low-grade gliomas, early adjuvant radiotherapy (soon after surgery, independent of symptoms or other signals of disease progression) in comparison with late radiotherapy (at tumor progression) improves progression free survival but not overall survival (24). They assigned 157 patients to the early radiotherapy group and 157 to the control group (late radiotherapy), and found that median progression-free survival was 5.3 (4.6-6.3) years in the early radiotherapy group and 3.4 years in the control group (HR (hazard ratio): 0.59, 95% CI: 0.45-0.77; $p < 0.0001$), while median overall survival in the early radiotherapy group was 7.4 years compared with 7.2 years in the control group

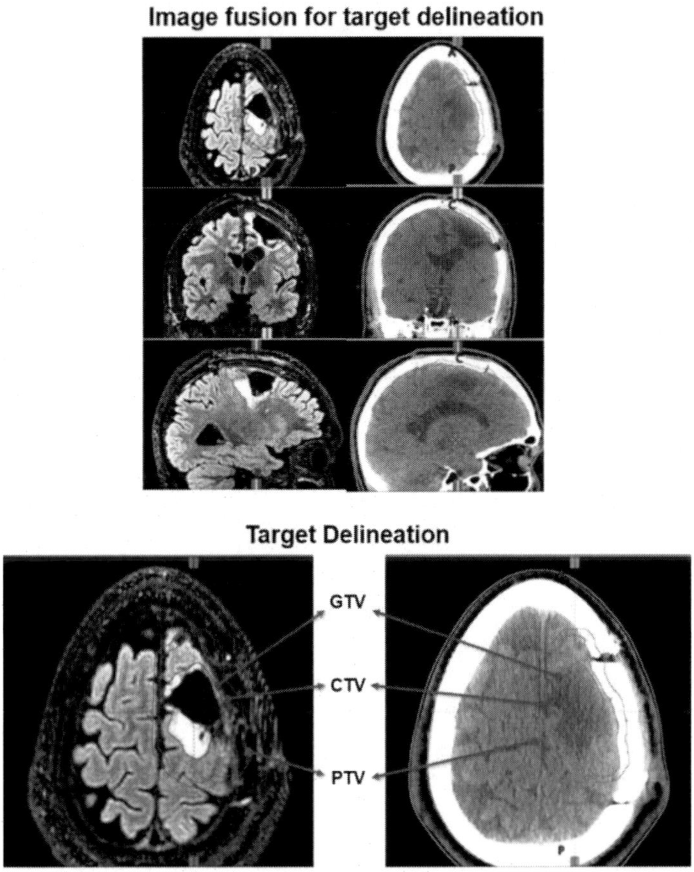

a. Treatment volume delineation: GTV: Hypersignal flair image; CTV: GTV plus 1.0 - 1.5 cm; PTV: CTV plus 0.3 - 0.5 cm.

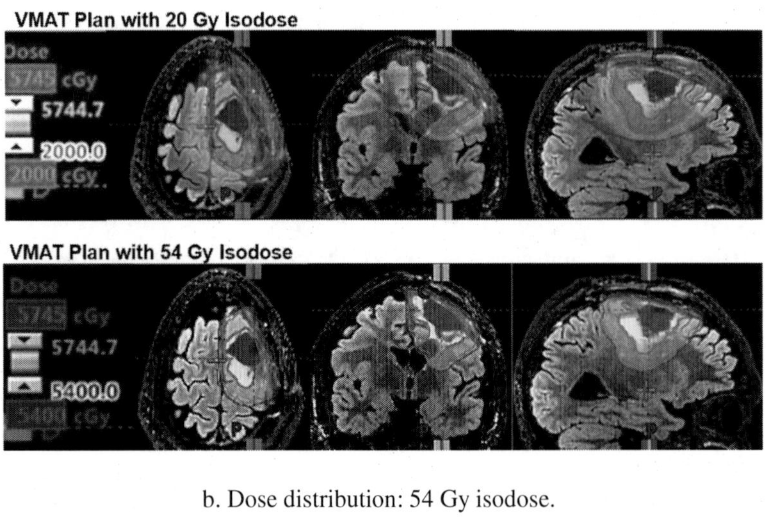

b. Dose distribution: 54 Gy isodose.

Figure 1(a-d). (Continued).

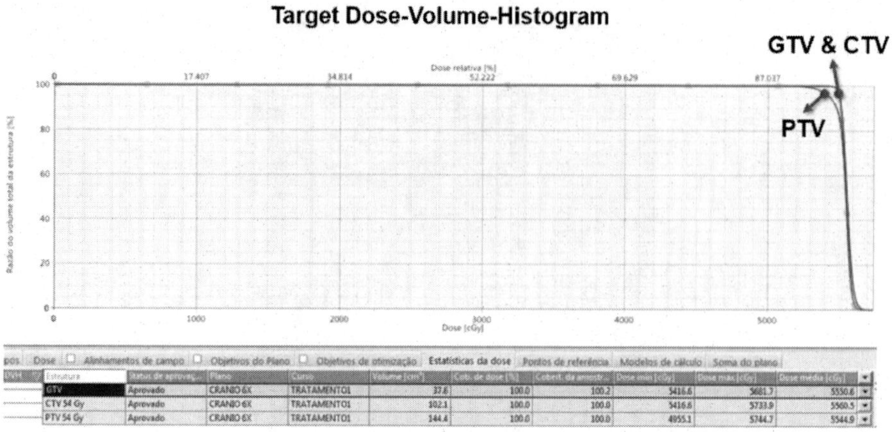

c. Dose-volume histogram for GTV, CTV, and PTV.

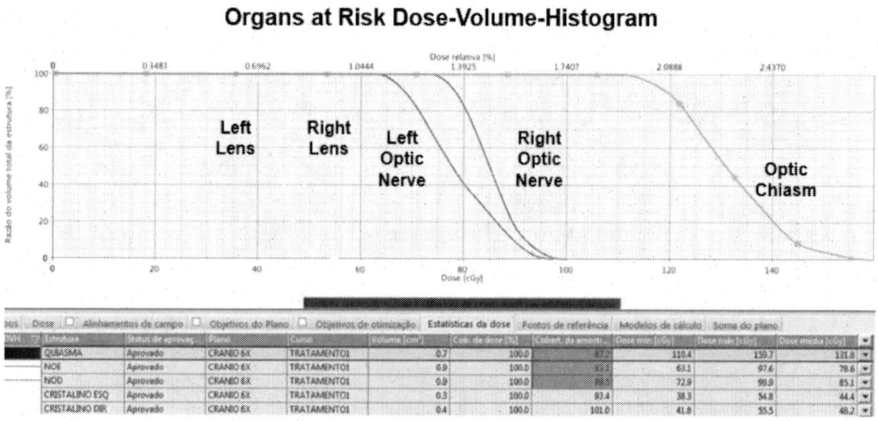

d. Dose-volume histogram for GTV, CTV, and PTV.

Figure 1(a-d). Treatment volume and dose distribution in a low-grade glioma radiation therapy.

(HR: 0.97, 95% CI: 0.71-1.34; p = 0.872). Also, according to the authors, seizures were better controlled in the early radiotherapy group as measured by year 1 whereas. At baseline there were no differences between the two groups in seizure control (p = 0.8701), but after one year, and among patients who were still progression-free, 26 of 102 (25%) patients who were irradiated had seizures in contrast to 29 of 71 (41%) patients who had not been irradiated (p = 0.0329). Post-hoc analysis found no differences between the two groups for cognitive deficit, focal neurological deficit, performance-status or headaches. With such results, radiotherapy has shown to be a reliable early adjuvant treatment for patients regardless of symptoms and should not be delayed out of fear of "losing treatment options," so to speak, after later progression. However, this still didn't bring to light an adjuvant treatment that could stop or delay death from the disease, which is the foremost goal in treatment.

Chemo-radiation therapy

Chemotherapy and radiotherapy are being currently studied in the adjuvant setting as a part of the treatment of low-grade gliomas with high risk of recurring or turning into a more aggressive type of glioma. Therefore, before addressing the role of chemo-radiation therapy in low-grade gliomas, there must be an observation about literature divergence on the definition of what constitutes a high-risk patient. For example, RTOG 9802 defined high-risk patients as having either an age of 40 years or older regardless of the extent of resection, or incomplete resection regardless of age (10), while EORTC 22033-26033 requested at least the presence of one of four factors: age 40 years or older, radiologic evidence of progression, new or worsening neurological symptoms, or intractable seizures (25). In general, questions about the timing and sequence of radiation and chemotherapy are still not completely solved.

One must always be aware of the potential acute and late effects of each modality of treatment. Cognitive decline can take place in long-term survivors following radiation therapy after 8 to 12 years of follow-up. The concerns about the risk of late neurocognitive damage from radiotherapy, coupled with the recognition of an activity of alkylating agents (PCV, temozolomide) has led many clinicians to delay the use of radiotherapy in favor of initial chemotherapy alone. However, the risk of neurocognitive deficits with radiotherapy seems to be greatly reduced following regimens with daily fractions of no more than 2 Gy, while other therapeutic factors, such as prolonged use of antiepileptic drugs, may be of more concern (26).

The EORTC 22033-26033 phase III trial randomized high risk patients with grade II gliomas to either standard radiation therapy (3D-conformal RT up to 50.4 Gy in 1.8 Gy daily fractions, five days per week over a period of 5-6 weeks; intensity-modulated and stereotactically-guided RT were allowed with the same total dose prescription) or dose-dense temozolomide (TMZ: 75 mg/m^2 per day for 21 days, repeated every 28 days for up to 12 cycles or until tumor progression or unacceptable toxicity) with a design aiming to demonstrate a superiority of chemotherapy (25). Early results were published in 2017. No differences were detected in median PFS for the entire cohort and for patients with IDH mutations and 1p/19q codeletion (55.0 months for temozolomide vs. 61.6 months for radiotherapy) (25). In contrast, patients with tumors bearing mutated *IDH* and without 1p/19q co-deletion who received TMZ had a shorter PFS compared to those who received radiotherapy, with median PFS of 55 months (95% CI: 48 to 66) for RT versus 36 months (95% CI: 28.4-47) for TMZ, translating into a HR of 0.53 (95% CI:0.35-0.82; logrank p = 0.0043). Given that this subgroup of tumors was nearly 52% of the cases, represented most tumors in both age groups of patients (up to 40 and over 40 years old), and may be the most prevalent in the population, it's safe to say that one must consider the patient's situation carefully when deciding the most suitable adjuvant treatment. From a clinical point of view, these results suggest that in most patients with astrocytoma, radiotherapy is still to be preferred over chemotherapy as the initial adjuvant treatment in most settings. Data on overall survival from the EORTC 22033-26033 trial are still not mature, because the median OS has not yet been reached (16).

A recent retrospective analysis performed on the US National Cancer Database has suggested that chemotherapy alone is superior over RT alone in patients with oligodendroglial tumors, but not in those with astrocytomas (27).

Based on the success in combining radiation and chemotherapy in higher grade gliomas, this approach has been investigated in high risk grade II gliomas as well. RTOG (Radiation Therapy Oncology Group) 9802 is a prospective phase II/III trial that investigated the addition of PCV (procarbazine, lomustine, and vincristine) chemotherapy to RT for patients with WHO grade 2 glioma (10). The trial assigned patients either to radiation alone or radiation followed by PCV. The original publication of trial results in 2012 showed an improvement of PFS, but not OS with the addition of chemotherapy in the intention-to-treat analysis. However, after a longer follow-up of 6 years, a clear advantage for the combined treatment in terms of OS emerged as well. Median PFS was 4.0 vs. 10.4 years for radiation therapy alone vs. radiation followed by PCV, with a 10-year PFS of 21 and 51%, respectively. Median OS was 7.8 vs 13.3 years for radiation therapy alone vs radiation followed by PCV, and 10-year survival was 40 vs 60%, respectively, with a hazard ratio of death of 0.59 (logrank p = 0.002) for RT + PCV. This increase in survival was observed even though 77% of patients who progressed after RT alone received salvage chemotherapy. The treatment effect size was the largest in patients with oligodendrogliomas and tumors with IDH 1 mutations. However, the analysis by molecular subgroups was limited by inadequate tumor tissue availability.

What we have learned from recent phase III trials are two things. First, as PFS of patients receiving temozolomide alone in the EORTC trial is similar to that of patients receiving radiotherapy alone in EORTC and RTOG trials (3.2 and 4.0 years, respectively), temozolomide and radiotherapy are comparable as initial adjuvant treatments. Second, as PFS of patients receiving radiotherapy + PCV in the RTOG trial is clearly superior (10.4 years), if choosing radiotherapy as adjuvant treatment, PCV must be added (27).

Preliminary results of a relatively large single-arm phase II study (RTOG 0424) combining radiation and concomitant/adjuvant temozolomide have suggested an improved survival at three years compared to an historical control group receiving radiation therapy alone (36).

Whether temozolomide (a better tolerated agent) can replace the PCV regimen in association with radiotherapy in terms of efficacy is still unknown and will be clarified by the ongoing phase III study CODEL, which compares radiotherapy followed by PCV with radiotherapy and concomitant/sequential temozolomide in lower grade gliomas (grade I and II) with *IDH1* or two mutations and 1p/19q co-deletion. This trial had closed prematurely and then reopened with a different stratification due to positive findings of

EORTC 26951/RTOG 9402 trials during its accrual, where the previous arms were RT alone, RT plus TMZ and TMZ alone. Preliminary findings of the previous study design, including only 36 patients (12 in each arm), showed better PFS ($p < 0.001$) and OS ($p = 0.048$) for RT-arms compared to TMZ alone.

So far, no prospective or randomized trials have directly compared chemotherapy alone with chemoradiation. A retrospective analysis on the large US National Cancer Database has suggested that chemoradiation is not associated with a significant longer overall survival compared with chemotherapy alone. However, the median follow-up of this study is shorter (4.6 years) compared to that of RTOG 9802 (11.9 years), thus it is not able to capture the delayed major efficacy of adding chemotherapy to radiotherapy.

Pediatric populations

Gliomas in children pose an even bigger challenge than in adults, since more than half of them are infratentorial, such as brainstem gliomas and cerebellar astrocytomas. For tumors infiltrating the brainstem, broad resections are almost non-existent; while cerebellar tumors are resectable, they come with risks of neurological deficits caused by treatment. Brainstem gliomas account for approximately 10% of all pediatric brain tumors, and grade II astrocytomas count for 80% of them.

Chemoradiotherapy is the mainstay of treatment, but with a mere 3-year survival in the 5-10% of diffuse brainstem gliomas (accounting for grades II to IV), we still have a long way to go in identifying a reliable treatment (28). Radiotherapy regimens do not differ significantly from adult regimens, with the most common being 54 Gy over 1.8 Gy daily fractions using conformal EBRT, but with some cases using proton therapy. Concerning diffuse intrinsic pontine gliomas (DIPG), the use of concurrent/adjuvant temozolomide with radiotherapy failed to improve survival (29). Chemotherapy instead of radiotherapy is particularly recommended for younger children with low-grade gliomas, since these patients will live longer and therefore have a higher risk of developing radiotherapy-induced side effects later in life (from cognition impairment to second malignancies), especially for children with *neurofibromatosis type 1* (*NF1*) mutations as shown through the long-term follow up of the HIT-LGG-1996 trial (30). This German trial comprised of 1031 children and adolescents with low-grade gliomas randomized to 3 groups: 668 were just observed (following incomplete resection/biopsy or radiologic diagnosis for tumors deemed unresectable, all without threatening symptoms), 216 had vincristine-carboplatin adjuvant chemotherapy and 147 had adjuvant conventional radiotherapy/brachytherapy (both groups received treatment only after severe or progressive symptoms or radiologic progression). The chemotherapy arm was instituted with the aim of deferring or even avoiding radiotherapy in young patients, while radiation was recommended as standard treatment for children over 5 years of age.

The results showed that *NF1* mutation was a predictor factor for better PFS following chemotherapy regimen compared to wildtype *NF1* (HR: 0.58, 95% CI: 0.36-0.89, p = 0.021), and *NF1* mutant patients constituted 10.5% of their cohort, illustrating the substantial co-prevalence of this entity and low-grade glioma which is also found in other series (31). Patients under one year of age receiving radiotherapy had a worse PFS compared to patients between 1 and 4 years of age (p = 0.007). Ten-year PFS rates were 0.62 following radiotherapy and 0.44 following chemotherapy. Sixty-one of the 216 chemotherapy patients (28.2%) received salvage radiotherapy 0.3-8.7 years after initial diagnosis (median age of 7.2 years), meaning chemotherapy managed to delay radiotherapy for this subset of patients. Although children usually have a narrow therapeutic index and are prone to severe toxicity from most available drugs, metronomic chemotherapy (daily dosing of several medications in low dosage to target tumor endothelium as an anti-angiogenesis protocol instead of direct cytotoxic activity) is promising in reducing that toxicity profile (32).

CONCLUSION

Low grade gliomas are a heterogeneous group of neoplasms, and their natural history depends primarily on histopathologic type, genetic signature and tumor size. Most of these tumors behave in an aggressive way, even after surgery and radiation therapy, mostly due to malignant transformation. Still, low grade gliomas have a lower incidence and a better prognosis than other primary nervous system tumors. The medial survival of patients with low-grade gliomas is around 7 years, and 5-year OS rates consistently between 60% and 70% (33).

The prognostic factors of low-grade gliomas are not fully elucidated yet. So far, only *IDH* mutations, KPS score, age and the pathological type are recognized prognostic factors for low-grade gliomas, with growing evidence suggesting a positive effect of extent of resection on the prognosis of low-grade gliomas (9).

Over the last 15 years, several phase III randomized trials have investigated different paradigms of therapy intensification for this disease. These include immediate adjuvant radiation therapy (RT), increased dose of adjuvant RT, and addition of chemotherapy to adjuvant RT. The primary end point of most of these trials was overall survival (OS), but nearly all demonstrated either no difference between arms or a PFS benefit without an OS benefit, except for the RTOG-9802 trial (10). The effect of therapy intensification on cognitive function remains a concern in this population with substantial long-term survival (5).

Results from all these trials just give directions, so to speak, on how to manage these patients. However, many other factors may play a role. One can imagine that for a very small superficial tumor that could be almost completely resected, or otherwise treated with a small radiation field, perhaps five or six weeks of radiation is more appropriate, less toxic, and more practical for patients and health care systems than one year of temozolomide chemotherapy. Chemotherapy possibly makes more sense for patients with tumors demanding a large radiation field, more centrally localized, and when we want to avoid long-term neurocognitive deficits such as in children under 5 years of age (however, at the price of an increased risk of haematological adverse effects and infections after alkylating-agent chemotherapy) (16).

References

[1] Forst DA, Nahed BV, Loeffler JS, Batchelor TT. *Low-grade gliomas.* Oncologist 2014;19(4):403-13.

[2] Louis DN, Perry A, Reifenberger G, Von Deimling A, Figarella-branger D, Cavenee WK, et al. *The 2016 World Health Organization classification of tumors of the central nervous system: a summary.* Acta Neuropathol 2016;131(6):803-20.

[3] Hayhurst C. Contemporary management of low-grade glioma: a paradigm shift in neuro-oncology. Pract Neurol 2017;17(3):183-90.

[4] Capelle L, Fontaine D, Mandonnet E, Taillandier L, Golmard JL, Bauchet L, et al. *Spontaneous and therapeutic prognostic factors in adult hemispheric World Health Organization Grade II gliomas: a series of 1097 cases.* J Neurosurg 2013;118(6):1157-68.

[5] McGirt MJ, Chaichana KL, Attenello FJ, Weingart JD, Than K, Burger PC, et al. *Extent of surgical resection is independently associated with survival in patients with hemispheric infiltrating low-grade gliomas.* Neurosurgery 2008;63(4):700-8.

[6] Duffau H, Lopes M, Arthuis F, Bitar A, Sichez J-P, Van Effenterre R, et al. *Contribution of intraoperative electrical stimulations in surgery of low grade gliomas: a comparative study between two series without (1985-96) and with (1996-2003) functional mapping in the same institution.* J Neurol Neurosurg Psychiatry 2005;76(6):845-51.

[7] Smith JS, Chang EF, Lamborn KR, Chang SM, Prados MD, Cha S, et al. *Role of extent of resection in the long-term outcome of low-grade hemispheric gliomas.* J Clin Oncol 2008;26(8):1338-45.

[8] Xia L, Fang C, Chen G, Sun C. *Relationship between the extent of resection and the survival of patients with low-grade gliomas: A systematic review and meta-analysis.* BMC Cancer 2018;18(1):48.

[9] De Witt Hamer PC, Robles SG, Zwinderman AH, Duffau H, Berger MS. *Impact of intraoperative stimulation brain mapping on glioma surgery outcome: A meta-analysis.* J Clin Oncol 2012;30(20):2559-65.

[10] Buckner JC, Shaw EG, Pugh SL, Chakravarti A, Gilbert MR, Barger GR, et al. *Radiation plus procarbazine, CCNU, and vincristine in low-grade glioma.* N Engl J Med 2016; 374:1344-55.

[11] Cancer Genome Atlas Network, Brat DJ, Verhaak RG, Aldape KD, Yung WK, Salma SR, et al. *Comprehensive, integrative genomic analysis of diffuse lower-grade gliomas.* N Engl J Med 2015;372(14):2481-98.

[12] Everhard S, Kaloshi G, Crinière E, Benouaich-Amiel A, Lejeune J, Marie Y, et al. *MGMT methylation: a marker of response to temozolomide in low grade gliomas.* Ann Neurol 2006;60(6):740-3.

[13] Rivera AL, Pelloski CE, Gilbert MR, Colman H, De La Cruz C, Sulman EP, et al. *MGMT promoter methylation is predictive of response to radiotherapy and prognostic in the absence of adjuvant alkylating chemotherapy for glioblastoma.* Neuro Oncol 2010;12(2):116-21.

[14] Molenaar RJ, Maciejewski JP, Wilmink JW, van Noorden JCF. *Wild-type and mutated IDH1/2 enzymes and therapy responses*. Oncogene 2018;37(15):1949-60.

[15] Woehrer A, Sander P, Baberler C, Kern S, Maier H, Preusser M, et al. *FISH-based detection of 1p 19q codeletion in oligodendroglial tumors: procedures and protocols for neuropathological practice - a publication under the auspices of the Research Committee of the European Confederation of Neuropathological Societies (Euro-CNS).* Clin Neuropathology 2011;30(2):47-55.

[16] Baumert BG, Hegi ME, van den Bent MJ, von Deimling A, Gorlia T, Hoang-Xuan K, et al. *Temozolomide chemotherapy versus radiotherapy in high-risk low-grade glioma: A randomized phase III Intergroup study by EORTC/NCIC-TG/T ROG/MRC-CTU (EORTC 22033-26033).* Lancet Oncol 2016;17(11):1521-32.

[17] Wick W, Meisner C, Hentschel B, Platten M, Schilling A, Wiestler B, et al. *Prognostic or predictive value of MGMT promoter methylation in gliomas depends on IDH1 mutation.* Neurology 2013;81(17):1515-22.

[18] Muragaki Y, Chernov M, Maruyama T, Ochiai T, Taira T, Kubo O, et al. *Low-grade glioma on stereotactic biopsy: how often is the diagnosis accurate*? Minim Invasive Neurosurg 2008;51(5):275-9.

[19] Gusyatiner O, Hegi ME. *Glioma epigenetics: from subclassification to novel treatment options.* Semin Cancer Biol 2018;51:50-8.

[20] Spena G, Nava A, Cassini F, Pepoli A, Bruno M, D'Agata F, et al. *Preoperative and intraoperative brain mapping for the resection of eloquent-area tumors.* A prospective analysis of methodology, correlation, and usefulness based on clinical outcomes. Acta Neurochir (Wien) 2010;152(11):1835-46.

[21] Yordanova YN, Moritz-Gasser S, Duffau H. *Awake surgery for WHO grade II gliomas within "noneloquent" areas in the left dominant hemisphere: toward a "supratotal" resection.* Clinical article. J Neurosurg 2011;115(2):232-9.

[22] Shaw E, Arusell RM, Scheithauer B, O'Fallon J, O'Neill B, Dinapoli R, et al. *A prospective randomized trial of low versus high dose radiation in adults with a supratentorial low grade glioma: initial report of an NCCTG-RTOG-ECOG study.* J Clin Oncol 2002;20(9):2267-76.

[23] Grosshans DR, Mohan R, Gondi V, Shih HA, Mahajan A, Brown PD. *The role of image-guided intensity modulated proton therapy in glioma.* Neuro Oncol 2017;19(Suppl 2):ii30-7.

[24] Van den Bent MJ, Afra D, de Witte O, Ben Hassel M, Schraub S, Hoang-Xuan K, et al. *Long-term efficacy of early versus delayed radiotherapy for low-grade astrocytoma and oligodendroglioma in adults: the EORTC 22845 randomised trial.* Lancet 2005;366(9490):985-90.

[25] Baumert BG, Hegi ME, van den Bent MJ, von Deimling A, Gorlia T, Hoang-Xuan K, et al. *Temozolomide chemotherapy versus radiotherapy in high-risk low-grade glioma (EORTC 22033-26033): a randomised, open-label, phase 3 intergroup study.* Lancet Oncol 2016;17(11):1521-32.

[26] Klein M, Heimans JJ, Aaronson NK, van der Ploeg HM, Grit J, Muller M, et al. *Effect of radiotherapy and other treatment-related factors on mid-term to long-term cognitive sequelae in low-grade gliomas: a comparative study.* Lancet 2002;360 (9343):1361-68.

[27] Rudá R, Bruno F, Soffietti R. *What have we learned from recent clinical studies in low-grade gliomas*? Curr Treat Options Neurol 2018;20(8):33.

[28] Sridhar K, Sridhar R, Venkatprasanna G. *Management of posterior fossa gliomas in children.* J Pediatr Neurosci 2011;6(Suppl1):S72-7.

[29] Jalali R, Raut N, Arora B, Gupta T, Dutta D, Munshi A, et al. *Prospective evaluation of radiotherapy with concurrent and adjuvant temozolomide in children with newly diagnosed diffuse intrinsic pontine glioma.* Int J Radiat Oncol Biol Phys 2010;77(1):113-8.

[30] Gnekow AK, Falkenstein F, von Hornstein S, Zwiener I, Berkefeld S, Bison B, et al. *Long-term follow-up of the multicenter, multidisciplinary treatment study HIT-LGG-1996 for low-grade glioma in children and adolescents of the German Speaking Society of Pediatric Oncology and Hematology.* Neuro Oncol 2012;14(10):1265-84.

[31] Stokland T, Liu JF, Ironside JW, Ellison DW, Taylor R, Robinson KJ, et al. *A multivariate analysis of factors determining tumor progression in childhood low-grade glioma: a population-based cohort study (CCLG CNS9702).* Neuro Oncol 2010;12(12):1257-68.

[32] Kieran MW, Turner CD, Rubin JB. *A feasibility trial of antiangiogenic (metronomic) chemotherapy in pediatric patients with recurrent or progressive cancer.* J Pediatr Hematol Oncol 2005;27(11):573-81.

[33] Claus EB, Walsh KM, Wiencke J, Molinaro AM, Wiemels JL, Schildkraut JM, et al. *Survival and low-grade glioma: the emergence of genetic information.* Neurosurg Focus 2015;38(1):E6.

In: Cancer Management in Latin America II
Editors: Maurício F Silva et al.
ISBN: 978-1-53616-735-1

Chapter 6

MANAGEMENT OF MALIGNANT GLIOMAS

Felipe de Azevedo Rosas[1], MD, Gustavo Nader Marta[2], MD, PhD, Fiona Lim[3], MBBS, Bo Angela Wan[4], MD(C), Mauricio F Silva[5,6,7], MD, PhD and Douglas Guedes de Castro[1,*], MD, MSc

[1]Department of Radiation Oncology, AC Camargo Cancer Center, São Paulo, Brazil
[2]Hospital Sírio-Libanês, São Paulo, Brazil
[3]Department of Oncology, Princess Margaret Hospital, Hong Kong, PR China
[4]Odette Cancer Centre, Sunnybrook Health Sciences Centre, Toronto, Ontario, Canada
[5]Radiation Oncology Unit, Santa Maria Federal University, Santa Maria, Brazil
[6]Hospital de Caridade Astrogildo de Azevedo, Santa Maria, Brazil
[7]Latin America Cooperative Oncology Group, Porto Alegre, Brazil

ABSTRACT

Management of malignant gliomas is challenging e has evolved significantly. In the last decade, a solid body of evidence integrated molecular markers to the histological findings, severely changing the landscape of high-grade gliomas classification, helping carve more detailed subgroups with different prognosis and potential responsiveness to therapy. Moreover, technical development of surgery and radiotherapy and emergency of new systemic approaches have modified clinical practice both in the initial and recurrent setting. All these aspects are integrated and revised in this chapter.

* Corresponding Author's Email: douglas.castro@accamargo.org.br.

INTRODUCTION

Diffuse gliomas are infiltrative central nervous system neoplasms, historically classified by the WHO (World Health Organization) into morphological subtypes (astrocytomas, oligodendrogliomas, oligoastrocytomas and glioblastomas) as well as a grade system, based on the presence of necrosis, endothelium proliferation and mitosis. Grade II is considered to be low grade (slow growing tumors with better prognosis) while III and IV high-grade (fast growing tumors with significantly worse prognosis) (1). Regarding its incidence, high-grade gliomas, or so-called malignant gliomas, together account for almost half of all primary adult brain tumors, with an incidence of 5/100.000.

In the last decade, a solid body of evidence integrated molecular markers to the histological findings, severely changing the landscape of high-grade gliomas classification, helping carve more detailed subgroups with different prognosis and potential responsiveness to therapy. The most important tumor markers identified up until now are isocitrate-dehydrogenase (IDH) gene mutations, 1p/19q co-deletions, epidermal growth factor receptor (EGFR) gene amplifications or rearrangements and O6-methylguanine-DNAmethyl-transferase (MGMT) methylation status.

HIGH-GRADE GLIOMAS

Whether gliomas are product of a dedifferentiation of mature glial cells or originated from neural stem cells is still not clear. However, we have made important advances in understanding the molecular pathways to gliomagenesis. Numerous processes are involved in gliomas formation, and it is believed that the mutation of IDH1 and IDH2 are an early event when present. In addition, the existence of an IDH-independent process of mutation is now well known. Following then IDH mediated oncogenesis there are two distinct paths of malignant degeneration: astrocytic and oligodendrocytic. In the setting of development of an astrocytoma, frequently there are acquisitions of p53 and ATRX mutations whereas in the setting of an oligodendroglioma development co-deletion of chromosomes 1p/19q are generally observed. Continuous degeneration happens in both scenarios, but it is considered that only astrocytic lineages can culminate in a glioblastoma. The 2016 update on the WHO classification approached this more molecular-oriented scenario subdividing all histological subtypes depending on two parameters: co-deletion of 1p/19q and IDH mutation status, presenting then 3 groups; astrocytoma, IDH-mutant; astrocytoma, IDH-wild type; and oligodendroglioma, IDH-mutant and 1p/19q-codeleted. When molecular information is not available tumors can be classified as “not otherwise specified” (2).

Glioblastoma

Glioblastoma (GBM) accounts for approximately 15% of all central nervous system (CNS) tumors and 60% of all high-grade gliomas. It is 1.58 times more common in males than females and its incidence rates increase with age, being highest in the age 75-84 years. It is relatively rare among children with an incidence of 0.16/100.000 between ages 0-14 years. Comparatively the incidence rate between ages 75-84 is 15.2/100,000 (3). Despite constituting only 2% of all neoplasms it composes an important challenge due to its poor prognosis. It remains an incurable tumor with median survival of 14.6 months given the standard treatment and only 3 months if left untreated (4).

Being extremely fast-growing tumors, its diagnosis is most commonly due to the manifestation of clinical symptoms. These will depend on the location of the tumor within the brain. The most common symptoms are focal neurological deficits such as hemiparesia, confusion, aphasia, visual field impairment, seizures, cognitive impairment, headaches and behavioral changes.

Prognostic factors and molecular markers

The prognosis for patients with GBM remains extremely poor in spite of all research efforts. Receiving state of the art treatment patients have a median survival time of 14.6 months. In 1993 Currant et al. (5) published a recursive partitioning analysis (RPA) of prognostic factors based on 3 RTOG trials including 1,578 patients with malignant gliomas treated from 1974 and 1985 consistently identifying pretreatment and treatment related variables that significantly impacted overall survival (5). Among the 26 analyzed pre-treatment variables, age was the most important, with patients under 50 years faring best. Tumor histology, with GBM patients showing worse survival for younger patients, Karnofsky performance score (KPS) for older patients and mental status also exhibited impact on survival. Extent of surgery and radiotherapy dose were the only treatment related variables showing impact. In 2011 Li et al. (6) updated the previous RPA involving only GBM patients from the expanded RTOG glioma database. This model resulted in 3 distinct prognostic groups defined by age, performance score, extent of resection and neurologic function. Group III (patients under 50 years, with KPS>90%) had median survival time of 16.3 months. Group IV (patients under 50 years with KPS<90% or over 50 years, KPS>70%, submitted to partial or total tumor resection and with good neurological function) had median survival time of 11.3 months). Group V (patients over 50 years with KPS<70%, KPS>70% but submitted only to biopsy or KPS>70%, submitted to partial or total tumor resection but not able to work due to impaired neurological function) had median survival time of 6.7 months.

GBM can also be divided into primary, or *de novo*, predominant in patients aged over 55 years old and secondary, usually with a history of prior lower grade diffuse glioma, mostly occurring in younger patients (7).

Lately biomarkers such as EGFR, IDH 1/2 and MGMT methylation status, have been under investigation as prognostic tools (8, 9). MGMT encodes a DNA-repair protein that hinders the effectiveness of treatment by removing alkyl groups from guanine, a target site for alkylating chemotherapy agents. Epigenetic silencing of the MGMT may suppress this repair mechanism, therefore increasing the cytotoxicity of chemotherapy, and radiotherapy (9). Hegi et al. (8) tested the relationship between MGMT silencing in the tumor and survival of patients enrolled in the EORTC trial 26981 comparing radiotherapy alone and radiotherapy with concomitant and adjuvant temozolamide. The MGMT promoter was methylated in 45% of the patients and was considered an independent favorable prognostic factor. Among the patients treated with radiotherapy and temozolamide who contained methylated MGMT promoter, the median survival time was 21.7 months, compared with 15.3 months of non-methylated patients. Mutations on IDH genes are commonplace on lower grade diffuse gliomas, being found on 70-80% of grade II and III gliomas and secondary glioblastomas being very rare in primary glioblastomas (10). Being so, mutations on IDH1 and IDH2 when found on GBM are positively correlated to secondary GBM arising from a prior lower grade glioma. Hartmann et al, retrospectively analyzed 382 patients with GBM and anaplastic gliomas from NOA-04 trial and from a prospective translational cohort study of the German Glioma Network and found that IDH1 mutations were the most prominent single prognostic factor, trumping even tumor histology (11). Other studies have confirmed this association between IDH mutation and improved survival outcomes compared to IDH wild-type (12). This prognostic importance of IDH genes mutation was reflected on the 2016 WHO classification of CNS tumors, now dividing GBM into 3 groups:

1) GBM, IDH wild type, (90% of the cases)
2) GBM, IDH-mutant (10% of the cases)
3) GBM NOS, when no IDH evaluation can be performed.

Concomitant loss of chromosomes 1p and 19q is another molecular alteration that correlates with favorable outcomes. Frequently associated with IDH mutations and therefore secondary GBM, 1p19q co-deletion could predict a better response to chemotherapy.

Treatment

Despite significant research effort, GBM still is an incurable tumor imposing enormous social and medical burden. The standard of care for newly diagnosed GBM stands on a

2005 landmark study by Stupp et al. and consists of maximum safe resection, radiotherapy with concomitant temozolamide (TMZ) followed by adjuvant TMZ (13). The median survival from diagnosis is 14.6 months as opposed to 12.1 months with radiotherapy alone and the 2-year survival rate was 26%. The association of tumor treating fields should be considered for newly diagnosed patients with no contraindications. Progression is expected with very limited options towards recurrent GBM and no standard of care.

The role of surgery

Surgery is the initial therapeutic approach in treating GBM and its primary objectives are maximum safe resection, tissue sampling for pathological analysis, improving quality of life and relieving possible mass effect. It is responsible for the most important treatment related prognosis factor: extent of resection (14). Although the goal is to achieve gross total tumor resection the surgeon must balance between an aggressive removal and the neurological preservation. On a worst-case scenario, the tumor may occupy an eloquent area making the surgery unfeasible. When close to eloquent cortical regions pose a distinct challenge to the surgeon due to high risk of postsurgical neurological deficit. Therefore, it is not unusual for the oncologist to come across subtotal resections and biopsied only lesions. To shed light on this rather subjective classification of extent of resection Lacroix et al. analyzed 416 consecutive patients with surgically treated GBM and identified a significant survival advantage (13 months) with a resection of 98% or more of the tumor volume compared with less than 98% (8.8 months). Another study conducted by Chaichana et al. (15) retrospectively reviewed 259 patients who underwent primary GBM surgery found that the minimum extent of resection associated with prolonged survival was 70%.

Radiotherapy

Adjuvant radiotherapy has been the standard of care for patients with GBM for the last decades. A controlled, prospective study published on 1978 (BTSG 69-01 trial) successfully demonstrated that the addition of adjuvant radiotherapy importantly improved the median overall survival (OS) of patients with anaplastic gliomas (16). Later in 1981 the Scandinavian Glioblastoma Study Group published their results from a trial comparing post-op radiotherapy with and without bleomycin with best supportive care for patients with grade III and IV gliomas. Their results showed no benefit from bleomycin but a significant improvement in median OS with the addition of radiotherapy (10.8 months vs. 5.2 months) (17). These two studies demonstrated that adjuvant radiotherapy nearly doubled median OS crystalizing its place among the components of standard treatment. Currently it is delivered concomitant to TMZ (75 mg/m2/day for 6 weeks) and followed by six maintenance cycles of TMZ. Optimal dose-fractionation schedule is 60Gy in 30 fractions, following Stupp protocol, for patients under 70 years with good clinical and neurological performance. Numerous others dose schedules have been investigated without clear benefits. Concerning the technique, treatment is usually performed with conformal 3D radiotherapy (3DRT) or Intensity modulated radiotherapy (IMRT). There are no evidence suggesting better disease control with IMRT, however has been shown that IMRT reduces the dose to organs at risk by allowing inhomogeneous dose plans reflecting in less toxicity (18).

Target volume delimitation

Although GBM and other diffuse gliomas are widely infiltrating there are no benefits in treating the whole brain, so localized irradiation volumes are recommended. Hochberg et al, had 35 GBM patients CT scans evaluated and compared with their autopsy results and found that recurrence occurred within a 2cm margin in 78% of the patients with 56% of them recurring within a 1cm margin of the initial tumor volume (19). These findings were confirmed in different studies adding body to the evidence that treatment could be more localized (20-21). The two most important guidelines on delineation of target volume for the treatment of GBM follow this rationale. The RTOG guideline divides the treatment in two phases. Phase 1 delivering 46 Gy in 2 Gy fractions to contrasting enhancing lesion, plus peritumoral edema, plus 2-cm margin to PTV and phase 2 delivering a 14 Gy boost in 2 Gy fractions to contrast enhancing lesion (preoperative MR imaging), plus 2.5-cm margin to PTV (22). The EORTC guideline delivers the treatment in a single phase of 60 Gy in 2 Gy fractions to contrast enhancing lesion (GTV), plus 2-cm (or 3-cm) to CTV (13).

Dose definition

Nowadays the standard dose for treating GBM is 60 Gy in 30 fractions of 200 cGy. The Brain Tumor Study Group examined 621 patients who entered three protocols between 1966 and 1975 and were treated with surgery following radiotherapy with different doses. The median OS for patients with no radiotherapy was 18 weeks. Those who received a dose of 50Gy had a median OS of 28 weeks, and those receiving 55 Gy and 60 Gy respectively 36 and 42 weeks (23), showing that 60 Gy was associated with 2.3 times longer survival. Dose escalation above 60 Gy with three-dimensional conformal therapy, brachytherapy and stereotaxic radiosurgery failed to show prognostic improvement (24-26) and were related to increased toxicity. However, all these studies were conducted in the pre-TMZ era. More recently, investigation concerning escalating dose and dose per fraction using IMRT concomitant with TMZ suggested improved results with doses up to 75 Gy (30 x 2.5 Gy) without prohibitive toxicity. In addition, attention must be paid to keep dose to critical structures (brainstem, optical nerve and optical chiasms) within the acceptable limits. Nevertheless, more data from ongoing trials is still needed.

Treatment of the elderly

As previously stated, age is an important independent prognostic factor in GBM patients with older patients fairing significantly worse. As so, maximum therapeutic benefit must be provided with minimum toxicity for this subgroup. Although Stupp trial demonstrated a benefit in OS with concomitant TMZ and radiotherapy followed by adjuvant TMZ, patients older than 70 years were excluded from the study (13). Moreover, on a subgroup analysis, patients between 65-70 years had no survival advantage with combined therapy. Following this rationale Keime-Guibert et al. investigated if best supportive care after surgery could have reasonable outcomes compared to adjuvant radiotherapy for this subgroup. Eighty-one patients over 70 years (KPS>=70%) were randomized between involved field adjuvant radiotherapy with 50.4 Gy in 28 fractions and BSC. The arm receiving adjuvant radiotherapy had a substantial benefit in survival, causing the trial to be closed early (27). In a subsequent study Roa et al. compared then a short course radiation treatment for the elderly versus standard radiotherapy. In this prospective randomized study, 95 patients with at least 60 years and KPS >= 50% received either adjuvant radiotherapy with 40 Gy in 15 fractions or 60 Gy in 30 fractions. This trial was underpowered but it showed no difference in OS between both arms (28). A Nordic randomized phase III trial addressed the best treatment of this elderly population comparing survival, quality of life and safety among 3 treatment strategies: single agent TMZ chemotherapy, hypofractionated radiotherapy (34 Gy in 10 fractions) and standard radiotherapy (60 Gy in 30 fractions). They concluded that TMZ chemotherapy and hypofractionated radiotherapy were potential alternatives for treatment of elderly and frail patients (4). Exploring yet an alternative hypofractionated schedule, a randomized, prospective, multicenter, phase 3, noninferiority trial compared short course radiotherapy with 25 Gy in 5 fractions with 40 Gy in 15 fractions. A total of 98 patients were stratified by age, KPS and extent of resection. Median OS and PFS were not statistically significantly different between arms suggesting that 25 Gy in 5 fractions is another acceptable and shorter treatment option for patients aged > 65 years mainly those with poor performance (29, 30). Finally, a 2017 trial explored if the addition of concomitant TMZ to the short course radiotherapy could improve outcomes in patients older than 65 years compared to short course alone. The patients receiving concomitant TMZ exhibited better OS and PFS especially those with methylated MGMT (31). Nowadays we have a solid enough body of evidence allowing us to manage elderly and frail patients with a hypofractionated adjuvant radiotherapy be it with 40 Gy/15, 34 Gy/10 or 25 Gy/5 in non-methylated, while methylated patients can be treated with TMZ alone (32) sparing them the burden of multiple daily visits and more toxic treatments as well as improving the treatment cost effectiveness (33). Treatment with concurrent and adjuvant TMZ are an option for older patients with good performance.

Systemic treatment

Since the Stupp trial, the main systemic treatment for non-recurrent GBM is TMZ, nevertheless, in the course of GBM treatment history, other therapeutic agents were studied and used. Active agents also include nitrosureas (carmustine and lomustine), etoposide, irinotecan, cisplatin and the PCV (procarbazine, lomustine and vincristine) scheme. Regardless of not being first choice in primary treatment, alternative treatment schemes often have a place in recurrent disease. The first evidence that chemotherapy could benefit these patients arose at late 60's with BTSG 69-01 showing a greater survival rate at 18 months among patients receiving carmustine with radiotherapy (16). Unfortunately, subsequent studies showed only a marginal benefit or none at all with the use of nitrosureas (16, 34-36). Another technique explored for drug delivering were carmustine wafers applied locally at the time of the primary surgery. On a prospective, double blind study, Valtonen and col. compared the treatment with carmustine wafers against placebo. The study did not recruit as many patients as intended due to lack of carmustine on the market but for the 27 patients enrolled with grade IV tumors there was a statistically significant benefit from the active treatment group (37). Although they are safe the wafers treatment is related with complications such as delayed wound healing, intracranial infection, intracranial edema and seizures so they were not widely adopted (38). Platinum compounds demonstrated a mild efficacy as adjuvant therapy being used sometimes in the recurrence scenario. The PCV combination is commonplace in the grade III astrocytomas and oligodendrogliomas treatment but has shown no benefit in GBM patients even in relapsed disease (39).

TMZ is a modern alkylating agent with excellent penetration into central nervous system and acts promoting the methylation of O6 position of guanine. MGMT can repair this damage, so methylation of its promoter is associated with better outcomes after TMZ treatment. After 2005, it consolidated its place as a cornerstone in primary treatment being used concomitant and sequential to radiotherapy (13). Neoadjuvant treatment was also explored but with inferior results compared to the standard concomitant and sequential approach (40). Dosage is usually 75mg/m^2 daily while concurrent with radiotherapy followed by 150mg/m^2 daily for 5 days and later escalated to 200mg/m^2, if well tolerated, for five days in 28 days cycles. The toxicity is acceptable and includes mostly neutropenia, thrombocytopenia, nausea and asthenia with few patients experiencing grade III or IV toxic effects.

The addition of bevacizumab, a humanized anti-VEGF monoclonal antibody, was also explored on the setting of primary treatment. RTOG 08-25 evaluated 637 patients with GBM treated with standard treatment (radiotherapy plus concomitant and sequential TMZ) dividing them in two arms, with and without the addition of bevacizumab on the adjuvant therapy. The conclusion was that although the first line use of bevacizumab did not improve overall survival, but it has impact on progression free survival (10.7 months vs. 7.3 months) (41). Another important phase III trial, AVAglio, where 921 patients were randomized among radiotherapy with TMZ plus the addition of bevacizumab or placebo, and later after a 28-day break maintenance bevacizumab or placebo plus TMZ showed similar results. There was no benefit observed to overall survival, however the bevacizumab group showed an improvement on progression-free survival (10.6 months vs control 6.2 months) (42).

Tumor treating fields

Tumor treating fields (TTF) are low intensity alternating electrical fields created through the placement of noninvasive transducer arrays on the patient scalp. Its tumor cell killing effect consists on disrupting mitosis. During metaphase, the electrical fields impair the formation of microtubules and during telophase it induces intra-cellular dielectrophoresis of intracellular components resulting in apoptosis (43). Based on good results from pre-clinical trials a phase III (EF-11 trial) was conducted comparing TTF with standard chemotherapy in the recurrent disease scenario. Patients received either TTF monotherapy or standard care chemotherapy. The overall survival between groups was equivalent but with better toxicity profile on the TTF group (44). On the newly diagnosed disease scenario, the EF-14 trial compared TTF plus TMZ with TMZ alone as maintenance treatment following conventional radiochemotherapy. The TTF arm showed better overall survival and progression free survival than the TMZ arm (45) making it reasonable to assume that there is a place for TTF on GBM standard therapy.

Response assessment

Published in 1990, Macdonald et al. proposed the first neuro-oncology response assessment criteria. The Macdonald criteria was based on quantitative bidirectional measurements and accounted corticosteroids use and neurological status stratifying patients in four categories complete response (CR), partial response (PR), stable disease (SD), and progressive disease (PD) (46). Later on, 2010 the Response Assessment in Neuro-Oncology (RANO) was elaborated, addressing some deficiencies of the Macdonald criteria such as identification of "pseudoprogression" and "pseudoresponse" and now have largely outdated it. The RANO criteria also divide response in four types based on magnetic resonance imaging (MRI) and clinical features:

1) Complete response: Requires all of the following: complete disappearance of all enhancing measurable and non-measurable disease sustained for at least four weeks; no new lesions; stable or improved non-enhancing (T2/FLAIR) lesions; patients must be off corticosteroids (or on physiologic replacement doses only); and stable or improved clinically. Note: Patients with non-measurable disease only cannot have a complete response; the best response possible is stable disease.

2) Partial response: Requires all of the following: 50% decrease compared with baseline in the sum of products of perpendicular diameters of all measurable enhancing lesions sustained for at least four weeks; no progression of non-measurable disease; no new lesions; stable or improved non-enhancing (T2/FLAIR) lesions on same or lower dose of corticosteroids compared with baseline scan; the corticosteroid dose at the time of the scan evaluation should be no greater than the dose at time of baseline scan; and stable or improved clinically.
3) Stable disease: Requires all of the following: does not qualify for complete response, partial response, or progression; stable non-enhancing (T2/FLAIR) lesions on same or lower dose of corticosteroids compared with baseline scan. In the event that the corticosteroid dose was increased for new symptoms and signs without confirmation of disease progression on neuroimaging, and subsequent follow-up imaging shows that this increase in corticosteroids was required because of disease progression, the last scan considered to show stable disease will be the scan obtained when the corticosteroid dose was equivalent to the baseline dose.
4) Progression: Defined by any of the following: 25% increase in sum of the products of perpendicular diameters of enhancing lesions compared with the smallest tumor measurement obtained either at baseline (if no decrease) or best response, on stable or increasing doses of corticosteroids; significant increase in T2/FLAIR non-enhancing lesion on stable or increasing doses of corticosteroids compared with baseline scan or best response after initiation of therapy not caused by comorbid events; any new lesion; clear clinical deterioration not attributable to other causes apart from the tumor or changes in corticosteroid dose; failure to return for evaluation as a result of death or deteriorating condition; or clear progression of non-measurable disease (47).

Anaplastic gliomas

Anaplastic (WHO grade III) gliomas represent approximately 20% of adult gliomas. After the 2016 WHO brain tumor classification, the growing evidence on the prognostic importance of molecular markers changed the way we stratify and treat these tumors, even if a significant amount of the evidence available for treating these tumors are from trials that pooled together entities that we now understand and treat as different. Nowadays the classification of adult anaplastic gliomas is based on IDH and 1p/19q status. Anaplastic oligodendrogliomas are tumors defined by the existence of 1p/19q co-deletion frequently associated with IDH mutations. Anaplastic astrocytomas exhibit IDH mutations without 1p/19q co-deletions frequently associated with loss of ATRX expression. Regarding prognosis, anaplastic oligodendrogliomas with IDH mutations, which comprises the vast majority, have the best median outcomes, followed by IDH-mutant astrocytomas and finally IDH wild type anaplastic oligodendrogliomas having the worse prognosis among them all (2).

Treatment of anaplastic astrocytoma includes optimal safe resection and radiotherapy (60 Gy in 30 fractions). The NOA-04 trial randomized patients with grade III gliomas in 3 arms after surgery; adjuvant radiotherapy with 60 Gy in 30 fractions or adjuvant chemo. Patients who were randomized to the chemo arm were subsequently randomized between Vincristine, Procarbazine and lomustine (PCV) or TMZ. There was no difference in OS and PFS between the arms, so chemo and radiotherapy were both considered adequate adjuvant treatments (48). However, the later CATNON trial demonstrated that in the scenario of 1p/19q co-deleted anaplastic gliomas patients treated with adjuvant radiotherapy followed by 12 cycles of TMZ faired best.

Anaplastic oligodendrogliomas, in a similar way, are best treated with maximum safe resection followed by radiotherapy and chemotherapy. However, differently from the astrocytic lineage tumors, oligodendroglial tumors seem to respond better to PCV based chemo. The RTOG 9402 and EORTC 26951 results support this approach. The EORTC 26951 trial randomized 368 patients with anaplastic oligodendroglial tumors to receive either PCV (6 cycles) or observation after surgery and radiotherapy (59.4 Gy/33 fractions). An 11-years follow-up concluded that 1p/19q co-deleted tumors had significant better outcomes with the addition of PCV than non-co-deleted tumors (49). The possibility of replacing PCV for concomitant and adjuvant TMZ in this subset of patients will be responded by the ongoing CODEL trial, however we still lack evidence on the matter.

Recurrent malignant gliomas

Malignant gliomas almost inevitably relapse, irrespective of the initial treatment approach and all the evolution observed in the last 15 years. Management of the recurrence is challenging due to the balance risk of the salvage therapy toxicity and the lack of evidence from randomized trials of comparison between best supportive care and any active therapeutic approach.

The pattern of recurrence of malignant gliomas is predominantly local, having patients been treated in the pre or post-TMZ era (50, 51). Such pattern difficulties the initial evaluation and differentiation between progression and imaging changes induced by treatment. Pseudoprogression is defined as a new or enlarging area of contrast agent enhancement occurring early after the end of radiotherapy (e.g., within 3-4 months), in the absence of true tumor growth, which subsides or stabilizes without a change in therapy (52). Reported incidences range from 9-30% and patients with pseudoprogression tended to be less often clinically symptomatic than patients with early progressive disease (34% vs. 57%), and their tumors were more often MGMT promotor methylated. Radiation necrosis, although presents similar imaging features, emerges from around 6 months to several years posttreatment (53). Therefore, the first step in the management of recurrent glioma is define between actual progression and pseudo progression or radiation necrosis.

Regarding the therapeutic approach of recurrent gliomas, although different options are available, none is curative and it depends on the extent of disease and patient condition. The efficacy of treatment options remains poor and, therefore, enrollment in a clinical trial, whenever possible, is preferred (54).

Best supportive care only is often considered appropriate in patients with poor performance status (54). However, an active therapeutic approach may be beneficial for selected elderly and/or frail patients with recurrent glioma. Outcome analysis of patients with recurrent GBM from a prospective data collection and prognostically homogeneous study population showed a longer overall (55 versus 30 weeks) and progression-free survival (23 versus 9 weeks) in patients that received any treatment (chemotherapy, surgery or radiotherapy) than those who received best supportive care (see figure 1) (55).

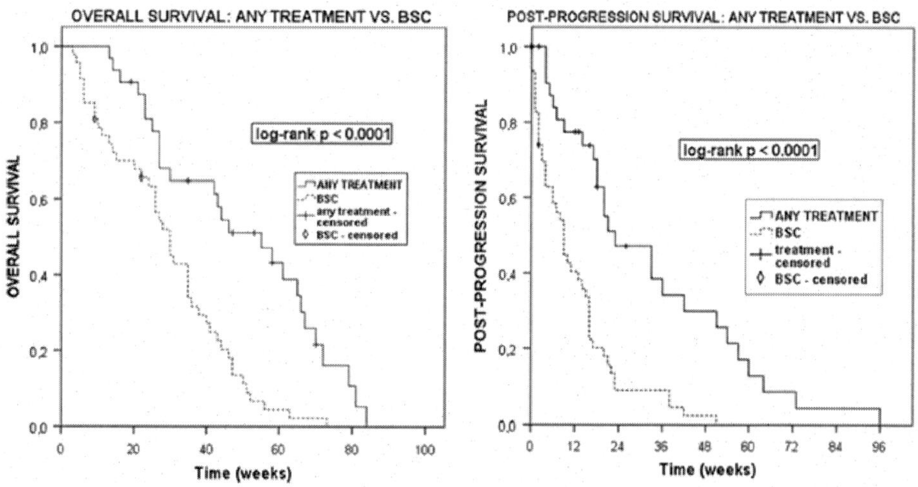

Figure 1. Overall and post-progression survival: any treatment versus best supportive care (BSC) in patients with recurrent GBM (55) (reproduced with permission, copyright 2018, Springer Nature).

Second surgery is considered for 20-30% of patients in clinical practice, commonly for symptomatic but circumscribed lesions and when the interval since the preceding surgery exceeds six months (32). However, data available on the impact of repeat surgery on overall survival are scarce. Evaluation of a prospectively collected clinical and imaging data of patients who underwent surgery for recurrent GBM from the DIRECTOR trial found that patients with complete resection of contrast-enhancing tumor was associated with improved post-recurrence survival (12.9 versus 6.5 months) when compared to patients with residual detection of contrast enhancement after surgery at first recurrence (56, 57).

Systemic treatment options, either cytotoxics or molecular targeted agents, may provide some benefit for patients with an adequate performance status who progressed after prior chemotherapy. The main options are nitrosoureas, TMZ rechallenge and bevacizumab. Alternative dosing regimens of TMZ showed similar results to lomustine, with progression-free survival rates at 6 months in the range of 15-25% (56).

Bevacizumab, a monoclonal antibody against vascular endothelial growth factor, alone or combined with irinotecan or lomustine have been associated with 6-month progression-free survival and 9-month overall survival far superior to TMZ or lomustine alone in phase II studies. In the BRAIN trial, the 6-month progression-free survival was 43% with bevacizumab and 50% with bevacizumab plus irinotecan in patients with recurrent GBM (57). The BELOB trial demonstrated the superiority of bevacizumab combined with lomustine versus either alone in terms of 9-month overall survival (38% for bevacizumab, 43% for lomustine alone and 63% for the combined bevacizumab and lomustine groups). The combination of bevacizumab and lomustine met prespecified criteria for assessment of this treatment in further phase 3 studies. However, the results in the bevacizumab alone group do not justified further studies of this treatment (58).

Re-irradiation (reRT) may be employed in selected patients with limited volume recurrences. Besides the volume of disease, additional factors have been evaluated in order to help selecting potential patients who benefit from reRT, as the current evidence is mainly from retrospective series. Combs et al. developed and validated a prognostic score system that uses primary histology, time between primary RT and reRT, age, KPS, tumor volume and re-resection. The "New Combs Prognostics Score" defined four prognostic groups, with a median overall survival ranging from 5.5 to 19.5 months, being 7.9 months for patients with GBM and 11.3 months for anaplastic glioma (59). The same group evaluated the role of early reRT after resection for recurrent GBM and found that median survival after surgery and reRT was 12 months (60). Currently, the NOA 17 trial is looking at the progression-free survival impact of early stereotactic fractionated reRT to the resection cavity of completely resected recurrent GBM.

Regarding the RT technique, hypofractionated RT and single fraction radiosurgery have both been shown to have an acceptable toxicity profile in a setting where maximising quality of life and reducing the overall time of radiotherapy are important (61). The largest series of patients with recurrent high-grade gliomas who underwent reRT was published by Fogh et al. In this series, 147 patients were treated to 35 Gy in 10 fractions with stereotactic hypofractionated RT and that approach was associated with a median survival time in excess of 10 months (62). Ho and Jena suggested as a reasonable approach to adopt single fraction radiosurgery for smaller tumors and hypofractionated stereotactic RT for either larger volumes or disease in an eloquent area and to keep the cumulative total dose normalized to 2 Gy/fraction below 100 Gy (61).

An exploratory approach in the recurrent glioma setting is the TTF. However, TTF were no superior to best physician's choice in a randomised phase III trial (44).

REFERENCES

[1] Louis DO, Ohgaki H, Wiestler OD, Cavenee WK, Burger PC, Jouvet A, et al. *WHO Classification of Tumours of Central Nervous System*. Acta Neuropathol 2007;14(2):97-109.

[2] Louis DN, Perry A, Reifenberger G, von Diemling A, Figarella-Branger D, Cavenee WK, et al. *The 2016 World Health Organization classification of tumors of the central nervous system: a summary*. Acta Neuropathol 2016;131:803-20.

[3] Ostrom QT, Gittleman H, Liao P, Vecchione-Koval T, Wolinsky Y, Kruchko C, et al. *CBTRUS Statistical Report: Primary Brain and Other Central Nervous System Tumors Diagnosed in the United States in 2010-2014*. Neuro Oncol 2017;18(s5):iv1-89.

[4] Malmstrom A, Gronberg BH, Marosi C, Stupp R, Frappaz D, Schultz H, et al. *Temozolamide versus standard 6-week radiotherapy versus hypo fractionates radiotherapy in patients older than 60 years with glioblastoma: The Nordic randomized, phase 3 trial*. Lancet Oncol 2012;13(9):916-26.

[5] Curran WJ Jr, Scott CB, Horton J, Nelson JS, Weinstein AS, Fischbach AJ, et al. *Recursive partitioning analysis of prognostic factors in three Radiation Therapy Oncology Group malignant glioma trials*. J Natl Cancer Inst 1993;85(9):704-10.

[6] Li J, Wang M, Won M, Shaw EG, Coughlin C, Curran WJ Jr, et al. *Validation and simplification of the Radiation Therapy Oncology Group recursive partitioning analysis classification for glioblastoma*. Int J Radiat Oncol Biol Phys 2011;81(3):623-30.

[7] Ohgaki H, Kleihues P. *The definition of primary and secondary glioblastoma*. Clinical Cancer Research 2013;19(4):764-72.

[8] Hegi ME, Diserens AC, Gorlia T, Hamou MF, de Tribolet N, Weller M, et al. *MGMT Gene Silencing and Benefit from Temozolomide in Glioblastoma*. N Engl J Med 2005;352(10):997-1003.

[9] Binabaj MM, Bahrami A, ShahidSales S, Joodi M, Joudi Mashhad M, Hassanian SM, et al. *The prognostic value of MGMT promoter methylation in glioblastoma: A meta-analysis of clinical trials*. Journal of Cellular Physiology 2017;233(1):378-86.

[10] Ichimura K, Pearson DM, Kocialkowski S, Bäcklund LM, Chan R, Jones DT, et al. *IDH1 mutations are present in the majority of common adult gliomas but rare in primary glioblastomas*. Neuro-Oncology 2009;11(4):341-7.

[11] Hartmann C, Hentschel B, Wick W, Capper D, Felsberg J, Simon M, et al. *Patients with IDH1 wild type anaplastic astrocytomas exhibit worse prognosis than IDH1-mutated glioblastomas, and IDH1 mutation status accounts for the unfavorable prognostic effect of higher age: implications for classification of gliomas*. Acta Neuropathol 2010;120(6):707-18.

[12] Cheng HB, Yue W, Xie C, Zhang RY, Hu SS, Wang Z. *IDH1 mutation is associated with improved overall survival in patients with glioblastoma: a meta-analysis*. Tumor Biology 2013;34(6):3555-9.

[13] Stupp R, Mason WP, van den Bent MJ, Weller M, Fisher B, Taphoorn MJ, et al. *Radiotherapy plus concomitant and adjuvant temozolomide for glioblastoma*. N Engl J Med 2005;352(10):987-96.

[14] Brown TJ, Brennan MC, Li M, Church EW, Brandmeir NJ, Rakszawski KL, et al. *Association of the extent of resection with survival in glioblastoma. a systematic review and meta-analysis*. JAMA Oncol 2016;2(11):1460-9.

[15] Chaichana, KL, Jusue-Torres I, Navarro-Ramirez R, Raza SM, Pascual-Gallego M, Ibrahim A, et al. *Establishing percent resection and residual volume thresholds affecting survival and recurrence for patients with newly diagnosed intracranial glioblastoma*. Neuro-Oncology 2013;16(1):113-22.

[16] Walker MD, Alexander E, Hunt WE, MacCarty CS, Mahaley MS Jr, Mealey J Jr, et al. *Evaluation of BCNU and/or radiotherapy in the treatment of anaplastic gliomas. Journal of Neurosurgery* 1978;49(3):333-43.

[17] Kristiansen K, Hagen S, Kollevold T. Combined modality therapy of operated astrocytomas grade III and IV. *Confirmation of the value of postoperative irradiation and lack of potentiation of bleomycin on survival time: a prospective multicenter trial of the Scandinavian Glioblastoma Study Group.* Cancer 1981;47(4):649-52.

[18] Thibouw D, Truc G, Bertaut A, Chevalier C, Aubignac L, Mirjolet C, et al. *Clinical and dosimetric study of radiotherapy for glioblastoma: three-dimensional conformal radiotherapy versus intensity-modulated radiotherapy.* Journal of Neuro-Oncology 2018;137(2):429-38.

[19] Hochberg FH, Pruitt A. *Assumptions in the radiotherapy of glioblastoma.* Neurology 1980;30(9):907-11.

[20] Halperin EC, Bentel G, Heinz ER, Burger PC. *Radiation therapy treatment planning in supratentorial glioblastoma multiforme: An analysis based on post mortem topographic anatomy with CT correlations.* Int J Radiat Oncol Biol Phys 1989;17(6):1347-50.

[21] Wallner KE, Galicich JH, Krol G, Arbit E, *Malkin MG. Patterns of failure following treatment for glioblastoma multiforme and anaplastic astrocytoma.* Int J Radiat Oncol Biol Phys 1989;16(6):1405-9.

[22] Colman H, Berkey BA, Maor MH, Groves MD, Schultz CJ, Vermeulen S, et al. *Phase II Radiation Therapy Oncology Group trial of conventional radiation therapy followed by treatment with recombinant interferon-beta for supratentorial glioblastoma: results of RTOG 9710.* Int J Radiat Oncol Biol Phys 2006;66(3):818-24.

[23] Walker MD, Strike TA, Sheline GE. *An analysis of dose-effect relationship in the radiotherapy of malignant gliomas.* Int J Radiat Oncol Biol Phys 1979;5(10):1725-31.

[24] Salazar OM, Philip Rubin MD, Feldstein ML, Pizzutiello R. *High dose radiation therapy in the treatment of malignant gliomas: final report.* Int J Radiat Oncol Biol Phys 1979;5(10):1733-40.

[25] Souhami L, Seiferheld W, Brachman D, Podgorsak EB, Werner-Wasik M, Lustig R, et al. *Randomized comparison of stereotactic radiosurgery followed by conventional radiotherapy with carmustine to conventional radiotherapy with carmustine for patients with glioblastoma multiforme: report of Radiation Therapy Oncology Group 93-05 protocol.* Int J Radiat Oncol Biol Phys 2004;60:853-60.

[26] Laperriere NJ, Leung PM, McKenzie S, Milosevic M, Wong S, Glen J, et al. *Randomized study of brachytherapy in the initial management of patients with malignant astrocytoma.* Int J Radiat Oncol Biol Phys 1998;41(5):1005-11.

[27] Keime-Guibert F, Chinot O, Taillandier L, Cartalat-Carel S, Frenay M, Kantor G, et al. *Radiotherapy for glioblastoma in the elderly.* N Engl J Med 2007;356(15):1527-35.

[28] Roa W, Brasher PM, Bauman G, Anthes M, Bruera E, Chan A, et al. *Abbreviated course of radiation therapy in older patients with glioblastoma multiforme: a prospective randomized clinical trial.* J Clin Oncol 2004;22(9):1583-8.

[29] Guedes de Castro D, Matiello J, Roa W, Ghosh S, Kepka L, Kumar N, et al. *Survival outcomes with short-course radiation therapy in elderly patients with glioblastoma: data from a randomized phase 3 trial.* Int J Radiat Oncol Biol Phys 2017;98(4):931-8.

[30] Roa W, Kepka L, Kumar N, Sinaika V, Matiello J, Lomidze D, et al. *International atomic energy agency randomized phase iii study of radiation therapy in elderly and/or frail patients with newly diagnosed glioblastoma multiforme.* J Clin Oncol 2015;33(35):4145-50.

[31] Perry JR, Laperriere N, O'Callaghan CJ, Brandes AA, Menten J, Phillips C, et al. *Short-Course Radiation plus Temozolomide in Elderly Patients with Glioblastoma.* N Engl J Med 2017;376(11):1027-37.

[32] Weller M, van den Bent M, Tonn JC, Stupp R, Preusser M, Cohen-Jonathan-Moyal E, et al. *European Association for Neuro-Oncology (EANO) guideline on the diagnosis and treatment of adult astrocytic and oligodendroglial gliomas*. Lancet Oncol 2017;18(6):e315-29.

[33] Ghosh S, Baker S, de Castro DG, Kepka L, Kumar N, Sinaika V, et al. *Improved cost-effectiveness of short-course radiotherapy in elderly and/or frail patients with glioblastoma*. Radiother Oncol 2018;127(1):114-20.

[34] Buckner JC, Ballman KV, Michalak JC, Burton GV, Cascino TL, Schomberg PJ, et al. *Phase III trial of carmustine and cisplatin compared with carmustine alone and standard radiation therapy or accelerated radiation therapy in patients with glioblastoma multiforme: North Central Cancer Treatment Group 93-72-52 and Southwest Oncology Group 9503 Trials*. J Clin Oncol 2006;24(24),3871-9.

[35] Nelson DF, Diener-West M, Horton J, Chang CH, Schoenfeld D, Nelson JS. *Combined modality approach to treatment of malignant gliomas--re-evaluation of RTOG 7401/ECOG 1374 with long-term follow-up: a joint study of the Radiation Therapy Oncology Group and the Eastern Cooperative Oncology Group*. NCI Monogr 1988;(6):279-84.

[36] Shapiro WR, Green SB, Burger PC, Mahaley MS Jr, Selker RG, VanGilder JC, et al. *Randomized trial of three chemotherapy regimens and two radiotherapy regimens in postoperative treatment of malignant glioma*. J Neurosurgery 1989;71(1):1-9.

[37] Valtonen S, Timonen U, Toivanen P, Kalimo H, Kivipelto L, Heiskanen O, et al. *Interstitial chemotherapy with carmustine-loaded polymers for high-grade gliomas: a randomized double-blind study*. Neurosurgery 1997;41(1):44-9.

[38] Nagpal S. *The role of BCNU polymer wafers (Gliadel) in the treatment of malignant glioma*. neurosurgery clinics of North America. Neurosurg Clin North Am 2012;23(2):289-95.

[39] Ajaz M, Jefferies S, Brazil L, Watts C, Chalmers A. *Current and investigational drug strategies for glioblastoma*. Clin Oncol 2014;26(7):419-30.

[40] Chinot OL, Barrié M, Fuentes S, Eudes N, Lancelot S, Metellus P, et al. *Correlation between o6-methylguanine-dna methyltransferase and survival in inoperable newly diagnosed glioblastoma patients treated with neoadjuvant temozolomide*. J Clin Oncol 2007;25(12):1470-5.

[41] Gilbert MR, Dignam, JJ, Armstrong TS, Wefel JS, Blumenthal DT, Vogelbaum MA, et al. *A randomized trial of bevacizumab for newly diagnosed glioblastoma*. N Engl J Med 2014;370(8):699-708.

[42] Chinot, OL, Wick W, Mason W, Henriksson R, Saran F, Nishikawa R, et al. *Bevacizumab plus radiotherapy-temozolomide for newly diagnosed glioblastoma*. N Engl J Med 2014;370(8):709-22.

[43] Zhu P, Zhu JJ. *Tumor treating fields: a novel and effective therapy for glioblastoma: mechanism, efficacy, safety and future perspectives*. Chin Clin Oncol 2017;6(4):41.

[44] Stupp R, Wong ET, Kanner AA, Steinberg D, Engelhard H, Heidecke V, et al. *NovoTTF-100A versus physician's choice chemotherapy in recurrent glioblastoma: A randomised phase III trial of a novel treatment modality*. Eur J Cancer 2012;48(14):2192-202.

[45] Stupp R, Taillibert S, Kanner AA, Kesari S, Steinberg DM, Toms SA, et al. *Maintenance therapy with tumor-treating fields plus temozolomide vs temozolomide alone for Glioblastoma: a randomized clinical trial JAMA* 2015;314(23):2535-43.

[46] Macdonald DR, Cascino TL, Schold SC, Cairncross JG. *Response criteria for phase II studies of supratentorial malignant glioma*. J Clin Oncol 1990;8(7):1277-80.

[47] Wen PY, Macdonald DR, Reardon DA, Cloughesy TF, Sorensen AG, Galanis E, et al. *Updated response assessment criteria for high-grade gliomas: response assessment in neuro-oncology working group*. J Clin Oncol 2010;28(11):1963-72.

[48] Wick W, Roth P, Hartmann C, Hau P, Nakamura M, Stockhammer F, et al. *Long-term analysis of the NOA-04 randomized phase III trial of sequential radiochemotherapy of anaplastic glioma with PCV or temozolomide*. Neuro Oncol 2016;18(11):1529-37.

[49] van den Bent MJ, Brandes AA, Taphoorn MJ, Kros JM, Kouwenhoven MC, et al. *Adjuvant procarbazine, lomustine, and vincristine chemotherapy in newly diagnosed anaplastic oligodendroglioma: long-term follow-up of EORTC Brain Tumor Group Study 26951*. J Clin Oncol 2013;31(3):344-50.

[50] Lee SW, Fraass BA, Marsh LH, Herbort K, Gebarski SS, Martel MK, et al. *Patterns of failure following high-dose 3-D conformal radiotherapy for high-grade astrocytomas: a quantitative dosimetric study*. Int J Radiat Oncol Biol Phys 1999;43(1):79-88.

[51] Oh J, Sahgal A, Sanghera P, Tsao MN, Davey P, Lam K, et al. *Glioblastoma: patterns of recurrence and efficacy of salvage treatments*. Can J Neurol Sci 2011;38(4):621-5.

[52] Wen PY, Macdonald DR, Reardon DA, Cloughesy TF, Sorensen AG, Galanis E, et al. *Updated response assessment criteria for high-grade gliomas: response assessment in neuro-oncology working group*. J Clin Oncol 2010;28(11):1963-72.

[53] Thust SC, van den Bent MJ, Smits M. *Pseudoprogression of brain tumors*. J Magn Reson Imaging 2018;48:571-89.

[54] *National Comprehensive Cancer Network*. Central Nervous System Cancers (Version 2.2018). URL:http://www.nccn.org/professionals/physician_gls/pdf/cns. Pdf.

[55] Socha J, Kepka L, Ghosh S, Roa W, Kumar N, Sinaika V, et al. *Outcome of treatment of recurrent glioblastoma multiforme in elderly and/or frail patients*. J Neurooncol 2016;126(3):493-8.

[56] Suchorska B, Weller M, Tabatabai G, Senft C, Hau P, Sabel MC, et al. *Complete resection of contrast-enhancing tumor volume is associated with improved survival in recurrent glioblastoma-results from the DIRECTOR trial*. Neuro Oncol 2016;18(4):549-56.

[57] Friedman HS, Prados MD, Wen PY, Mikkelsen T, Schiff D, Abrey LE, et al. *Bevacizumab alone and in combination with irinotecan in recurrent glioblastoma*. J Clin Oncol 2009;27(28):4733-40.

[58] Taal W, Oosterkamp HM, Walenkamp AME, Dubbink HJ, Beerepoot LV, Hanse MC, et al. *Single-agent bevacizumab plus lomustine versus a combination of bevacizumab plus lomustine in patients with recurrent glioblastoma (BELOB trial): a randomised controlled phase 2 trial*. Lancet Oncol 2014;15(9):943-53.

[59] Kessel KA, Hesse J, Straube C, Zimmer C, Schmidt-Graf F, Schlegel J, et al. *Modification and optimization of an established prognostic score after re-irradiation of recurrent glioma*. PLoS One 2017;12(7):e0180457.

[60] Combs SE, Kessel KA, Hesse J, Straube C, Zimmer C, Schmidt-Graf F, et al. *Moving second courses of radiotherapy forward: early re-irradiation after surgical resection for recurrent gliomas improves efficacy with excellent tolerability*. Neurosurgery 2018;83(6):1241-8.

[61] Ho ALK, Jena R. *Re-irradiation in the brain: primary gliomas*. Clin Oncol (R Coll Radiol) 2018;30(2):124-36.

[62] Fogh SE, Andrews DW, Glass J, Curran W, Glass C, Champ C, et al. *Hypofractionated stereotactic radiation therapy: An effective therapy for recurrent high-grade gliomas*. J Clin Oncol 2010;28(18):3048-53.

In: Cancer Management in Latin America II
Editors: Maurício F Silva et al.
ISBN: 978-1-53616-735-1

Chapter 7

MANAGEMENT OF HODGKIN'S LYMPHOMA

Lívia Alvarenga Fagundes Ferrigno[1,*], MD, Gustavo Nader Marta[2], MD, PhD, Fiona Lim[3], MBBS, Bo Angela Wan[4], MD(C) and Mauricio F Silva[5,6,7], MD, PhD

[1]Department of Radiation Oncology Hospital Beneficiência Portuguesa, São Paulo, Brazil
[2]Instituto de Câncer do Estado de São Paulo (ICESP), São Paulo, Brazil
[3]Department of Oncology, Princess Margaret Hospital, Hong Kong, PR China
[4]Odette Cancer Centre, Sunnybrook Health Sciences Centre, Toronto, Ontario, Canada
[5]Radiation Oncology Unit, Santa Maria Federal University, Santa Maria, Brazil
[6]Hospital de Caridade Astrogildo de Azevedo, Santa Maria, Brazil
[7]Latin America Cooperative Oncology Group, Porto Alegre, Brazil

ABSTRACT

The combined treatment with chemotherapy and radiotherapy is the standard of care in Hodgkin's disease. In 1992, introduction of the ABVD regimen consisting of doxorubicin, bleomycin, vinblastine and dacarbazine, marked a step improving survival and reducing toxic effects including infertility, second malignancies and myelosuppression. With early stage being cured in 90% of the cases and advanced disease in 70-80%, the focus now is reducing the treatment related morbidities by de-escalating and individualizing treatments. In the 1950's, Hodgkin's Lymphoma started to be cured with radiotherapy (RT) and since then, this tool has become a part of the standard therapy, balancing toxicity with chemotherapy. Specific to early-stage Hodgkin's Disease, a few cycles of cytotoxic therapy are combined with limited RT to eradicate local disease. In addition to dose reduction, modern RT technology has led to

* Corresponding Author's Email: livfagundes@hotmail.com.

radical changes in RT delivery, allowing more accurate targeting and conformal coverage while sparing normal tissues and avoiding unnecessary adverse effects. RT for lymphoma has developed from total nodal irradiation or involved-field RT to now involved-node and involved-site RT. For advanced stage Hodgkin's Lymphoma, the role of radiotherapy is limited to cases of bulky disease and partial response after chemotherapy. Future directions focus on maximizing the cure and minimizing collateral effects, de-escalating treatment, adapting PET response, and replacing toxic drugs effects by antibody-based drugs with promising results. In this chapter we review the clinical trials on management of, and the role of radiotherapy in early and advanced Hodgkin's disease.

INTRODUCTION

Introduction of the ABVD regimen consisting of doxorubicin, bleomycin, vinblastine and dacarbazine, marked a step improving survival and reducing toxic effects including infertility, second malignancies and myelosuppression (1, 2). Specific to early-stage Hodgkin's Disease, a few cycles of cytotoxic therapy are combined with limited radiotherapy (RT) to eradicate local disease (3, 4). RT for lymphoma has developed from total nodal irradiation or involved-field RT to now involved-node and involved-site RT (4-6).

The histopathological diagnosis of classical Hodgkin's disease is defined by the presence of the Reed-Stemberg cells, which is a binucleate cell with a well-delimited central nucleolus and an evident nuclear membrane (7). The histological classifications of Hodgkin's disease can be divided into classic and nodular lymphocytic predominance. The immunophenotype of the cells helps to distinguish these two forms:

1) Classical disease: In this subtype, Reed-Stemberg cells are present and generally express CD30 (85%) and CD15 (100%) antigens and generally don't express B cell (CD19, CD20, CD79a) and T cell antigens (CD3 and CD7). Some cases of Hodgkin's lymphoma express CD20. Depending on the hematoxylin-eosin analysis, it is possible to further divide into sub-types of: nodular sclerosis, mixed cellularity, lymphocyte rich or lymphocyte depleted.
2) Nodular lymphocytic predominant Hodgkin's lymphoma: "L and H" cells or "popcorn" cells with positive labeling for CD20 and CD45, but negative for CD15 and CD30. Reed-Stemberg cells are not present in this subtype.

This chapter focuses on classical Hodgkin's Lymphoma (HL) and presents summaries of major clinical trials in Table 1.

Table 1. Summary of included studies

Study	Stage	Chemo – RT	Result	Reference
DeVita et al. 1980	IIA, IVA	MOPP	The results of treatment of 198 patients with Hodgkin's disease with MOPP (mechlorethamine, vincristine, procarbazine, and prednisone) were analyzed. Complete remission: 80% Disease free beyond 10 years: 68% of patients achieving a complete remission have remained disease free beyond 10 years from the end of treatment. Results of autopsy on patients who died of other causes while in clinical complete remission did not show evidence of residual tumors except in one patient. The median number of cycles needed to achieve complete remission was three.	52
Canellos, et al, 1992	IIIE, IV	(1) MOPP alone given for 6 to 8 cycles, (2) MOPP alternating with ABVD (doxorubicin, bleomycin, vinblastine, and dacarbazine) for 12 cycles, and (3) ABVD alone for 6 to 8 cycles. Patients in a first relapse after radiation therapy were eligible.	Overall response rate: 93 percent Complete responses: 77 percent (67 percent in the MOPP group, 82 percent in the ABVD group, and 83 percent in the MOPP-ABVD group ($p = 0.006$ for the comparison of MOPP with the other two regimens, both of which contained doxorubicin). Failure-free survival at five years were 50 percent for MOPP, 61 percent for ABVD, and 65 percent for MOPP-ABVD. Overall survival at five years was 66 percent for MOPP, 73 percent for ABVD, and 75 percent for MOPP-ABVD ($p = 0.28$ for the comparison of MOPP with the doxorubicin regimens). MOPP had more severe toxic effects on bone marrow than ABVD and was associated with greater reductions in the prescribed dose.	1
HD6	IA or IIA non-bulky Hodgkin's lymphoma	ABVD x subtotal nodal irradiation Radiation therapy: 35 Gy in 20 daily fractions. ABVD: Both those with a favorable risk profile and those with an unfavorable risk profile received four cycles of ABVD,	10-year median follow-up. The median length of follow-up was 11.3 years. At 12 years, the rate of overall survival was 94% among those receiving ABVD alone, as compared with 87% among those receiving subtotal nodal radiation therapy	18

Table 1. (Continued)

Study	Stage	Chemo – RT	Result	Reference
		with restaging after two and four cycles of therapy. Restaging was CT scanning or gallium scanning. No patient underwent positron-emission tomography (PET). Patients who had a complete remission after two cycles received a total of four cycles of ABVD; those who did not have a complete remission or an unconfirmed complete remission after their second cycle received six cycles.	(hazard ratio (HR) for death with ABVD alone, 0.50; 95% confidence interval [CI], 0.25 to 0.99; p = 0.04); the rates of freedom from disease progression were 87% and 92% in the two groups, respectively (HR for disease progression, 1.91; 95% CI, 0.99 to 3.69; p = 0.05); and the rates of event-free survival were 85% and 80%, respectively (HR for event, 0.88; 95% CI, 0.54 to 1.43; p = 0.60). Among the patients randomly assigned to ABVD alone, 6 patients died from Hodgkin's lymphoma or an early treatment complication and 6 died from another cause; among those receiving radiation therapy, 4 deaths were related to Hodgkin's lymphoma or early toxic effects from the treatment and 20 were related to another cause.	
HD7	IA, IIB without risk factors	RT alone: 30 Gy EF-RT plus 10 Gy to the involved field (arm A) versus CTRT with two cycles of ABVD followed by the same radiotherapy (arm B).	FU = 120 Response rate: ns Arm A 94% e Arm B Overall survival at 15 years: OS did not differ significantly between trial arms (p = 0.3), with 15-year estimates of 77% versus 80% and an HR of 0.8 (95% CI: 0.6 to 1.2) Freedom from treatment failure was significantly different, with 15-year rates of 52% and 73% in arm B (HR of 0.5, 95% CI: 0.3 to 0.6), superiority of CMT compared with EF-RT was confirmed (p = 0.001). Second malignancies: 15-year estimates for the cumulative incidence of any SN were 16% and 14%, respectively, with a comparable distribution of solid and hematologic malignancies and SIRs of 2.7 (95% CI: 1.9 to 3.6) and 3.0 (95% CI: 2.2 to 4.0) Only a minority of deaths was HL-related (2% of analyzed patients in each arm) but instead attributed to SN (5% v 6%), cardiovascular disease (3% each), or respiratory disease (2% vs 1%)	15, 16

Study	Stage	Chemo – RT	Result	Reference
H8-F, H8-U	Ie, II favorable or unfavorable	538 patients (age 15 to 70 years) who had untreated stage I or II supradiaphragmatic Hodgkin's disease with favorable prognostic features (the H8-F trial) or unfavorable features (the H8-U trial). In the H8-F trial, we compared three cycles of mechlorethamine, vincristine, procarbazine, and prednisone (MOPP) combined with doxorubicin, bleomycin, and vinblastine (ABV) plus involved-field radiotherapy with subtotal nodal radiotherapy alone (reference group). In the H8-U trial, we compared three regimens: six cycles of MOPP-ABV plus involved-field radiotherapy (reference group), four cycles of MOPP-ABV plus involved-field radiotherapy, and four cycles of MOPP-ABV plus subtotal nodal radiotherapy.	H8-F Follow-up was 92 months. 5-year event-free survival rate was significantly higher after three cycles of MOPP-ABV plus involved-field radiotherapy than after subtotal nodal radiotherapy alone (98% vs. 74%, $p < 0.001$). 10-year overall survival estimates were 97% and 92%, respectively ($p = 0.001$). H8-U Follow-up was 92 months. 5-year event-free survival rates were similar in the three treatment groups: 84% after six cycles of MOPP-ABV plus involved-field radiotherapy, 88% after four cycles of MOPP-ABV plus involved-field radiotherapy, and 87% after four cycles of MOPP-ABV plus subtotal nodal radiotherapy. 10-year overall survival estimates were 88%, 85%, and 84%, respectively.	17
H9U	I, II unfavorable based on 4 prognostic factors: age, symptoms, number of involved areas, MT-ratio	6 cycles of ABVD *vs*4 cycles of ABVD *vs* 4 cycles of BEACOPP baseline, followed by 30 Gy IF-RT in all arms	808 patients were randomized in the H9-U trial. The 4-year EFS rates were 94%, 89% and 91% in the 3 arms, respectively ($p = 0.23$) and the 4-year OS rates 96%, 95% and 93% ($p = 0.89$). Chemotherapy-related toxicity (measured by antibiotics, transfusions, hospitalization, S.A.E.) was higher with BEACOPP compared to ABVD.	28
H9-F	I, II unfavorable based on 4 prognostic factors: age, symptoms, number of involved areas, MT-ratio	Compared 36 Gy involved field radiotherapy (IF-RT) *vs* 20 Gy IF-RT *vs* no RT in patients in complete remission (CR(u)) after 6 cycles of EBVP.	783 patients enrolled, 619 (79%) achieved a CR(u) and were randomized After a median follow-up of 33 months, the 4-year EFS rates were 87% in the 36 Gy and 84% in the 20 Gy arm; it was 70% in the no RT arm ($p < 0.001$). The 4-year OS rate was 98% in all 3 arms	28
HD 10	Oldervoll et al. (34)	2 ABVD – 20Gy IFRT 2 ABVD – 30Gy RT 4 ABVD – 20Gy 4 ABVD – 30Gy	Freedom from treatment failure not different ($p = 0.39$) Overall survival not different ($p = 0.61$).	16,29

Table 1. (Continued)

Study	Stage	Chemo – RT	Result	Reference
			At 5 years, the rates of freedom from treatment failure were 93.0% (95% confidence interval [CI], 90.5 to 94.8) with the four-cycle ABVD regimen and 91.1% (95% CI, 88.3 to 93.2) with the two-cycle regimen. Freedom from treatment failure when the effects of 20-Gy and 30-Gy doses of radiation therapy were compared, there were also no significant differences in freedom from treatment failure (p = 1.00) or overall survival (p = 0.61). Adverse events and acute toxic effects of treatment were most common in the patients who received four cycles of ABVD and 30 Gy of radiation therapy (group 1). Secondary cancers: Over a median follow-up period of 7.5 years (90 months), secondary cancers were diagnosed in a total of 55 patients (4.6%): 38 solid tumors, 15 cases of non-Hodgkin's lymphoma, and 2 cases of acute myeloid leukemia. There were no significant differences in the occurrence of secondary cancers among the four treatment groups (p = 0.59), the pooled chemotherapy groups (p = 0.89), or the pooled radiation therapy groups (p = 0.34) Long – FU – 53 months 10-year PFS estimates of 87% each and an HR of 1.0 (95% CI, 0.6 to 1.5 within the calculated margin for noninferiority of 2.2). The 10-year OS estimates were excellent, with 94% each and an HR of 0.9 (95% CI, 0.5 to 1.6; With SIRs (standardized incidence ratios for SN) of 2.1 each and a 10-year cumulative incidence of 8% and 9% in arms A and D, respectively, no difference in terms of incidence and type of SN was observed. SN accounted for the majority of deaths (2% of analyzed patients), whereas HL-related death was reported in 1% of patients.	

Study	Stage	Chemo – RT	Result	Reference
H10 EORTC 20051	I, II; 15 to 70 years	Favorable: 1) 2ABVD →PET → 1ABVD + INRT 30Gy 2) 2ABVD → PET negative → 2ABVD 3) 2ABDV → PET positive → 2 BEACOPPesc + INRT 30Gy +/- 6Gy Unfavorable: 4) 2ABVD →PET → 2ABVD + INRT 30Gy +/- 6Gy 5) 2ABVD → PET negative → 4ABVD 6) 2ABDV → PET positive → 2 BEACOPPesc + INRT 30Gy =/- 6Gy	1,137 patients. - Favorable subgroup, 85.8% had a negative early PET scan (standard arm, one event *v* experimental arm, nine events). PFS rates at 1 year were 100.0% and 94.9% in the standard and experimental arms, respectively. - Unfavorable subgroup, 74.8% had a negative early PET scan (standard arm, seven events *v* experimental arm, 16 events). PFS rates at 1 year were 97.3% and 94.7% in the standard and experimental arms, respectively - Futility analysis showed statistical significance for PFS in both favorable and unfavorable early PET–negative groups, the IDMC recommended closing the study for continued accrual in the early PET–negative experimental arm. Moreover, it recommended changing treatment in patients with early PET–negative scans who were randomly assigned to the experimental arm and had not yet completed treatment from chemotherapy alone to the standard combined-modality approach, if possible.	25
RAPID Trial	IA,IIA; no bulky disease	PET adapted Trial. Stage IA or stage IIA Hodgkin's lymphoma received three cycles of ABVD and then underwent PET scanning. Patients with negative PET findings were randomly assigned to receive involved-field radiotherapy or no further treatment; patients with positive PET findings received a fourth cycle of ABVD and radiotherapy.	On the basis of a maximum allowable difference of 7 percentage points, this study did not show noninferiority of the strategy of no further treatment; although the measured difference was 3.8 percentage points, the 95% confidence interval included a possible difference of up to 8.8 percentage points. Nevertheless, the results of RAPID suggest a rationale for taking a more individualized approach to the treatment of early-stage Hodgkin's lymphoma.	24
HD 11	Early unfavorable	4 arms: - 4ABVD + 20Gy IFRT - 4ABVD + 30Gy IFRT - 4BEACOPP + 20Gy - 4BEACOPP + 30Gy (IFRT)	All groups had equivalent overall response rate and overall survival, apart from those who had four cycles of ABVD plus 20 Gy whose overall response rate was significantly worse. Long FU – 106 months	16, 30

Table 1. (Continued)

Study	Stage	Chemo – RT	Result	Reference
			Superiority of bleomycin, etoposide, doxorubicin, cyclophosphamide, vincristine, procarbazine, and prednisone at baseline over ABVD was not observed. After BEACOPP baseline, 20 Gy IF-RT was noninferior to 30 Gy (10-year PFS, 84% v 84%; HR, 1.0; 95% CI, 0.7 to 1.5). Progression free survival: PFS was inferior in ABVD-treated patients receiving 20 Gy instead of 30 Gy IF-RT (10-year PFS, 76% v 84%; HR, 1.5; 95% CI, 1.0 to 2.1). Overall Survival: No differences in OS or second neoplasias were observed in in both trials. Conclusion: Moderate dose escalation using BEACOPP (baseline) did not significantly improve outcome in early unfavorable HL. Four cycles of ABVD should be followed by 30 Gy of IFRT.	
HD 12	Advanced	Eight cycles of BEACOPP (escalated) was compared with four cycles of BEACOPP (escalated) followed by four cycles of the baseline dose of BEACOPP (BEACOPP (baseline); 4 + 4), and RT with no RT in the case of initial bulk or residual disease.	1,670 patients age 16 to 65 years were enrolled onto the HD12 study. At 5 years, FFTF was 86.4% in the BEACOPP (escalated) arm and 84.8% in the 4 + 4 arm (difference, -1.6%; 95% CI, -5.2% to 1.9%), and overall survival was 92% versus 90.3% (difference, -1.7%; 95% CI, -4.6% to 1.1%). Deaths related to acute toxicity of chemotherapy were observed in 2.9% of patients (BEACOPP (escalated), n = 19; 4 + 4, n = 27). FFTF was inferior without RT (90.4% v 87%; difference, -3.4%; 95% CI, -6.6% to -0.1%), particularly in patients who had residual disease after chemotherapy (difference, -5.8%; 95% CI, -10.7% to -1.0%), but not in patients with bulk in complete response after chemotherapy (difference, -1.1%; 95% CI, -6.2% to 4%). Conclusion: The reduction of BEACOPP to the 4 + 4 regimen did not substantially reduce severe toxicity but might decrease efficacy.	40

Study	Stage	Chemo – RT	Result	Reference
			Our results do not support the omission of consolidation RT for patients with residual disease.	
HD13	Classic or nodular, lymphocyte predominant	Randomised, multicentre trial (HD13) we compared two cycles of ABVD with two cycles of ABV (doxorubicin, bleomycin, and vinblastine), AVD (doxorubicin, vinblastine, and dacarbazine), and AV (doxorubicin and vinblastine). In each treatment group, 30 Gy involved-field radiotherapy (IFRT) was given after both cycles of chemotherapy were completed	Compared with ABVD, inferiority of the dacarbazine-deleted variants was detected with 5 year differences of −11·5% (95% CI −18·3 to −4·7; HR 2·06 [1·21 to 3·52]) for ABV and −15·2% (−23·0 to −7·4; HR 2·57 [1·51 to 4·40]) for AV. Non-inferiority of AVD compared with ABVD could also not be detected (5 year difference −3·9%, −7·7 to −0·1; HR 1·50, 1·00 to 2·26). 178 (33%) of 544 patients given ABVD had WHO grade III or IV toxicity, compared with 53 (28%) of 187 given ABV, 142 (26%) of 539 given AVD, and 40 (26%) of 151 given AV. Leucopenia was the most common event, and highest in the groups given bleomycin.	23
HD14	Early unfavorable	Randomly assigned to either four cycles of ABVD or an intensified treatment consisting of two cycles of escalated BEACOPP (bleomycin, etoposide, adriamycin, cyclophosphamide, vincristine, procarbazine, and prednisone) followed by two cycles of ABVD (2 + 2). Chemotherapy was followed by 30 Gy IFRT in both arms. The primary end point was freedom from treatment failure (FFTF); secondary end points included progression-free survival (PFS) and treatment-related toxicity.	With a total of 1,528 qualified patients included, the 2 + 2 regimen demonstrated superior FFTF compared with four cycles of ABVD (P < .001; hazard ratio, 0.44; 95% CI, 0.30 to 0.66), with a difference of 7.2% at 5 years (95% CI, 3.8 to 10.5). The difference in 5-year PFS was 6.2% (95% CI, 3.0% to 9.5%). There was more acute toxicity associated with 2 + 2 than with ABVD, but there were no overall differences in treatment-related mortality or secondary malignancies.	32
HD 15	Advanced	182 patients with newly diagnosed advanced stage Hodgkin's lymphoma aged 18-60 years were randomly assigned to receive either eight cycles of BEACOPP (escalated) (8×B(esc) group), six cycles of BEACOPP(escalated) (6×B(esc) group), or eight cycles of BEACOPP(14)	2126 patients were included in the intention-to-treat analysis set,. 705 in the 8×B(esc) group, 711 in the 6×B(esc) group, and 710 in the 8×B(14) group. Freedom from treatment failure was sequentially non-inferior for the 6×B(esc) and 8×B(14) groups as compared with 8×B(esc). 5-year freedom from treatment failure rates were 84·4% (97·5% CI 81·0-87·7) for the	33

Table 1. (Continued)

Study	Stage	Chemo – RT	Result	Reference
		(8×B(14) group). Randomisation (1:1:1) was done centrally by stratified minimisation. Non-inferiority of the primary endpoint, freedom from treatment failure, was assessed using repeated CIs for the hazard ratio (HR) according to the intention-to-treat principle. Patients with a persistent mass after chemotherapy measuring 2·5 cm or larger and positive on PET scan received additional radiotherapy with 30 Gy; the negative predictive value for tumour recurrence of PET at 12 months was an independent endpoint	8×B(esc) group, 89·3% (86·5-92·1) for 6×B(esc) group, and 85·4% (82·1-88·7) for the 8×B(14) group (97·5% CI for difference between 6×B(esc) and 8×B(esc) was 0·5-9·3). Overall survival in the three groups was 91·9%, 95·3%, and 94·5% respectively, and was significantly better with 6×B(esc) than with 8×B(esc) (97·5% CI 0·2-6·5). The 8×B(esc) group showed a higher mortality (7·5%) than the 6×B(esc) (4·6%) and 8×B(14) (5·2%) groups, mainly due to differences in treatment-related events (2·1%, 0·8%, and 0·8%, respectively) and secondary malignancies (1·8%, 0·7%, and 1·1%, respectively). The negative predictive value for PET at 12 months was 94·1% (95% CI 92·1-96·1); and 225 (11%) of 2126 patients received additional radiotherapy. CONCLUSION: Treatment with six cycles of BEACOPP (escalated) followed by PET-guided radiotherapy was more effective in terms of freedom from treatment failure and less toxic than eight cycles of the same chemotherapy regimen. Thus, six cycles of BEACOPP (escalated) should be the treatment of choice for advanced stage Hodgkin's lymphoma. PET done after chemotherapy can guide the need for additional radiotherapy in this setting.	
EORTC	Advanced	333 patients to consolidation RT or observation after the achievement of a CR with a MOPP/ABV hybrid regimen 247 patients achieved a PR after MOPP/ABV	The omission of RT for patients who achieve a CR with ABVD (EORTC) trial that randomly assigned 333 patients to consolidation RT or observation after the achievement of a CR with a MOPP/ABV hybrid regimen. When compared with patients who received RT, patients who did not receive RT had similar rates of event-free survival (77 versus 73%) and overall survival (85 versus 78%) at eight years.	38

Study	Stage	Chemo – RT	Result	Reference
			Patients who received RT had a nonsignificant trend towards a higher rate of secondary cancer at eight ears (13 versus 6%). However, there are several limitations to this trial: the chemotherapy regimen (MOPP/ABV hybrid) is no longer in use due to its excessive toxicity; most patients received eight cycles of chemotherapy and still the fraction of patients randomized in CR was only 65%, and, most patients with bulky disease were not randomized. It is also unexplained why the excess in leukemia cases that was reported only in CR patients who received low-dose radiation consolidation has not been observed in the larger group of partial responders who have all received radiation as well. Partial response — EORTC trial described above. In this same trial, 247 patients achieved a PR after MOPP/ABV, 227 of whom were given consolidation RT. When compared with those who had achieved a CR after MOPP/ABV, those patients who received RT after achieving a PR had similar rates of event-free survival (76%) and overall survival (84%) at eight years. In this trial, response was determined using computed tomography (CT) criteria. It is likely that a percentage of patients who achieve a PR by CT criteria had fibrosis rather than residual HL suggesting that some of these patients were potentially overtreated. Response criteria now incorporate findings from PET scans.	
LY09 trial	Advanced	A nonrandomized study of RT embedded within a randomized trial of chemotherapy (ABVD x two other multidrug regimens) advanced stage HL 222 patients who received RT mostly due to bulky disease or incomplete response	Although the radiation group included mostly patients with these unfavorable features, the addition of consolidation RT resulted in superior progression-free survival (hazard ratio [HR] 0.40, 95% CI 0.23-0.69). Overall survival was also significantly better for those who received RT (HR, 0.47; 95% CI 0.29-0.77). Median follow-up was seven years.	39

Selection of initial treatment for Hodgkin's Lymphoma is usually based upon presenting stage and prognostic factors. They are staged according to Ann Arbor, based on laparotomy and lymphangiogram (8) and modified by Cotswolds (9) to include modifications regarding the presence of bulky disease and imaging studies. In 2014 Lugano proposed revisions based on positron emission tomography (PET) and extranodal involvement (10, 11). For treatment purposes, Hodgkin's disease is commonly classified into early stage (I to II) or advanced disease (III to IV). Patients with early stage are sub-classified into favorable and unfavorable prognoses based on the number of sites involvement, number of lymph node regions involved, presence or absence of systemic symptoms or of bulky extended disease. Waldeyer's ring, spleen and tonsils are considered nodal tissue.

Ann Arbor stage (8, 9)

I. Involvement of one lymph node region or lymphoid structure
II. Involvement of two or more lymph node regions on the same side of the diaphragm
III. Involvement of lymph nodes on both side of the diaphragm
IV. Involvement of extra nodal sites other than one contiguous or proximal extra nodal site

Modifying features

A: No symptoms
B: Unexplained fever >38°C in the absence of infection, drenching night sweats and unexplained loss of >10% of body weight over the preceding 6 months
X: Bulky disease (mediastinal mass larger than a third of thoracic diameter, or any nodal mass >10 cm in diameter)
E: Involvement of one contiguous or proximal extranodal site. Extensive extranodal is designated stage IV.
Fatigue, pruritus and alcohol induced pain are associated with lymphoma but not considered B symptoms

For advanced Hodgkin's lymphomas, simple staging is not sensitive enough to arrive at an accurate prognosis. Prognostic factors delineate groups at high risk for first relapse and this group could benefit from more intensive therapy. The strongest predictor of outcome is the International Prognostic Score (IPS) which incorporates seven predictive factors: serum albumin < 4g/dl (1 point), Hemoglobin < 10,5g/dl (1 point), male sex (1 point), staged IV according to the Anne Arbor Classification (1 point), age ≥ 4s (1point), leukocyte count ≥ 15,000/mm^3 (1 point), lymphocyte count < 600/mm^3 or < 8% of white blood cell count (1 point). From the presence of these potentially unfavorable factors, 6 groups are defined with different survival disease-free and overall survival (12, 13).

For the initial stages, prognostic factors are also used to categorize patients with initial disease in two groups, favorable and unfavorable, and enable them to be divided into clinical trials and thus to be treated appropriately according to the risk of relapse. These differed according to the different onco-hematology groups, which are described below (14):

EORTC (European Organization for the Research and Treatment of Cancer) unfavorable prognosis criteria

- Age greater than or equal to 40 years.
- Erythrocyte sedimentation rate greater than 30 mm/h with B symptoms (if no B symptoms, use the 50 mm/h mark).
- Ratio of a chest X-ray to a T5-T6 height and the extent of mediastinal bulky disease greater than 0.35.
- Involvement of 4 or more nodal sites.

GHSG (Germain Hodgkin's Study Group) unfavorable prognostic criteria

- Erythrocyte sedimentation rate greater than or equal to 30 mm/h with symptoms B or greater or equal to 50 mm/h without symptoms B.
- Extension of the large mediastinal mass (at least 1/3 of the diameter of the thorax).
- Involvement of 3 or more nodal sites.
- Involvement of extranodal disease.

NCIC (National Cancer Institute of Canada) unfavorable prognostic criteria

- Age greater than or equal to 40 years.
- Aggressive histologies such as lymphocyte depletion or mixed cellularity.
- Erythrocyte sedimentation rate greater than 50 mm/h.
- B symptoms.

- Ratio between the maximum measure of thoracic disease and the patient's thorax greater than or equal to 0.33.
- 4 or more compromised nodal sites.

Stanford unfavorable prognostic criteria

- B symptoms.
- Bulky disease defined as conglomerate greater than 10 cm or ratio between the maximum measure of thoracic disease and the patient's thorax greater or equal to 0.33.

Early stage favorable risk

Combined-modality treatment (CMT) is the treatment of choice for early stage Hodgkin's lymphoma. Results from the HD7 trial showed that the combined modality was superior to extended-field radiotherapy (15, 16). The chemotherapy regimen known as ABVD is preferred for patients with early stage Hodgkin's disease (17-19). This scheme includes applications of ABVD (doxorubicin, bleomycin, vimblastine and dacarbazine) every 14 days in a 28-day cycle. Two administrations are considered 1 cycle. For initial Hodgkin's Lymphoma with favourable prognoses, there are few randomized studies comparing different chemotherapy regimens.

The preference for ABVD over other regimens (containing alkylating agents) comes from studies that compared MOPP versus ABVD for Hodgkin's lymphoma with unfavorable prognosis (advanced or initial stage) (20). Trials for early favorable disease focused on maintaining excellent cure rates, while de-escalating therapy. The landmark HD10 trial suggested that the standard of care in patients who fit the GHSG prognostic criteria is two cycles of ABVD followed by 20 Gy IFRT (16,21,22). It achieved excellent cure rates (>90%) equivalent to four cycles of ABVD plus 30 Gy IFRT.

The effects of ABVD include: hair loss, myelosuppression with risk of infection, dose-dependent cardiotoxicity with adriamycin, pulmonary toxicity with bleomycin, and autonomic neuropathy with vinblastine (19). A reduction of chemotherapy intensity by omission of dacarbazine and/or bleomycin from ABVD cannot be generally recommended because of poorer tumor control observed in the GHSG HD13 trial (23).

It is not standard to suppress consolidation radiotherapy except in specific situations. Despite the HD6 trial reporting 10-year median follow-up comparing mantle-field RT-containing treatment with ABVD alone, long-term follow-up analyses of large randomized prospective trials evaluating current treatment strategies with regard to long-term efficacy and safety have not been published thus far (18).

There are no conclusive data that support a response-adapted, PET-guided RT approach to date (16); both the UK National Cancer Research Institute RAPID trial (24) and the EORTC/Group des Etudes des Lymphomes de l'Adulte (GELA)/Fondazione Italiana Linfomi (FIL) H10 trial (25) failed to demonstrate noninferiority in patients who were PET negative after chemotherapy and did not receive RT. Currently, the GHSG HD16 and HD17 trials are evaluating a similar PET-guided RT approach.

The impact of consolidating RT on outcome is supported by a National Cancer Database analysis of 20,600 patients with early stage HL and by a Cochrane analysis, both showing inferior tumor control and OS with chemotherapy alone compared with CMT (26, 27). Two cycles of ABVD followed by 20 Gy IFRT are still considered standard of care in early-stage favorable HL patients who fit the GHSG criteria (15, 16, 28). Omission of RT in patients who are PET negative and have a favorable risk profile can be justified only in selected individual patients after weighing the risk-benefit ratio of tumor control and toxicity.

Early Stage Unfavorable Risk

Studies show that four cycles of ABVD combined with IFRT or involved site radiotherapy (ISRT) appear to be sufficient. There is no difference in disease-free survival or overall survival in adding two more cycles of chemotherapy. This has been demonstrated in the EORTC H8U and EORTC H9U trials (20, 24). Most the UK clinicians consider four cycles of ABVD plus 30 Gy to be the standard of care in this subgroup.

The HD11 trial (16, 29, 30) randomized four cycles of ABVD plus 20 Gy or 30 Gy IFRT with four cycles of BEACOPP (bleomycin, etoposide, doxorubicin, doxorubicin, cyclophosphamide, vincristine, procarbazine and prednisone) plus 20 Gy or 30 Gy IFRT. All groups had equivalent overall response rate and overall survival, apart from those who had four cycles of ABVD plus 20 Gy whose overall response rate was significantly worse. There is still a lack of international consensus with some clinicians favoring six cycles of ABVD with no IFRT and others using BEACOPP regimens, but BEACOPP has higher toxicity (mainly acute myelogenous leukemia and myelodysplastic syndrome) and lack of benefit in terms of disease-free survival or relapse-free survival as demonstrated in studies GHSG HD11 and EORTC H9U.

It is better combining fewer cycles of cytotoxic therapy and limited RT instead of exposing the body to longer courses of cytotoxic therapy. An intensification of chemotherapy in early-stage unfavorable Hodgkin's Lymphoma was evaluated in the recent HD14 trial which showed that two cycles of BEACOPP escalated and two cycles of ABVD resulted in a significant PFS advantage compared with four cycles of ABVD at

5 years. Although there has been more acute toxicity and no improvement in OS so far, the improved tumor control is a relevant outcome parameter for patients (31, 32).

ADVANCED STAGE

There is no consensus regarding the optimal first-line treatment for advanced stage Hodgkin's Lymphoma. The ABVD regimen is favored in the UK, some parts of Europe and USA while BEACOPP is favoured in Germany. The BEACOPP regimen is intensive (especially escalated BEACOPP) and consist of bleomycin, etoposide, doxorubicin, doxorubicin, cyclophosphamide, vincristine, procarbazine and prednisone. It is administered on days 1 and 8 of a 21-day cycle with scheduled growth factor support for a total time of chemotherapy ranging from 18 to 24 weeks. Six cycles of escalated BEACOPP is considered the 'gold standard' by the German Hodgkin's Study Group (GHSG). The GHSG HD15 study (22, 33) found that six cycles of escalated BEACOPP is likely better than eight. Although efficacy is similar, six cycles improved overall survival (91.9% *vs* 95.3%) by reducing acute toxicities and secondary cancers.

Other studies (34, 35, 36) compared different strategies: 6-8 cycles of ABVD with 8 cycles of BEACOPP (four cycles of the dose-intense escalated regimen followed by four standard cycles depending on the response) in stage IIB–IV. When compared with ABVD, BEACOPP is associated with higher rates of toxicity including reversible bone marrow suppression, secondary malignancies, and sterility. Toxicities are particularly severe in the elderly. Escalated BEACOPP programs have shown advantages in freedom from progression when compared with ABVD and overall survival when compared with COPP/ABVD. These advantages are most marked among patients with higher risk IPS scores (IPS ≥ 4) and this more intense regimen is a reasonable alternative to ABVD for younger patients (< 50 years) with the highest risk of relapse.

One study randomized 331 patients to ABVD or BEACOPP (34). Localized radiotherapy as consolidation and autologous stem cell transplantation in those who relapse was permitted within the study. The trial found that the 7-year progression-free survival was better with BEACOPP (85 *vs* 73% $p = 0.004$). More patients therefore required salvage treatment and an autologous stem cell transplant after ABVD, but the 7-year overall survival was not significantly different (89% for BEACOPP *vs* 84% for ABVD, $p = 0.39$). BEACOPP toxicity was significantly higher with severe adverse events seen in 6% compared with 1% in the ABVD group. Similar results were confirmed in the HD2000 trial (35) and a Cochrane review (36). It is unknown whether this advantage will be lost over longer follow-up due to an increase in second malignancies and cardiac toxicities, which account for the majority of late deaths.

There is a paucity of data regarding response-adapted therapy through checking a positron emission tomography with computed tomography (PET/CT) mid-treatment.

There are limited data regarding the efficacy of treatment escalation in those without an early response. It was evaluated in the RATHL randomized trial (37) of 1214 patients with advanced stage HL defined as those with stage IIB to IV disease or stage IIA with adverse features (bulky disease or at least three involved sites). The results suggest that patients who attain a PET score of 1, 2, or 3 after two cycles of ABVD may reasonably complete therapy with four additional cycles of AVD without bleomycin. The decision for an individual patient must consider the risk of pulmonary toxicity with further bleomycin versus the potentially small increase in relapse with bleomycin omission.

While this approach is an option for all patients with advanced stage HL, it is most attractive for those with additional risk factors for bleomycin toxicity (ex. older age, underlying pulmonary disease, active smokers). Younger patients who wish to minimize their chance of relapse may choose to complete therapy with four more cycles of ABVD (14). There is a paucity of data regarding the preferred approach for patients with a PET score of 4 or 5 after two cycles of ABVD. Outside of a clinical trial, many clinicians will continue with ABVD therapy with modifications based on further imaging and/or biopsy samples. Nonrandomized trials have evaluated treatment escalation in this population (14).

The use of radiotherapy following chemotherapy in advanced stage disease is controversial. Its use is acceptable in partial response or initial bulky disease (14, 22). The HD15 trial showed that when six cycles of escalated BEACOPP-based chemotherapy are used, consolidation radiotherapy can be omitted with no adverse outcomes in patients with a residual PET-negative mass. This approach reduces the numbers requiring consolidation radiotherapy. Whether omission of radiotherapy based on PET-negativity after ABVD is safe remains unanswered, although this practice is being increasingly adopted. In the RATHL trial, consolidation radiotherapy was left to the treating clinician's discretion and was administered to 2.6 and 4.3 percent of those receiving ABVD and AVD, respectively (37). The data are not clear and most still advocate consolidation radiotherapy following ABVD to sites of bulky disease at presentation or residual masses, regardless of PET signal.

The omission of radiotherapy for patients who achieve complete response with ABVD is supported by the EORTC trial (phase III) that showed similar rates of event free survival and overall survival in patients who achieved complete responses with MOPP/ABV who may or may not have received consolidation radiotherapy (38). The use of radiotherapy in patients who achieve partial response is based on the same EORTC trial. It showed that patients with partial response who received consolidation radiotherapy had similar rates of event-free survival and overall survival when compared with those who had achieved complete response to MOPP/ABV.

Bulky mediastinal disease (> 10cm or > 1/3 the chest diameter) is an adverse prognostic factor. The use of consolidation radiotherapy in bulky disease is supported by largely retrospective analysis. The LY09 trial (39), a retrospective non-randomized analysis, demonstrated that in patients treated with ABVD, the 5-year progression-free survival and the 5-year overall survival were significantly better across all prognostic groups who received consolidation radiotherapy (87% *vs* 93% and 71% *vs* 86%, respectively). However, the PET assessments were not part of this study.

After BEACOPP, the addition of RT improves freedom from treatment failure rates in patients with advanced stage HL who have residual disease after the completion of BEACOPP (39, 40). However, patients with advanced stage HL who still have residual disease on CT scan after escalated BEACOPP but are PET-negative maintain a progression-free survival rate of 94 to 96% without receiving additional RT (33).

RADIATION FIELD

In the late 1960s, studies by Peters (41) and Kaplan (42) advocated curative treatment of lymphoma by irradiating all sites of known disease and adjacent uninvolved sites. Treatment fields became larger and terms such as "mantle," "inverted Y," "extended field" radiation therapy (EFRT) and "total lymphoid irradiation" were introduced to describe these fields, which contrasted with the previous limited-field treatment current known as "involved-field" radiation therapy (IFRT) (43). Beginning in the mid-1970s, however, combined modality therapy became more common in the treatment of the lymphomas and marked the renaissance of IFRT (17, 19, 20, 43-46). The volume of IFRT is based on the Ann Arbor-defined lymphoid regions and radiation treatment planning includes 2-dimensional (2D) simulation using bony landmarks to define the borders of the lymphoid regions. Outside its use in prospective clinical trials, IFRT was more variably defined. Yahalom and Mauch (47) published guidelines for the design of IFRT fields based upon 2D imaging.

Reducing radiation volumes in the treatment of lymphomas, especially in the context of combined modality therapy, can reduce the risk of late effects. Evidence support a reduction from EFRT to IFRT (17, 44-46). However, over the last decade, there was an improved in diagnostic imaging with PET/CT and the use of 3-dimensional (3D) planning. In response to these changes in modern radiation oncology practices, Girinsky et al. (48) developed guidelines for "involved-node RT" (INRT) to be used with European Organization for Research and Treatment of Cancer Groupe d'Etude des Lymphomes de l'Adulte (EORTCGELA) trials.

Results have been quite promising in successfully reducing the field size without impacting event-free survival (49), but most centers are unable to meet the stringent criteria of INRT, which requires pre-chemotherapy evaluation by a radiation oncologist and a PET-CT scan performed in the radiation treatment position and obtained before chemotherapy. In response, the International Lymphoma Radiation Oncology Group (ILROG), an international group of radiation oncologists with special expertise in the treatment of lymphoma, developed the concept of "involved-site" RT (ISRT) and published guidelines (5) to help bridge the differences between IFRT and INRT. The difference between ISRT and INRT is the "precision." Involved node radiotherapy needs the PET-CT scan to be performed in the radiation treatment position and obtained before chemotherapy. The ISRT needs pre-chemotherapy image exams well documented, but not necessarily in the same position, and PET is not necessary.

In ISRT, clinical judgment in conjunction with the best available imaging is used to contour a clinical target volume (CTV) that will accommodate the uncertainties in defining the prechemotherapy gross tumour volume (GTV) in each individual case. For these reasons, ISRT is a slightly larger irradiated volume than INRT (42). ISRT is based on the initial involved volume in the treated site and reduced in consideration of the node regression after chemotherapy such that most uninvolved normal organs are spared of radiation. For most cases, ISRT results in significantly smaller radiation fields than the IFRT used previously.

IFRT and ISRT are nowadays standard and preferred over larger radiation fields. If the pre-chemotherapy image exams are well documented, ISRT is preferred over IFRT.

Field definitions

1) **Total lymphoid irradiation**: frequently used in the past but no longer recommended for the treatment of Hodgkin's disease. It consists of the delineation of all nodal chains including Waldeyer's ring, cervical, supraclavicular, infra clavicular, axilla, mediastinum, para aortic, spleen, iliac, inguinal and femoral nodes bilaterally. It was often treated with opposite anterior-posterior parallel fields.
2) **Extended field irradiation or subtotal lymphoid irradiation**: rarely used nowadays. This technique consists of the identification of the disease as supra or infra diaphragmatic and the systematic treatment only on the affected side: mantle (Waldeyer, cervical, supra and infra clavicular fossa, axilla and mediastinum) for supra diaphragmatic and inverted Y disease (paraaortic, spleen, iliac, inguinal and femoral) for infra diaphragmatic disease.
3) **Involved field irradiation (IFRT)**: current standard technique. It consists of contouring only the affected areas (only cervical and right armpits, for example), and a proportional decrease of the classic fields for the treatment of lymphomas according to the anatomical chains (20).
4) **Involved site irradiation (ISRT)**: accurate technique. It consists of the systematic fusion of staging images, notably 18-FDG PET, with simulation tomography, in order to delimit only the sites affected, avoiding radiation to areas previously unaffected by the disease. The ISRT needs pre-chemotherapy image

exams to be well documented, but not necessarily in the same position, and PET is not necessary (5).

5) **Involved node irradiation (INRT):** the most precise technique that delineates only the previously affected lymph nodes, maintaining a minimum field size (45). It needs the pre-chemotherapy PET/CT to be performed in the same position as the CT planning radiotherapy.

CONCLUSION

While the majority of patients with lymphoma will be cured, treatment-related toxicities have become a competing cause of late mortality. The selection of therapy must balance the desire to maintain a high rate of cure and the need to minimize long-term complications. For early stage disease with favourable prognosis, combined modality treatment remains the treatment standard of care, emphasizing that "minus is more." In patients with the favorable characteristics defined by the GHSH group, combined modality therapy with abbreviated chemotherapy and low dose ISRT is the treatment of choice (two cycles of ABVD with ISRT of 20 Gy). Three to four cycles of ABVD followed by 30 Gy ISRT can be used for patients with favorable risk early stage disease that would not fit the enrollment criteria for the GHSG study. A reduction of chemotherapy intensity by omission of dacarbazine and/or bleomycin from ABVD cannot be generally recommended because of poorer tumor control observed. It is not recommended to suppress consolidation radiotherapy even in those patients with negative PET after two cycles of ABVD. There are no conclusive data that support a response-adapted, PET-guided RT approach to date. The treatment choice needs to be always individualized to minimize the toxic effects while maximizing cure.

For advanced stages, the most widely used regimen is ABVD. Some groups prefer BEACOPP, but there is no consensus of the optimal first line regimen. BEACOPP and escalated BEACOPP programs have shown advantages in freedom from progression among patients with higher risk IPS scores, but the toxicity is high and must be considered when choosing this therapy. It is not known if this gain will be lost over the long-term follow up through increased risk of malignancies and cardiac toxicities. Despite the increasing availability of guidelines for the treatment of HL, there must remain room for individualization of treatment. In particular, patient preference must be considered in balancing risk of relapse and risk of toxicities. Some options result in a higher recurrence risk at the gain of a less toxic initial treatment while other treatment choices result in a higher risk of acute and/or late complications (14).

The role of consolidation radiotherapy after chemotherapy induction for advanced stage HL is controversial. RT appears to improve freedom from progression but not overall survival. Its use depends primarily on the initial chemotherapy administered and the patient's response to chemotherapy. The decision to proceed with adjuvant radiation after ABVD must be individualized. Consolidation with radiotherapy cannot be omitted in patients with partial response and bulky disease. Those who focus on minimizing toxicity favor the use the of PET/CT approach, reducing the number of cycles of chemotherapy and using radiotherapy for advanced stage disease. PET/CT is an excellent staging modality in Hodgkin's lymphoma, and there are data suggesting its value as an early marker of treatment response and prognosis. PET positivity after two cycles of ABVD appears highly predictive of relapse and worse overall survival (22). The negative predictive value for PET at 12 months was 94.1% in one study (33).

Future directions focus on PET-adapting approaches and on the use of brentuximab, which is an exciting antibody-drug conjugate which links a monoclonal antibody against CD30 (expressed strongly on Hodgkin's cells) to a microtubule toxin (monomethyl auristatin E). Studies showed promising results in refractory and advanced stage Lymphoma. As a single agent, it has displayed an excellent overall response rate (75%) with 34% complete response in phase II studies in relapsed, refractory Hodgkin's lymphoma post autologous stem cell transplantation (22,50-52). The ECHELON-1 study, a multi Institution, international randomized control trial compared ABVD with AVD plus brentuximab vedotin. AVD + bretuximab showed 4.9 percentage-point lower combined risk of progression, death, or non-complete response and use of subsequent anticancer therapy at 2 years.

REFERENCES

[1] Canellos GP, Anderson JR, Propert KJ, Nissen N, Cooper MR, Henderson ES, et al. *Chemotherapy of advanced Hodgkin's Disease with MOPP, ABVD or MOPP alternating with ABVD*. N Engl J Med 1992;327(21):1478-84.

[2] Eyre TA, King AJ, Collins GP. *Classical Hodgkin's Disease: past, present and future perspective*. Br J Hosp Med (Lond) 2013;74(11):612-8.

[3] Bentzen SM, Harari PM, Bernier J. *Exploitable mechanisms for combining drugs with radiation: Concepts, achievements and future directions*. Nat Clin Pract Oncol 4:172-80.

[4] Ng AK, Dabaja B, Hoppe RT, Illidge T, Yahalom J. *Re-examining the role of radiation therapy for diffuse large b-cell lymphoma in the modern era*. J Clin Oncol 2016;34(13):1443-7.

[5] Specht L, Yahalom J, Illidge T, Berthelsen AK, Constine LS, Eich HT, et al. *Modern radiotherapy for Hodgkin's lymphoma field and dose guidelines from the International Lymphoma Radiation Oncology Group (ILROG)*. Int J Radiat Oncol Biol Phys 2014;89:854-62.

[6] Girinsky T, van der Maazen R, Specht L, Aleman B, Poortmans P, Lievens Y, et al. *Involved-node radiotherapy (INRT) in patients with early Hodgkin's lymphoma: Concepts and guidelines*. Radiother Oncol 2006;79:270-277.

[7] Schmitz R, Stanelle J, Hansmann ML, Küppers R. *Pathogenesis of classical lymphocyte-predominant Hodgkin's lymphoma*. Annu Rev Pathol 2009;4:151-74.

[8] Carbonne PP, Kaplan HS, Musshoff K, Smithers DW, Tubiana M. *Report of The Committee on Hodgkin's Disease Staging classification*. Cancer RES 1971;31: 1860-1.

[9] Lister TA; Crowther D; Sutcliffe SB, Glatstein E, Canellos GP, Young RC, et al. *Report of a committee convened to discuss the evaluation and staging of patients with Hodgkin's disease: Costwolds meeting*. J Clin Oncol 1987;7(11):1630-6.

[10] Cheson BD, Fisher RI, Barrington SF, Cavalli F, Schwartz LH, Zucca E, et al. *Recommedations for initial evaluation, staging, and response assessment of Hodgkin's and non-Hodgkin's lymphoma: the Lugano classification*. J. Clin Oncol 2014;32(27):3059-68.

[11] Barrington SF, Mikhaeel NG, Kostakoglu L, Meignan M, Hutchings M, Müeller SP, et al. *Role of imaging in the staging and response assessment of lymphoma: consensus of the International Conference on Malignant Lymphomas Imaging Working Group*. J Clin Oncol 2014;32(27):3048-58.

[12] Hasenclever D, Diehl V. *A prognostic score for advanced Hodgkin's disease: International Prognostic Factors Project on Advanced Hodgkin's disease*. N Engl J Med 1998;339(21):1506-14.

[13] Moccia AA, Donaldson J, Chhanabhai M, Hoskins PJ, Klasa RJ, Savage KJ, et al. *International prognostic score in advanced-stage hodgkin's lymphoma: Altered utility in the modern era*. J Clin Oncol 2012;30(27):3383-8.

[14] UpToDate 2017. URL: https://www.uptodate.com.

[15] Engert A, Franklin J, Eich HT, Brillant C, Sehlen S, Cartoni C, et al, *Two cycles of doxorubicin, bleomycin, vinblastine, and dacarbazine plus extended-field radiotherapy is superior to radiotherapy alone in early favorable Hodgkin's lymphoma: Final results of the GHSG HD7 trial.* J Clin Oncol 2007;25(23):3495-502.

[16] Sasse S, Brockelmann PJ, Goergen H, Plütschow A, Müller H, Kreissl S, et al. *Long-term follow-up of contemporary treatment in early-stage Hodgkin's lymphoma: updated analyses of the German Hodgkin's Study Group HD7, HD8, HD10, and HD11 Trials*. J Clin Oncol 2017; 35(18):1999-2007.

[17] Fermé C, Eghbali H, Meerwaldt JH, Rieux C, Bosq J, Berger F, et al. *Chemotherapy plus involved-field radiation in early-stage Hodgkin's disease.* N Engl J Med 2007;357(19):1916-27.

[18] Meyer RM, Gospodarowicz MK, Connors JM, Pearcey RG, Wells WA, Winter JN, et al. *ABVD alone versus radiation-based therapy in limited-stage Hodgkin's lymphoma*. N Engl J Med 2012;366(5): 399-408.

[19] Noordijk EM, Carde P, Dupouy N, Hagenbeek A, Krol AD, Kluin-Nelemans JC, et al. *Combined-modality therapy for clinical stage I or II Hodgkin's lymphoma: long term results of the European Organisation for Research and Treatment of Cancer H6 randomized controlled trials*. J. Clin Oncol 2006;24(19):3128-35.

[20] Engert A, Schiller P, Josting A, Herrmann R, Koch P, Sieber M, et al. *Involved-field radiotherapy is equally effective and less toxic compared with extend-field radiotherapy after four cycles of chemotherapy inpatients with early-stage unfavourable Hodgkin's Lymphoma: results of the HD8 trial of German Hodgkin's Lymphoma Study Group*. J Clin Oncol 2003;21(19):3601-8.

[21] Canellos GP, Anderson JR, Propert KJ, Nissen N, Cooper MR, Henderson ES, et al. *Chemotherapy of advanced Hodgkin's disease with MOPP, ABVD, or MOPP alternating with ABVD*. N Engl J Med 327(21):1478-84.

[22] Eyre TA, King AJ, Collins GP. *Classical Hodgkin's lymphoma: past, present and future perspectives.* Br J Hosp Med (Lond). 2013;74(11):612-8.

[23] Behringer K, Goergen H, Hitz F, Zijlstra JM, Greil R, Markova J, et al: *Omission of dacarbazine or bleomycin, or both, from the ABVD regimen in treatment of early-stage favourable Hodgkin's lymphoma (GHSG HD13): an open-label, randomised, non-inferiority trial.* Lancet 2015; 385(9976):1418-27.

[24] Radford J, Illidge T, Counsell N, Hancock B, Pettengell R, Johnson P, et al. *Results of a trial of PET-directed therapy for early-stage Hodgkin's lymphoma*. N Engl J Med 2015;372(17):1598-607.

[25] Raemaekers JM, André MP, Federico M, Girinsky T, Oumedaly R, Brusamolino E, et al: *Omitting radiotherapy in early positron emission tomography-negative stage I/II Hodgkin's lymphoma is*

associated with an increased risk of early relapse: Clinical results of the preplanned interim analysis of the randomized EORTC/LYSA/FIL H10 trial. J Clin Oncol 2014;32(12):1188-94.

[26] Olszewski AJ, Shrestha R, Castillo JJ. *Treatment selection and outcomes in early-stage classical Hodgkin's lymphoma: Analysis of the National Cancer Data Base*. J Clin Oncol 2015;33(6):625-33.

[27] Herbst C, Engert A. *Meta-analyses of early-stage Hodgkin's lymphoma*. Acta Haematol 2011;125(1-2):32-8.

[28] E. M. Noordijk, J. Thomas, C. Fermé, van 't Veer MB, Price P, Divine M, et al. *First results of the EORTC-GELA H9 randomized trials: the H9-F trial (comparing 3 radiation dose levels) and H9-U trial (comparing 3 chemotherapy schemes) in patients with favorable or unfavorable early stage Hodgkin's lymphoma (HL)*. J Clin Oncol 2005;23(16 suppl):6505.

[29] Engert A., Plütschow A, Eich H, Lohri A, Dörken B, Borchmann P, et al. *Reduced treatment intensity in patients with early-stage Hodgkin's lymphoma*. N Engl J Med 2010;363(7):640-52.

[30] Eich HT, Diehl V, Görgen H, Pabst T, Markova J, Debus J, et al. *Intensified chemotherapy and dose-reduced involved-field radiotherapy in patients with early unfavorable Hodgkin's lymphoma: final analysis of the German Hodgkin's Study Group HD11 trial*. J Clin Oncol 2010;28(27):4199-206.

[31] Buerkle C, Goergen H, Muller H, Paul Bröckelmann, Stefanie Kreissl, *Michael Fuchs, et al. Patient preferences - survey of Hodgkin's lymphoma survivors on treatment-associated burden and side effects*. European Hematology Association, Copenhagen, Denmark, 2016 June 10.

[32] Von Tresckow B, Plütschow A, Fuchs M, Klimm B, Markova J, Lohri A, et al. *Dose-intensification in early unfavorable Hodgkin's lymphoma: final analysis of the German Hodgkin's Study Group HD14 trial*. J Clin Oncol 2012;30(9):907-13.

[33] Engert A, Haverkamp H, Kobe C, Markova J, Renner C, Ho A, et al. *Reduced-intensity chemotherapy and PET-guided radiotherapy in patients with advanced stage Hodgkin's lymphoma (HD15 trial): a randomised, open-label, phase 3 non-inferiority trial*. Lancet 2012;379(9828):1791-9.

[34] Viviani S, Zinzani PL, Rambaldi A, Brusamolino E, Levis A, Bonfante V, et al. *ABVD versus BEACOPP for Hodgkin's lymphoma when high-dose salvage is planned*. N Engl J Med 2011;365(3):203-12.

[35] Bauer K, Skoetz N, Monsef I, Engert A, Brillant C. *Comparison of chemotherapy including escalated BEACOPP versus chemotherapy including ABVD for patients with early unfavourable or advanced stage Hodgkin's lymphoma*. Cochrane Database Syst Rev 2011;8:CD007941.

[36] Federico M, Luminari S, Iannitto E, Polimeno G, Marcheselli L, Montanini A, et al. *ABVD compared with BEACOPP compared with CEC for the initial treatment of patients with advanced Hodgkin's lymphoma: results from the HD2000 Gruppo Italiano per lo Studio dei Linfomi Trial*. J Clin Oncol 2009;27(5):805-11.

[37] Johnson P, Federico M, Kirkwood A, Fosså A, Berkahn L, Carella A, et al. *Adapted treatment guided by interim PET-CT Scan in advanced Hodgkin's lymphoma*. N Engl J Med 2016;374(25):2419-29.

[38] Aleman BM, Raemaekers JM, Tomiŝiĉ R, Baaijens MH, Bortolus R, Lybeert ML, et al. *Involved-field radiotherapy for patients in partial remission after chemotherapy for advanced Hodgkin's lymphoma*. Int J Radiat Oncol Biol Phys 2007;67(1):19-30.

[39] Johnson PW, Sydes MR, Hancock BW, Cullen M, Radford JA, Stenning SP. *Consolidation radiotherapy in patients with advanced Hodgkin's lymphoma: survival data from the UKLG LY09 randomized controlled trial (ISRCTN97144519)*. J Clin Oncol 2010;28(20):3352-9.

[40] Borchmann P, Haverkamp H, Diehl V, Cerny T, Markova J, Ho AD, et al. *Eight cycles of escalated-dose BEACOPP compared with four cycles of escalated-dose BEACOPP followed by four cycles of baseline-dose BEACOPP with or without radiotherapy in patients with advanced-stage Hodgkin's lymphoma: final analysis of the HD12 trial of the German Hodgkin's Study Group*. J Clin Oncol 2011;29(32):4234-42.

[41] Peters MV. *Prophylactic treatment of adjacent areas in Hodgkin's disease*. Cancer Res 1966;26(6):1232-43.

[42] Kaplan HS. *The radical radiotherapy of regionally localized Hodgkin's disease.* Radiology 1962;78:553-61.

[43] Hoppe BS, Hoppe RT. *Expert radiation oncologist interpretations of involved-site radiation therapy guidelines in the management of Hodgkin's lymphoma.* Int J Radiat Oncol Biol Phys 2015;92(1):40-5.

[44] Noordijk EM, Carde P, Mandard AM, Mellink WA, Monconduit M, Eghbali H, et al. *Preliminary results of the EORTC-GPMC controlled clinical trial H7 in early-stage Hodgkin's disease.* Ann Oncol 1994;5(Suppl 2):107-12.

[45] Bonadonna G, Bonfante V, Viviani Simonetta, Di Russo A, Villani F, Valagussa P. *ABVD plus subtotal nodal versus involved-field radiotherapy in early-stage Hodgkin's disease: long-term results.* J Clin Oncol 2004;22(14):2835-41.

[46] Sasse S, Klimm B, Gorgen H, Fuchs M, Heyden-Honerkamp A, Lohri A, et al. *Comparing long-term toxicity and efficacy of combined modality treatment including extended- or involved-field radiotherapy in early-stage Hodgkin's lymphoma.* Ann Oncol 2012;23(11):2953-9.

[47] Yahalom J, Mauch P. *The involved field is back: Issues in delineating the radiation field in Hodgkin's disease.* Ann Oncol 2002;13(Suppl 1):79-83.

[48] Girinsky T, van der Maazen R, Specht L, Aleman B, Poortmans P, Lievens Y, et al. *Involved-node radiotherapy (INRT) in patients with early Hodgkin's lymphoma: Concepts and guidelines.* Radiother Oncol 2006;79(3):270-7.

[49] Maraldo MV, Aznar MC, Vogelius IR, Petersen PM, Specht L. *Involved node radiation therapy: an effective alternative in early-stage Hodgkin's lymphoma.* Int J Radiat Oncol Biol Phys 2013;85(4):1057-65.

[50] Younes A, Gopal AK, Smith SE, Ansell SM, Rosenblatt JD, Savage KJ, et al. *Results of a pivotal phase II study of brentuximab vedotin for patients with relapsed or refractory Hodgkin's lymphoma.* J Clin Oncol 2012; 30(18):2183-9.

[51] Connors JM, Ansell SM, Fanale M, Park SI, Younes A. *Five-year follow-up of brentuximab vedotin combined with ABVD or AVD for advanced-stage classical Hodgkin's lymphoma.* Blood 2017;130(11):1375-7.

[52] DeVita VT Jr, Simon RM, Hubbard SM, Young RC, Berard CW, Moxley JH, et al. *Curability of advanced Hodgkin's disease with chemotherapy.* Long-term follow-up of MOPP-treated patients at the National Cancer Institute. Ann Intern Med 1980;92(5):587-95.

In: Cancer Management in Latin America II
Editors: Maurício F Silva et al.
ISBN: 978-1-53616-735-1

Chapter 8

MANAGEMENT OF NON-HODGKIN LYMPHOMA

Paulo Renato Figueiredo Ferreira[1,*], MD, PhD,
Tahiane de Brum Soares[2], MD, MSc,
Bernardo Pinatti Pinto[1], MD and Tiago Pereira de Leão[1], MD
[1]Department of Radiation Oncology, Hospital de Clinicas de Porto Alegre, Brazil
[2]Department of Hematology,
Irmandade da Santa casa de Misericordia de Porto Alegre, Brazil

ABSTRACT

The non-Hodgkin lymphomas (NHL) are a heterogeneous group of B-cell and T-cell neoplasms that arise primarily in the lymph nodes. NHL accounts for less than 5% around the world. Although some of the observed patterns in NHL have been related to HIV/AIDS, these conditions cannot fully explain the magnitude of the changes, neither do changes in classification systems nor improved diagnostic capabilities. Inverse associations with ultraviolet radiation exposure and alcohol and fish intake, and positive associations with meat and saturated fat intake have been reported in several studies; additional studies are needed to confirm or refute these associations. Family history of NHL or other hematolympho-proliferative cancers and personal history of several autoimmune disorders are associated with increased risk of NHL, but are not likely to account for a large proportion of cases. HIV and other infectious agents, such as human herpesvirus 8 and Epstein-Barr, appear to be associated with differing types of NHL, such as some B-cell lymphomas. The extent to which the etiology of NHL types may differ is important to resolve in ongoing and future studies.

* Corresponding Author's Email: prferreira@hcpa.edu.br.

INTRODUCTION

Non-hogdkin's Lymphomas (NHL) are a heterogenous group of neoplastic transformations of mature B, T, and natural killer (NK) cells. In adults, NHL are seven times more common and have a mortality rate twenty times higher than Hodgkin´s Lymphoma (1). The median age is 55 to 65 years old (2).

In most cases, the cause of NHL is unknown. Some infectious agents, like the Epstein-Barr virus (Burkitt´s lymphoma), human herpes 8 virus (cavity lymphoma), human T cell leukemia virus-HTLV (T cell leukemia/lymphoma), hepatitis C virus (B cell monocytoid lymphoma and lymphoplasmacitoid lymphoma), and the gram-negative bacteria Helicobacter pylori (MALT lymphoma - "mucosa-associated lymphoid tissue") are correlated as causative factors. Patients with rheumatoid arthritis, celiac disease, systemic lupus erythematosus, Sjogren's syndrome and other autoimmune disorders also appear to have an increased risk. Some occupational exposures may be considered as possible causes to to NHL, as herbicides, especially phenoxy herbicides, fungicides, arsenic, lead, pesticides, dyes, organic solvents, asbestos, high levels of nitrates in water, and vinyl chloride. NHL may be also related to previous radiation and chemotherapy.

An increased incidence of NHL has been observed since the end of the last century. The possible factors are related advances in molecular diagnostic techniques, aging of the population, immunosuppression from human immunodeficiency virus (HIV), infectious agents, and occupational/ environmental exposures (3).

The prognosis in NHL is more related on histology and clinical parameters than the stage.

Some few indolent lymphomas can be treated with radiotherapy alone. However, In general, the treatment for early stages aggressive lymphomas and, under certain conditions, also in advanced stages, is similar and usually combines chemotherapy and radiotherapy. More recently, the development of new modalities, such as target therapy, high dose chemotherapy followed by stem cell transplantation and immunotherapy have changed this context.

In this chapter we discuss the most relevant topics in clinical aspects, pathological characteristics, diagnostic workup, staging, treatment and response assessment in general, and specific treatment topics in particular, for the most prevalent NHL subtypes.

Clinical aspects

NHL may involve lymph nodes in almost any anatomic region and also be present at extra nodal sites. Clinically, around 2/3 of NHL present as a nodal involvement at initial diagnosis (2). The presentation may be related to the histology, e.g., in patients with primarily nodal disease, presentation is typically an asymptomatic lump in a lymphatic region.

Table 1. Frequencies of the most prevalent histologic types of NHL according to the International Lymphoma Study Group Classification of Non-Hodgkin's Lymphoma - The Non-Hodgkin's Lymphoma Classification (4)

Histological type	% in NHL	Median age	% of stages I, II vs III, IV	% B symptoms	% extra nodal localization	IPI			% 5-year survival
						0/1	2/3	4/5	
Diffuse large B cell	33	-	-	-	-				
Primary mediastinal	2,4	37	66/34	38	56	52	37	11	
All other subtypes	31	64	54/46	33	71	35	46	19	70-85
Follicular	22	-	-	-	-				70-80
Grades 1 and 2	16	-	-	-	-				
Grade 3	6	59	33/67	28	64	45	48	7	
Marginal zone	10								
MALT	8	60	67/33	19	31	44	48	8	
Nodal	2	58	26/74	37	16	60	27	13	
Peripheral T cell	7	61	20/80	50	45	17	52	31	20-90
Anaplastic T large cell	2	34	51/49	53	59	61	18	21	
B cell chronic lymphocytic Leukemia/ small B cell lymphocytic lymphoma	7	65	9/91	33	80	23	64	13	50
Mantel cell	6	63	20/80	28	81	23	54	23	27

Table 1 presents general data of the most prevalent NHL subtypes and their related frequency, median and overall survival (OS), B symptoms, extra nodal localization, stage prevalence and a prognostic factor index. Most nodal presentations of NHL are asymptomatic. Typical B symptoms are defined as unexplained fevers ($\geq 38.3^{o}$ C), night sweats, and more than 10% weight loss, but they are much less frequently encountered in NHL than in Hodgkin´s Lymphoma. They usually do not influence treatment choice. Patients with extra nodal lymphomas usually have localized disease (stages I and II), mainly in the gastrointestinal (25% a 35%) and head and neck (18% a 28%). Around 50% of DBLCL are extra nodal, and 15% are associated with B symptoms. Prognosis for nodal and extra nodal lymphomas is equivalent for the same stage, histology and other variables.

Table 2. 2016 revision of the World Health Organization classification of lymphoid neoplasms (7)

Mature B-cell Neoplasms
Chronic lymphocytic leukemia/small lymphocytic lymphoma
Monoclonal B-cell lymphocytosis
B-cell prolymphocytic leukemia
Splenic marginal zone lymphoma
Hairy cell leukemia
Splenic B-cell lymphoma/leukemia, unclassifiable
Splenic diffuse red pulp small B-cell lymphoma
Hairy cell leukemia variant
Lymphoplasmacytic lymphoma
Waldenstrom macroglobulinemia
Monoclonal gammopathy of undetermined significance (MGUS), IgM
μ Heavy chain disease
γ Heavy chain disease
α Heavy chain disease
Monoclonal gammopathy of undetermined significance (MGUS), IgG/A
Plasma cell myeloma
Solitary plasmacytoma of bone
Extraosseous plasmacytoma
Monoclonal immunoglobulin deposition diseases
Extra nodal marginal zone lymphoma of mucosa-associated lymphoid tissue (MALT lymphoma)
Nodal marginal zone lymphoma
Pediatric nodal marginal zone lymphoma
Follicular lymphoma
In situ follicular neoplasia
Duodenal-type follicular lymphoma
Large B-cell lymphoma with IRF4 rearrangement
Primary cutaneous follicle center lymphoma
Mantle cell lymphoma
In situ mantle cell neoplasia
Diffuse large B-cell lymphoma (DLBCL), NOS
Germinal center B-cell type
Activated B-cell type
T-cell/histiocyte-rich large B-cell lymphoma
Primary DLBCL of the central nervous system (CNS)
Primary cutaneous DLBCL, leg type
EBV+ DLBCL, NOS
EBV+ mucocutaneous ulcer
DLBCL associated with chronic inflammation
Lymphomatoid granulomatosis
Primary mediastinal (thymic) large B-cell lymphoma
Intravascular large B-cell lymphoma
ALK+ large B-cell lymphoma

Plasmablastic lymphoma
Primary effusion lymphoma
HHV8+ DLBCL, NOS
Burkitt lymphoma
Burkitt-like lymphoma with 11q aberration
High-grade B-cell lymphoma, with MYC and BCL2 and/or BCL6 rearrangements
High-grade B-cell lymphoma, NOS
B-cell lymphoma, unclassifiable, with features intermediate between DLBCL and classical
Hodgkin lymphoma
Mature T and NK Neoplasms
T-cell prolymphocytic leukemia
T-cell large granular lymphocytic leukemia
Chronic lymphoproliferative disorder of NK cells
Aggressive NK-cell leukemia
Systemic EBV+ T-cell lymphoma of childhood
Hydroa vaccineformelike lymphoproliferative disorder
Adult T-cell lymphoma/leukemia
Extra nodal NK/T-cell lymphoma, nasal type
Enteropathy-associated T-cell lymphoma
Monomorphic epitheliotropic intestinal T-cell lymphoma
Indolent T-cell lymphoproliferative disorder of the GI tract
Hepatosplenic T-cell lymphoma
Subcutaneous panniculitislike T-cell lymphoma
Mycosis fungoides
Sezary syndrome
Primary cutaneous CD30+ T-cell lymphoproliferative disorders
Lymphomatoid papulosis
Primary cutaneous anaplastic large-cell lymphoma
Primary cutaneous γδ T-cell lymphoma
Primary cutaneous CD8+ aggressive epidermotropic cytotoxic T-cell lymphoma
Primary cutaneous acral CD8+ T-cell lymphoma
Primary cutaneous CD4-positive small/medium T-cell lymphoproliferative disorder
Peripheral T-cell lymphoma, NOS
Angioimmunoblastic T-cell lymphoma
Follicular T-cell lymphoma
Nodal peripheral T-cell lymphoma with TFH phenotype
Anaplastic large-cell lymphoma, ALK+
Anaplastic large-cell lymphoma, ALK−
Breast implant-associated anaplastic large-cell lymphoma
aExcludes Hodgkin lymphoma, posttransplant lymphoproliferative disorders, and histiocytic/dendritic cell neoplasms.

Pathology

The histological classification and immunophenotyping of NHL has substantially evolved over the last decades. In 1982, the utilized pathologic classification of NHL was the Working Formulation (5), which subdivided NHL into low-grade, intermediate-grade, high-grade, and miscellaneous. It was clinically useful but represented an oversimplification. In 2008, the World Health Organization (WHO) classification system (6) defined five main categories for lymphoid neoplasms: precursor B- and T-cell neoplasms, mature B-cell neoplasms, mature T/NK cell neoplasms, HL, and immunodeficiency associated lymphoproliferative disorders. In 2016, the WHO classification was again updated (see Table 2) (7) and described approximately 70 distinct NHL entities. By the current standards, combining pathologic findings with clinical presentation is required to distinguish some entities. The specific diseases described may be either indolent or aggressive in behavior, or even there may be a range of behaviors within a specific disease entity (e.g., follicular lymphoma).

Lymphocytes at various stages in ontologic development can be defined and differentiated by the detection of certain antigens on the cell surface. This antigen footprint is referred to as the immunophenotyping. It can be detected by a flow cytometric analysis of single cell suspensions from whole blood, bone marrow, body fluids, or by immunohistochemistry. These techniques have become fundamental in diagnosing and monitoring NHL.

Of the approximately 80,000 new cases of NHL that are annually diagnosed in the US, approximately 70,000 will have B-cell lymphoma and 10,000 will have T-cell lymphoma. The most common NHL subtypes are diffuse large B cell lymphoma (DLBCL) and follicular lymphoma (FL), accounting for approximately 50% to 60% of all NHL cases (4).

Diagnosis and pre-treatment evaluation

The diagnosis of LNH is based upon an excisional biopsy, which aims a comprehensive morphologic, molecular and immunohistochemical evaluation. When appropriate, flow cytometry has special utility in searching malignant cells in peripheral blood, bone marrow or cerebrospinal fluid. A Lumbar puncture is advised in particular situations with high risk of CNS involvement, such as in patients with Burkitt´s lymphoma, testicular lymphoma or aggressive B cell lymphoma involving paranasal sinuses. By the same reasons, it can be advisable to consider candidates for lumbar puncture patients with DLBCL involving multiple sites, high levels of lactate dehydrogenase and poor performance status.

The clinical evaluation of patients with NHL should include questions about growth history of any lymph node enlargement and any specific symptoms suggestive of extra nodal disease or B symptoms and establishing performance status. All enlarged nodes, peripheral nodal areas, including epitrochlear lymph nodes and Waldeyer´s ring, as well as potential extra nodal sites, as spleen and liver should be palpated. Relevant laboratory exams are complete and differential blood count, lactic dehydrogenase (LDH), complete metabolic panel, hepatitis B testing (due to the risk of reactivation with immunotherapy or chemotherapy), pregnancy tests, echocardiogram in patients intended to receive anthracyclines, pelvic, abdominal and thoracic contrast computerized tomography (CT) and or whole body CT with fluorodeoxyglucose (FDG) positron emission tomography (PET-CT). PET-CT should be recommended for routine staging of FDG-avid, nodal lymphomas (essentially all histologies, except chronic lymphocytic leukemia/small lymphocytic lymphoma, lymphoplasmacytic lymphoma/Waldenstrom's macro-globulinemia, mycosis fungoides, and marginal zone NHLs, unless there is a suspicion of aggressive transformation) as the gold standard (8). CT is preferred for low or variable FDG avidity. Additional work up depends on the NHL histology and its natural history. For example, bone marrow biopsy and aspirate may be recommended in apparent stage I or II FL, as well in aggressive NHL, but it may be questioned in negative PET-CT patients with diffuse large B cell lymphoma (9). If a PET-CT indicates marrow involvement in DLBCL, a confirmatory bone marrow biopsy is not recommended. A guideline of essential work up for NHL patients, related to the subtype, is available (10).

Table 3. The Lugano classification:
Revised staging system for primary nodal lymphomas (9)

Stage	Involvement	Extra nodal (E) Status
LIMITED		
I	One node or a group of adjacent nodes	Single extra nodal lesions without nodal involvement
II	Two or more nodal groups on the same side of the diaphragm	Stage I or II by nodal extent with limited contiguous extra nodal involvement
II bulky*	II as above with "bulky" disease	Not applicable
ADVANCED		
III	Nodes on both sides of the diaphragm; nodes above the diaphragm with spleen involvement	Not applicable
IV	Additional noncontiguous extralymphatic involvement	Not applicable

NOTE. Extent of disease is determined by positron emission tomography-computed tomography for avid lymphomas and computed tomography for nonavid histologies. Tonsils, Waldeyer's ring, and spleen are considered nodal tissue.

*Whether stage II bulky disease is treated as limited or advanced disease may be determined by histology and a number of prognostic factors.

Staging

Over the last decades, staging systems for lymphomas were the Ann Arbor system and the Cotswolds modification (11). The increased use of systemic and multimodality approaches has made Ann Arbor stage less relevant in directing the choice of therapy and motivated a recent updating, knew as the Lugano Classification (9) (see Table 3). As a result, PET-CT is formally incorporated into standard staging for FDG-avid lymphomas. A modification of the Ann Arbor descriptive terminology is recommended for anatomic distribution of disease extent, but the suffixes A or B for symptoms are suggested only to be included for Hodgkin´s Lymphoma. A bone marrow biopsy is no longer indicated for the routine staging of most DLBCL. However, regardless of stage, general practice is to treat patients based on limited (stages I and II, nonbulky) or advanced (stage III or IV) disease, with stage II bulky disease considered as limited or advanced disease based on histology and a number of prognostic factors. Tumor bulk is no longer a part of the staging system because of the lack of consensus of its definition, as well as the uncertain influence of bulk on prognosis in the current therapeutic era.

Table 4. International prognostic index (IPI)*

Age > 60 years
LDH > upper limit normal
ECOG Performance Status ≥2
Ann Arbor Stage III or IV
Number of extra nodal disease sites >1

Nº of Factors	Risk Group	3-year EFS (%)	3-year PFS (%)	3-year OS (%)
0-1	Low	81	87	91
2	Low Intermediate	69	75	81
3	High Intermediate	53	59	65
4-5	High	50	50	59

*ECOG, Eastern Cooperative Oncology Group; EFS, event-free survival; PFS, progression-free survival; OS, OS. Adapted from Ziepert M et al. (13).

Prognostic factors

NHL subtypes have been traditionally divided into indolent (low grade-slow growing), aggressive (intermediate grade - fast growing), and highly aggressive types (high grade - very rapidly growing). The principles of this classification are the cell lineage (B, T, NK), stage of differentiation (e.g.: precursor vs mature) and clinical presentation (nodal vs extra nodal). Examples of Indolent NHL include: FL (grade 1, 2, and 3a), chronic lymphocytic leukemia/small lymphocytic, lymphoma (CLL/SLL), marginal zone, and lymphoplasmacytic (Waldenström) lymphoma. They grow slowly but are considered incurable. An example of intermediate NHL is mantle cell lymphoma (MCL), although this subtype more often behaves more aggressively and is incurable. Aggressive lymphomas include: DLBCL, Burkitt lymphoma, lymphoblastic, and double hit large cell lymphomas and B-cell lymphoma unclassifiable. These subtypes grow rapidly and require treatment. However, they can be curable with treatment.

NHL in extra lymphatic organs like testis, ovary, eye, central nervous system (CNS) and liver have a particular poor prognosis. In these sites, some secondary prognostic factors are more important than the staging (12). Since the last decade, the International Prognostic Index (IPI) (13) has been utilized in almost all NHL. It is based on five independent prognostic factors for OS: staging (I-II versus III-IV), age (<60 years versus ≥60 years), performance status (0-1 versus ≥2), LDH concentration (normal versus altered) and the number of extra nodal sites (1 versus >1) (Table 4). The number of factors is added and adjusted for age. In patients younger than 60 years old, the index composition includes only three factors: stage, LDH and performance status. Based on the number of factors present in the age-adjusted IPI (IPI-AA), patients may have a score 0 to 5, and may classified in three risk categories:

- Low risk: no factors IPI-AA.
- Intermediate risk: one factor IPI-AA.
- High risk: two or more factors IPI-AA.

A distinguished classification is related to the FL, which has particular prognostic factors. This risk classification is the Folllicular Lymphoma International Prognostic Index (FLIPI) (Table 5) (14).

Response assessment

In the current PET-CT era, a complete metabolic response, even with a persistent mass, is considered a complete response. In aggressive NHL, the estimated negative predictive value is of 80% to 100% and a lower positive predictive value is considered from 50% to 100% (15). Either biopsy or follow-up scan is advised if further treatment based on residual metabolically active disease on PET-CT is being considered.

The Lugano Classification (see Table 3) also has recommendations for response assessment after treatment based on a 5-point scale, both for clinical trials including interim analysis and for end-of-treatment assessment (9). Interim PET-CT is used to assess early treatment response and, at end of treatment, to establish remission status. A score of 1 or 2 is considered to represent complete metabolic response at interim and end of treatment. FDG uptake declines during therapy in chemotherapy-sensitive disease, and residual FDG uptake higher than normal liver uptake is frequently seen at interim in patients who achieve complete metabolic response at the end of treatment. Recent data suggest that most patients with uptake higher than mediastinum but less than or equivalent to liver (score of 3) have good prognosis at the end of treatment with standard therapy in DLBCL (15) and follicular lymphoma (16). Interpretation of a score of 3 depends on the timing of assessment, the clinical context, and the treatment. A score of 4 or 5 at interim suggests chemotherapy-sensitive disease, provided uptake has reduced from baseline, and is considered to represent partial metabolic response. At the end of treatment, residual metabolic disease with a score of 4 or 5 represents treatment failure even if uptake has reduced from baseline. A score of 4 or 5 with intensity that does not change or even increases from baseline and/or new foci compatible with lymphoma represents treatment failure at interim and at the end-of-treatment assessment.

For histologies with low or variable FDG avidity and in areas where PET-CT is unavailable, CT-based response is preferred. Nevertheless, in the absence of a PET-CT scan, a mass that has decreased in size but is still present is considered a partial response in the absence of biopsy documenting absence of lymphoma (17).

There is insufficient data to support routine surveillance scans in NHL (18); besides, the false-positive rate with PET scans is greater than 20%. By the other hand, follow-up scans should be prompted by clinical indications. The Lugano Classification has recommendations for follow-up in patients with NHL. For indolent lymphomas, asymptomatic intra-abdominal or retroperitoneal disease progression may be a concern in patients with residual disease in those areas after therapy. Then, judicious use of scans can be considered. Attempts should be made to limit the number of scans to which a patient is exposed. For potentially curable subtypes, such as DLBCL, the likelihood of relapse decreases over time; thus, the follow-up frequency can decrease proportionally and be annual after 5 years. For FL, mantle-cell lymphoma (MCL), and other incurable histologies, the likelihood of recurrence continues or increases over time, and patients should be observed every 3 to 6 months, determined by pretreatment risk factors, whether the patient is being managed conservatively, and whether treatment has achieved a complete or less than complete response (9).

Follicular Lymphoma

Diagnosis and clinical presentation

Follicular lymphoma (FL) is the most common indolent NHL, and second most common subtype (approximately 20% of all NHL) (19). The median age in 60-65 years old. There are no specific risk factors for FL beyond the known relationships between exposures and

NHL. Patients with FL usually have a history of waxing and waning of lymph nodes, sometimes for a few years. Retroperitoneal lymph node masses and splenomegaly are common, and symptoms develop gradually. They usually grow slowly, respond well to therapy for several years, but are considered incurable. It is not uncommon that patients with nodal presentations may initially appear to have localized disease, but subsequent evaluation detects a more advanced stage. PET-CT) is now considered the gold-standard imaging technique for staging FL (8), but some authors believe bone marrow biopsy to be the standard of care (20).

It is believed that FL is a malignancy arising from follicular germinal center B cells and express a number of antigens and chromosomal translocation. It is assigned grades 1, 2 and 3 by the WHO classification. Grade 3 is further subdivided into 3A and 3B. It is of particular relevance to the clinician to be aware that FL Grade 1, 2, and 3A are all closely related and have similar biologic behavior and response to therapy. However, FL grade 3B, has a clinical course very similar to DLBCL and is usually managed as such (21).

The FLIPI (14) (see Table 5) has been used as an important tool for the pre therapeutic assessment of prognosis and the adaptation of treatment strategies in distinct groups of patients. Depending on the number of present factors, patients are classified as low, intermediate and high risk. In patients with good prognosis (0-1 adverse factor), 10 year OS is 71%, indicating that treatment should aim quality of life and avoid excessive toxicity. More recently, an updated version, known as FLIPI-2 has been utilized (21) (see Table 5). Not all patients with FL require immediate intervention. Indications of treatment are suggested by a nomogram proposed by The Groupe d'Etude des Lymphomes Folliculaires (GELF) is (21).

Table 5. The Follicular Lymphoma International Prognostic Index (FLIPI) and FLIPI-2 (14)

FLIPI	**FLIPI-2**
Age ≥60	Age > 60
Ann Arbor stage III-IV	Bone marrow involvement
Hemoglobin < 12 g/dL	Hemoglobin < 12g/dL
LDH > ULN	Beta-2 microglobulin > ULN
# of nodal sites > 4	Diameter of largest LN > 6cm
Original FLIPI	
Score	Risk Group
0 - 1	Low
2	Intermediate
3 or more	High
FLIPI-2	
Score	Risk Group
0	Low
1-2	Intermediate
3 or more	High

Treatment of stages I or II FL

Only 15-30% of FL patients are stage I or II. Patients with initial stage FL can be potentially cured and should receive initial treatment with radiation therapy alone. Radiation therapy alone results in a 5, 10, and 15-year freedom from treatment failure of 72%, 46%, and 39%, and an OS at 5-, 10-, and 15-year rates of 93%, 75%, and 62%, respectively, with a median survival of approximately 19 years (22). In the current PET-CT era, these results can be even better. Radiation therapy is the treatment of choice for limited stage FL in doses of 24 to 30 Gy to the involved lymphoid region. Randomized studies of higher (e.g., 40-45 Gy) or lower doses (e.g., 4 Gy) of radiation for indolent NHLs have shown no superiority over 24 Gy (23). In general, there appeared to be no dose response demonstrated. However, higher doses of 30-36 Gy should be considered for grade 3 FL.

Prospectively studies with the addition of systemic therapy to radiation therapy for limited stage FL have failed to improve outcomes. By the other hand, patients with limited stage FL grade 3A and 3B FL should be treated according to treatment for DLBCL, i.e., with the R-CHOP regimen (rituximab, cyclophosphamide, doxorubicin, vincristine, and prednisone), plus radiation therapy, when appropriate.

Patients who are not ideal candidates for radiation therapy, or have disease sites that are unfeasible to irradiate, or with bulky disease in whom significant toxicity would be expected with radiation therapy, observation or systemic therapy with rituximab alone or chemoimmunotherapy can be considered.

Treatment of stages III or IV FL

The majority of patients with FL present with advanced stage disease (III - IV) and most are considered incurable. A phase III trial showed no survival advantage to early therapy in comparison to systemic therapy in patients with asymptomatic, advanced stage NHL (mostly FL) (24, 25). These patients should be observed until symptoms or complications of the disease require treatment. Observed patients can be evaluated by a history, physical exam, and laboratory studies performed every 3 months, and a CT scan obtained every six months. When indicated, outcomes can be improved with multiple effective therapeutic agents. The Groupe d'Etude des Lymphomes Folliculares (GELF) (21) proposes a policy to treat advanced stage FL, which generally reserve treatment for patients with one or more of the following factors present: tumor mass > than 7 cm in diameter; three or more lymph node sites involved with diameter > 3cm; systemic symptoms present; substantial splenomegaly; pleural or pericardial effusion; organ compression; performance status ECOG more than 1; peripheral blood involvement or cytopenias; and LDH or beta-2 microglobulin > upper limit of normal.

The choice of initial regimen depends on a patient's general health and symptoms intensity. Single-agent rituximab can be utilized in patients with a low tumor burden who requires therapy or in patients with co-morbidities that make them inadequate for chemoimmunotherapy.

In chemotherapy-naïve patients with low grade FL and a relatively low tumor burden, the overall response rate following a course of weekly rituximab ranges from 66-80% (25, 26). When indicated, most patients with advanced stage FL receive chemoimmunotherapy. Rituximab combined to chemotherapy confers a clear survival benefit and should be included as part of first-line therapy (27). The overall response rate to regimens with bendamustine alone, cyclophosphamide, doxorubicin, vincristine, and rednisone (CHOP), or cyclophosphamide, vincristine, and prednisone (CVP) combined with rituximab ranges from 88-97% (28, 29).

Relapsed and transformed FL

The choice of regimen in patients with relapsed FL who require therapy depends on the duration of initial response and the type of initial treatment used. Patients with relapsed disease who are asymptomatic and have a low tumor burden can be observed. When a patient previously treated with rituximab has maintained responses, this agent can be reincorporated alone, with 40-60% of response rates (26). Patients with a short remission duration after rituximab alone or patients who relapse after first-line chemoimmunotherapy are generally treated with an alternative non-crossresistant regimen.

FL can transform to a more aggressive lymphoma, typically DLBCL, at a rate of 2-3% per year. Approximately 10-20% of patients undergo transformation at 10 years (30).

Hematopoietic stem cell transplantation (HSCT) for FL, including both autologous stem cell transplantation (ASCT) and allogeneic HSCT, can be utilized in patients with relapsed or refractory disease to prolong remission duration and potentially provide durable responses and cures (31).

Diffuse Large B Cell Lymphoma

Diagnosis and clinical presentation

Diffuse large B cell lymphoma (DLBCL) encompasses many entities under the same denomination (see Table 1). The frequencies of stages I-II and stage IV are 30% to 40% and 40%, respectively. Extra nodal sites are common, occurring in 40% of cases, including GI tract, testis, bone, thyroid, skin, CNS, and bone marrow. Bone marrow involvement initially is found in only 10% to 20% of patients and has a strong correlation with the risk of spread to the CNS (32). Testicular, paranasal sinus, epidural, and the presence of multiple extra nodal sites, are also sites with risk for CNS dissemination. DLBCL can arise as a histologic transformation from any indolent B-cell NHL or CLL.

Treatment

Treatment guidelines for patients with DLBCL is based on clinical stage. Over the last 15 years, randomized studies have shown that rituximab significantly improves survival when combined with standard combination chemotherapy and improves prognostic significantly (33). The addition of rituximab has resulted in a 10-15% increase in OS as compared with chemotherapy alone (34). This difference has been confirmed in subsequent clinical trials that randomized R-CHOP versus CHOP alone. At 10 years, OS was reported to be 44%, while patients younger than 60 years of age had an event-free survival (EFS) of 79% after three years with 93% OS rates at 6 years (35).

These outcomes favor R-CHOP as the standard regimen for most cases of DLBCL. In patients with stage I-II, the treatment is usually abbreviated and includes combination chemoimmunotherapy plus involved field radiotherapy, or combination chemoimmunotherapy alone. The benefit of adding radiotherapy to 6 to 8 cycles of chemotherapy remains unclear. The SWOG randomized trial compared eight cycles of CHOP to three cycles of CHOP plus involved field radiotherapy in patients with localized diffuse aggressive lymphoma (36). Patients treated with three cycles of CHOP plus radiotherapy had a significantly better OS than patients treated with eight cycles of CHOP alone (82% versus 72%). Overall toxicity and cardiac toxicity were significantly higher in the patients receiving CHOP alone. The Mabthera International phase III trial (33) randomized CHOP versus R-CHOP-R. All patients with IPI 0 or IPI 1 and masses >7.5 cm received 30 to 40 Gy of involved field radiation to those sites. Those patients with IPI of 0 and bulk disease had a 10% to 15% lower pathological free survival (PFS) than patients without bulk. Currently, the most appropriate management of patients with early stage DLBCL with bulk disease remains controversial. New agents added to R-CHOP, like bortezomib (37) and lenalidomide (38) are under investigation.

The IPI, that originally predicted patient outcomes treated with CHOP, was recently revised after the advent R-CHOP. The revised IPI (rIPI) is a better predictor of outcome in patients treated with R-CHOP (39). Four-year OS for the very good (IPI = 0), good (IPI 1 or 2), and poor (IPI 3 or more) risk groups is 94, 79, and 55%, respectively. By the other hand, PET-CT also carries prognostic importance both during as well as after systemic therapy evaluations. PET-CT has been assigned in the Deauville scale (Table 6), based on FDG uptake criteria (40). In a number of studies, residual PET-positive disease after the completion of chemotherapy alone in aggressive NHLs (mostly DLBCL) is associated with a high risk of disease progression (4142). A negative PET-CT achieved early in the course of therapy is associated with improved progression-free survival (PFS), but not always OS, compared with a positive interim PET-CT. When compared with interim response assessment, postchemotherapy PET-CT response appears to be more prognostic, particularly in terms of the positive predictive value.

Risk of central nervous system relapse

Some authors recommend adding CNS prophylaxis with high-dose methotrexate or intrathecal methotrexate ot cytarabine in patients with high-risk lymphoma and specific extra nodal localizations, such as renal, adrenal, and nasopharingeal (43). Relapsed DLBCL in the CNS receive high-dose methotrexate containing regimens, usually in combination to high dose cytarabine (44). Primary DLBCL of the testis can be treated with R-CHOP and CNS prophylaxis. Irradiation of the contralateral testis is also recommended (38).

Double hit DLBCL

Double hit lymphomas with MYC and BCL2 rearrangement are aggressive and carry poor outcomes when treated with R-CHOP (45). There is no standard treatment for these patients. In a retrospective study, the R-EPOCH regimen resulted in higher rate of complete responses in comparison to R-CHOP (46).

Table 6. Deauville criteria (40)

Score	FDG Uptake
1	No uptake at disease sites
2	Uptake in disease site≤ uptake in mediastinum
3	Uptake in disease site > uptake in mediastinum but ≤ uptake in liver
4	Uptake in disease site>uptake in liver
5	Uptake in disease site markedly increased at any site or new disease sites.

Relapsed and refractory DLBCL

Relapsed or refractory to therapy patients can still be cured with appropriate salvage chemotherapy and ASCT. However, ASCT can be curative only in patients who are chemosenstive to salvage therapy. Several regimens are currently available, including R-DHAP (rituximab, dexamethasone, cytarabine, and cisplatin), RICE (rituximab, ifosfamide, carboplatin, and etoposide), R-ESHAP (rituximab, etoposide, metilprednisolone, cytarabine, and cisplatin) and R-GDP (rituximab, dexamethasone, gemcitabine, and cisplatin). In a randomized study, both R-DHAP and R-ICE demonstrated similar efficacy. In a phase III study that evaluated second-line therapy of relapsed or refractory DLBCL with R-ICE versus R-DHAP, the 3-year OS was 49% (47). Allogeneic transplant may be considered an alternative in patients with a suitable matched donor. Myeloablative chemotherapy may be preceded by full-dose allogeneic transplantation designed to have not an antitumor effect as well as to condition the patient for the infusion of the donor cells. It may also be preceded by a nonmyeloablative or reduced intensity conditioning program designed to enable the recipient to accept the donor stem cells. Nonmyeloablative allogeneic transplants are associated with a much lower treatment-related mortality (10% to 20%) compared with myeloablative allogeneic transplants (40% to 50%) (48). Frequently, total-body irradiation is a component of the conditioning program. Recent guidelines for transplantation concerning autologous and allogeneic transplantation is available (49).

Primary mediastinal large b-cell lymphoma

Primary mediastinal large b-cell lymphoma (PMLBCL) is a distinct presentation from DLBCL. It is a rare disease occurring in young patients and its treatment is not standard. Traditional regimens such as MACOP-B (methotrexate, leucovorin, doxorubicin, cyclophosphamide, vincristine and bleomycin) or VACOP-B (etoposide, doxorubicin, cyclophosphamide, vincristine, prednisone and bleomycin) were superior in comparison to CHOP regimen. The benefit of adding rituximab to CHOP (R-CHOP) in PMLBCL is less clear at the present time. The role of mediastinal radiotherapy following induction immunochemotherapy is being evaluated by a phase III trial of the international extra nodal Lymphoma Study Group (IELSG) in patients achieving complete metabolic PET response after systemic therapy (50).

DLBCL in older patients

Patients with significant co-morbidities or older than 80 years may be treated with rituximab in combination with attenuated chemotherapy, regimens such as the R-miniCHOP (51).

MANTLE CELL LYMPHOMA

Diagnosis and clinical presentation

Mantle cell lymphoma (MCL) a proliferation of monomorphic small to medium-sized B cells and has heterogeneous outcomes. Most cases of MCL are associated with chromosome translocation t(11;14) (q13;q32). The molecular consequence of translocation is overexpression of the protein cyclin D1 (52). Morphologic variants include the blastoid and pleomorphic types, as well as small cell and marginal zone-like variants, an indolent subtype, and in situ lesions (53). In the International Lymphoma Classification Project, it accounted for 8% of all NHL. Approximately 70% of patients have stage IV disease and B symptoms are observed in approximately one-third of patients. It has an increased prevalence in men above the age of 60 years. Patients with MCL present globally a median OS of 36 months that drops to 18 months for the blastoid variant (54).

MCL has also deserved an individual prognostic classification adapted from IPI, the Mantle Cell lymphoma International Prognostic Index (MIPI) (55), which includes age, performance status, serum LDH, complete blood count (WBC). The classification distinguishes three groups in relation to survival in 5 years, reaching 60% in low risk, 51% in medium and 29% in high risk.

Lymph nodes, spleen, gastrointestinal tract, Waldeyer's ring and bone marrow are the most frequent sites involved. Approximately 10% of the patients present with an indolent or localized disease (56). In asymptomatic patients, with low MIPI or elderly MCL patients, a watchful waiting approach should be considered and does not compromise survival (52). Other characteristics of MCL are presented in table 1.

Treatment

Chemotherapy and rituximab are the mainstay of treatment, which is dependent on patients age and performance status. The chemoimmunoitherapy ranges from R-hyperCVAD in patients with better performance and R-CHOP or BR (bendamustine plus rituximab) in patients with some limitation (28). Hyper-CVAD consists of two combinations of drugs (courses A and B) given in an alternating fashion. The term 'hyper' refers to the hyperfractionated nature of the treatment, which is given in smaller doses given frequently in order to minimize toxicity. Course A regimen consists of cyclophosphamide, vincristine, doxorubicin and dexamethasone. Course B consists of methotrexate and cytarabine. The alternative regimen uses cycles of R-CHOP and cycles of R-DHAP in younger or fit patients. (57).

High dose chemotherapy and ASCT are often used in patients who have complete responses to the first line of treatment. For patients not eligible for transplantation, maintenance with rituximab should be considered (58).

Radiation therapy given to the primary lesion in association with systemic treatment is recommended in rare patients presenting with localized disease. In a small series of patients with limited stage I or II disease, the authors (59) observed that patients receiving 30 Gy radiation therapy with or without chemotherapy had a 5-year PFS of 68%, compared with 11% for those not receiving radiation therapy (P = 0.002). Although OS for the whole group was 53% at 6 years, it was 71% for those initially treated with RT, but only 25% for those not given RT (P = 0.13). The authors suggest a potentially role for RT in limited-stage MCL.

In patients who are refractory to systemic treatment or progression, the use of low-dose radiation therapy (10-20 Gy) has good results for palliation, since MCL is one of the most radiation-sensitive tumors (60).

Relapse treatment

Recurrence of MCL occurs in the majority of patients after primary treatment. There are currently three systemically-restricted treatment drugs in this context: bortezomib, lenalidomide and ibrutinib (61, 62). Bortezomib has also been combined with other agents such as Bendamustine and rituximab in the BVR regimen which also had excellent activity or in monotherapy. Bendamustine rituximab (BR) regimen has also been tested in relapsed MCL patients. The mTOR inhibitor, temsirolimus, was tested in a phase II study of patients with relapsed/refractory MCL. Allogeneic stem cell transplantation is felt to be the only potentially curative treatment for advanced MCL and can be considered in some cases (52).

SMALL LYMPHOCYTIC LYMPHOMA/B-CELL CHRONIC LYMPHOCYTIC LEUKEMIA

Diagnosis and clinical presentation

Small lymphocytic lymphoma (SLL) and B-cell chronic lymphocytic leukemia (BCCLL) are variants of the same disease, which manifest as a proliferation of mature B cells. Peripheral blood flow cytometry analysis is determinant in the diagnosis, presenting CD5 positive, CD10 negative, CD20 low positive and CD23 positive. Fluorescence in situ Hybridization (FISH analysis) for t(11:14) is useful in distinguishing MCL. Their clinical characteristics are presented in table PRF. Patients with 60 year old or more are the most affected. Around 80% of patients present as stage IV. Patients are usually diagnosed at routine health care visits because of elevated lymphocyte counts. Most of the patients are asymptomatic. The most common symptom of CLL is lymphadenopathy, while difficulty exercising and fatigue are common complaints (63). Rare clinical signs can be infection, anemia, B symptoms or bleeding, all suggestive of advanced stage.

SLL usually is limited to rare lymph node involvement estimated at less than 10%. The differentiation between SLL and CLL occurs through the analysis of peripheral blood, being the existence of more than 5 x 10^9/L the definition criterion for CLL. The diagnosis of SLL requires lymph node or splenic involvement, in the absence of lymphocytosis described above (64).

Although uncommon, SLL/BCCLL can transform in DLBCL (Richter Syndrome) and it is associated with a shorter survival. PET-CT can be useful in case of suspected transformation (65). The Binet's prognostic classification separates patients by the number of sites involved; stage A includes two or fewer sites, stage B includes three or more, stage C includes cytopenias (66). The Rai classification is similar to Binet's and presents the same prognosis (67).

Treatment

Systemic therapy may consist of monotherapy or combination therapy involving glucocorticoids, alkylating agents, and purine analogs. Fludarabine may be the most effective single drug treatment currently available in patients fit and without del 17p or TP53 mutation. The use of ibrutinib in monotheraphy, at first line, is available and demonstrate better outcomes in patients with del 17p or TP53 mutation (68). Combination therapy protocols have not been shown to be more effective than fludarabine alone. As no cure is yet available, new therapies are required. Experimental treatments include allogeneic stem cell transplant, mini-allogeneic transplants, and monoclonal antibodies (e.g., alemtuzumab against CD52; rituximab against CD20) (63).

Radiation therapy with curative intent therapy is indicated in rare patients with initial localized presentation utilizing dose ranges from 24-30Gy in involved fields. Palliatively, 2Gy in two fractions can be used, with a response rate close to 80% at 14 months. If necessary, this treatment can be repeated (68).

MARGINAL ZONE LYMPHOMAS AND MUCOSA ASSOCIATED LYMPHOMA TISSUE

Diagnosis and clinical presentation

Marginal zone lymphomas (MZL) are indolent NHLs including three different histologies: nodal MZL, splenic MZL, and extra nodal MZL of mucosa-associated lymphoid tissue (MALT). They comprise approximately 10% of all lymphomas. The stomach is the most common extra nodal site, followed by eye/adnexa, lung, skin, and salivary glands (69). MALT lymphoma represents approximately 75% of all MZL and is the main focus of this topic. It was first described in 1983 (70) and is characterized primarily by a infiltrate of marginal zone B-cells, small lymphocytes, monocytoid B cells, and plasma cells, among other subtypes. The tumor cells express pan B-cell-associated antigens including CD19, CD20, CD22, and CD79a, but there is no specific marker for MALT at present. However, lack of CD5 (positive in CLL/SLL and MCL), CD10 (positive in FL), and cyclin D1 (positive in MCL) expression helps distinguish MALT from other small B-cell lymphomas (71). Translocation t(11;18)(q21;q21) is found in around 30% of MALT lymphomas (72). When present, the t(11;18) translocation predicts for a limited response to H. pylori-directed therapies in gastric MALT lymphoma (73).

General clinical characteristics of MALT lymphomas are presented in Table 1. The most frequent initial presentation of MALT lymphoma is stage I or II in approximately 70% of cases, affecting mainly patients around 60 years of age. It is usually an indolently lymphoma. Fifty percent of all MALT lymphomas arise from the stomach. Non-gastric MALT lymphomas occur in the lung, salivary gland, skin, and other organs. Initial bone marrow involvement has been reported in 23.5% to 37% of cases (74). It has been described a related risk of monoclonal gammopathy in patients with MALT lymphomas and some authors recommend paraprotein analysis and flow cytometric studies in the pretherapeutic workup (75). When affecting the stomach, MALT lymphoma is associated with H pylori infection in up to 92% of cases (76).

Because three fourths of the patients have localized disease, the natural history of MALT lymphomas allows to stage each site separately. Localized MZL is mainly represented by extra-nodal MZL of MALT type, that can, however, be disseminated in 25% of the cases (77). Besides the routine blood tests for patients with NHL, additional laboratory tests should include HCV (given its association with MALT lymphoma), HIV, β2-microglobulin and protein electrophoresis and serum light chains. Imaging exams include chest, abdomen, and pelvis CT scans. A bone marrow biopsy should be considered for patients with multifocal disease. Evaluation of the gastric mucosa is reasonable for all patients with non-gastric MALT lymphoma given the risk of gastric involvement in these patients.

Treatment

Management of MALT lymphoma depends both on stage and site of disease. Helicobacter pylori eradication therapy must be given to all gastric MALT lymphomas, independently of stage or histological grade (77). For gastric presentation, omeprazole, metronidazole, and clarithromycin are the recommended initial therapy (78), with a complete response rates of approximately 80% (79). H pylori eradication should be documented at least 6 weeks after the antibiotic treatment (77). Gastric MALT lymphoma associated with an H pylori infection that do not harbor a t(11;18) translocation, eradication of H pylori results in good long-term disease control and OS (79). Radiation therapy is the treatment of choice in patients with H pylori-negative patients who fail to respond to H pylori therapy, and in patients with t(11;18) translocation (80). Radiation therapy, in the dose of 24 to 30Gy, is effective when indicated. Control rates higher than 90% in 5 years have been reported (81). Relapses are not infrequent, and may occur in approximately 25% of cases (82).

Chemotherapy, immunotherapy, or chemoimmunotherapy are generally reserved for patients with relapsed or refractory disease to antibiotic therapy or radiation therapy, or in patients with more advanced stage or aggressive disease (83). Available options and their respective complete response rates include single-agent therapy with chlorambucil, cyclophosphamide, cladribine, bortezomib, and rituximab. Multiagent anthracycline-based chemotherapy are appropriate for younger patients with more aggressive disease. Expected response rates are approximately 75% (83, 84).

Nodal Marginal Zone Lymphoma and Splenic Marginal Zone Lymphoma

Nodal marginal zone lymphoma (NMZL) is usually disseminated. Treatment should follow the therapeutic principles adopted for FL (85). Patients with strictly localized disease may be considered for localized radiation therapy. Involved Field Radiotherapy may be a reasonable option only for localized stage. In cases of low tumor burden, a watchful and waiting strategy is usually employed. Rituximab plus chemotherapy with or without an anthracycline is considered an appropriate option in disseminated-stage disease (86). Patients with t(11;18) will most probably be unresponsive to alkylating agents (77).

Criteria for initiating treatment in splenic marginal zone lymphoma (SMZL) include progressive or painful splenomegaly, and symptomatic/progressive cytopenias (77). Patients with SMZL can be treated, with splenectomy, chemotherapy, rituximab alone, or rituximab-chemotherapy (bendamustine, chlorambucil).

PRIMARY CENTRAL NERVOUS SYSTEM LYMPHOMAS (PCNL)

Diagnosis and clinical presentation

Most Primary Central Nervous System Lymphomas (PCNSL) are of B-cell lineage, typically DLBCL (about 90% of cases). The remainder consists of T-cell lymphoma, and poorly characterized lymphomas of low grade or Burkitt's lymphoma, in 10%. The occurrence of PCNSL is rare in immunocompetent patients, and in immunocompromised patients it is associated with EBV (87). The disease is more common in men (the male-to-female ratio is 2:1) and in elderly persons. PCNSL comprises all primary intracerebral and intraocular lymphomas. The incidence of PCNSL has been increasing in recent decades, not only in the immunocompromised population. Neurocognitive symptoms are the first clinical manifestation, Generic symptoms, such as altered mental status, seizures and manifestations of increased intracranial pressure, such as headache, nausea, and vomiting may occur. Immunocompetent patients are more likely to have localized neurological deficits.

The diagnosis can often be suggest by radiologic imaging. In comparision to other primary brain tumors or metastatic lesions, PCNSL is usually isodense or hyperdense on nonenhanced CT scans. The preferred imaging modality for PCNSL is MRI, which can detect up to 10% of lesions missed by CT. Lesions appear isointense to hypointense on T1-weighted images, and approximately 50% are hyperintense on T2-weighted imaging. Homogeneous contrast enhancement in commonly seen in immunocompetent patients (88). Lesions are multifocal in 50% of patients with AIDS, whereas only 25% of immunocompetent patients have multifocal disease at presentation (89). In patients with HIV infection, disease is often multifocal in the brain and may be difficult to distinguish from CNS infections (90).

In the presence of leptomeningeal and ocular involvement, the evaluation should include lumbar puncture (if the intracranial pressure is not increased) and full ophthalmologic examination. Evaluate for extracranial disease is also appropriate. Stereotactic-guided biopsy is the chosen method to diagnose PCNSL.

A prognostic model for PCNSL developed at Memorial Sloan is based on age and Karnofsky performance status and divides patients into three prognostic classes (91). Class 1: patients < 50 years with a median survival of 8.5 years. Class 2: patients ≥ 50 years with good performance status (KPS ≥ 70) with median survival of 3.2 years. Class

3: patients ≥ 50 years with poor performance status (KPS < 70) with median survival of 1 year.

Treatment

Historically, the treatment of PCNSL was whole-brain radiation therapy (WBRT), but results were poor. Reported median survivals were 12.2 to 17 months, and 5-year survival rates of 10% to 20% (92). Dose escalation beyond 50 Gy resulted in high toxicity rates without improvements in survival (93). Given the poor results achieved with radiation therapy alone, evaluation of systemic chemotherapy was in order. CHOP and its variations, the efficacy in PCNSL disappointing (94). Antimetabolites such as MTX and cytarabine (ara-C) constitute the backbone of most anti-PCNSL regimens with proven efficacy in prospective trial (95).

Methotrexate particularly in high doses, is known to penetrate the brain barrier. There has been much variability in dosage, scheduling, and combinations with intrathecal methotrexate and other cytotoxics such as cytarabine, vincristine, thiotepa, temozolomide, and rituximab. Chemotherapy has been evaluated in combination with WBRT. The Memorial Sloan- Kettering evaluated WBRT with 23.4 Gy for patients achieving complete response to rituximab and MTX-based chemotherapy (96). Median PFS and OS for all patients enrolled on the study were 3.3 and 6.6 years, respectively. For those patients who achieved a complete response and received reduced-dose WBRT, the 5-year OS was 80%. Significant post-WBRT neurotoxicity was not observed. Nevertheless, the exact role of WBRT after high-dose MTX is controversial, particularly in patients achieving a complete response to chemotherapy and in those patients >60 years old. It is clear that 45-Gy WBRT has high toxicity. Low-dose WBRT (23.4 Gy) after chemotherapy for patients achieving a complete response remains a promising approach.

NHL in elderly

Elderly patients have a higher incidence of lymphoma in comparison to younger patients. The prevalence of serious comorbidities in NHL patients aged 60-69 years or over 70 years of age was 43 and 61%, respectively, in one series (97) The IPI classification showed a lower overall survival in patients over 60 years than 60 years of age or younger, which may be explained by the dose reduction in treatment. Complete remission rate was reported to be 52% using full-dose chemotherapy in younger patients, and 37% in patients 65 years of age or older who receive initial 50% dose reduction of cyclophosphamide and doxorrubicin (98).

Fit elderly patients are candidates for standard chemotherapy, while frail elderly patients often receive palliative care (99). The chemoimmunotherapy for DLBCL have clearly demonstrated a significant survival benefit in patients over age of 60 years. Many regimens have been reported with the concern of decrease the toxicity of treatment in elderly patients. In a cohort of 149 patients with 80 years or older, authors reported 58 deaths, 33 of which were secondary to lymphoma progression; 12 deaths were attributed to treatment toxicity. The most frequent side-effect was hematological toxicity (100). Two year OS and PFS were 59% and 47%, respectively. As dose reductions and delays may well result in lower response rates in the elderly population, the administration of full-dose CHOP therapy in these patients has been advocated. Myeloid growth factor support should be considered for patients over 60 years of age (99).

Regimens such PEPC and BR can be useful for palliation in elderly patients who are not considered for CHOP, with over 50% RRs and median PFS over 6 months (101).

REFERENCES

[1] Jemal A, Thomas A, Murray T, Thun M. *Cancer statistics*, 2002. CA Cancer J Clin 2002;52(1):23-47.

[2] d'Amore F, Christensen BE, Brincker H, Pedersen NT, Thorling K, Hastrup J, et al. *Clinicopathological features and prognostic factors in extranodal non-Hodgkin lymphomas*. Danish LYFO Study Group. Eur J Cancer 1991;27(10):1201-8.

[3] Torre LA, Bray F, Siegel RL, Ferlay J, Lortet-Tieulent J, Jemal A. *Global cancer statistics, 2012*. CA Cancer J Clin 2015;65(2):87-108.

[4] *National Cancer Institute sponsored study of classifications of non-Hodgkin's lymphomas: summary and description of a working formulation for clinical usage*. The Non-Hodgkin's lymphoma pathologic classification project. Cancer 1982;49(10):2112-35.

[5] Swerdlow SH, Campo E, Harris NL, Jaffe ES, Pileri SA, Stein H, Thiele J. *WHO classification of tumours of haematopoietic and lymphoid tissues*. Lyon: International Agency for Research on Cancer, 2008

[6] Swerdlow SH, Campo E, Pileri SA, Harris NL, Stein H, Siebert R, et al. *The 2016 revision of the World Health Organization classification of lymphoid neoplasms*. Blood 2016;127(20):2375-90.

[7] Armitage JO, Weisenburger DW. *New approach to classifying non-Hodgkin's lymphomas: clinical features of the major histologic subtypes*. Non-Hodgkin's Lymphoma Classification Project. J Clin Oncol 1998;16:2780-95.

[8] Barrington SF, Mikhael NG, Kostakoglu L, Meignan M, Hutchings M, Müeller SP, et al. *Role of imaging in the staging and response assessment of lymphoma: Consensus of the International Conference on Malignant Lymphomas Imaging Working Group*. J Clin Oncol 2014;32(27):3048-58.

[9] Cheson BD, Fisher SF, Barrington SF, Cavalli F, Schwartz LH, Zucca E, et al. *Recommendations for initial evaluation, staging, and response assesment of Hodgkin and non-Hodgkin lymphoma: The Lugano Classification*. J Clin Oncol 2014;32:3059-68.

[10] National Comprehensive Cancer Network. *National Comprehensive Cancer Network Guidelines Version 5. 2018, Non-Hodgkin´s Lymphomas*. URL: https://www.nccn.org/professionals/physician_gls/pdf/b-cell.pdf

[11] Lister TA, Crowther D, Sutcliffe SB, Glatstein E, Canellos GP, Young RC, et al. *Report of a committee convened to discuss the evaluation and staging of patients with Hodgkin's disease: Cotswolds meeting*. J Clin Oncol 1989;7(11):1630-6.

[12] Tsang R, Gospodarowicz M, O'Sullivan B. *Staging and management of localized non-Hodgkin's lymphomas: variations among experts in radiation oncology*. Int J Radiat Oncol Biol Phys 2002;52(3):643-51.

[13] Ziepert M, Hasenclever D, Kuhnt E, Glass B, Schmitz N, Pfreundschuh M, et al. *Standard international prognostic index remains a valid predictor of outcome for patients with aggressive CD20+ B-cell lymphoma in the rituximab era.* J Clin Oncol 2010;28(14):2373-80.

[14] Solal-Celigny P, Roy P, Colombat P, White J, Armitage JO, Arranz-Saez R, et al. *Follicular lymphoma international prognostic index*. Blood 2004;104(5):1258-65.

[15] Pregno P, Chiapella A, Bellò M, Botto B, Ferrero S, Franceschetti S, et al. Interim 18-FDG-PET/CT failed to predict the outcome in diffuse large B-cell lymphoma patients treated at the diagnosis with rituximab-CHOP. Blood 2012;119(9):2066-73.

[16] Dupuis J, Berriolo-Riedinger A, Julian A, Brice P, Tychyj-Pinel C, Tilly H, et al. *Impact of [(18)F] fluorodeoxyglucose positron emission tomography response evaluation in patients with high-tumor burden follicular lymphoma treated with immunochemotherapy: A prospective study from the Groupe d'Etudes des Lymphomes de l'Adulte and GOELAMS.* J Clin Oncol 2012;30(35):4317-22.

[17] Cheson BD, Pfistner B, Juweid ME, Gascoyne RD, Specht L, Horning SJ, et al. *Revised response criteria for malignant lymphoma*. J Clin Oncol 2007;25(5):579-86.

[18] Zinzani PL, Stefoni V, Tani M, Fanti S, Musuraca G, Castellucci P, et al. *Role of [18F] fluorodeoxyglucose positron emission tomography scan in the follow-up of lymphoma.* J Clin Oncol 2009;27(11):1781-7.

[19] Siegel R, DeSantis C, Virgo K, Stein K, Mariotto A, Smith T, et al. *Cancer treatment and survivorship statistics, 2012.* CA Cancer J Clin 2012;62(4):220-41.

[20] Brady JL, Binkley MS, Hajj C et al. *Definitive radiotherapy for localized follicular lymphoma staged by ^{18}F-FDG PET-CT: a collaborative study by ILROG.* Blood. 2019 Jan 17;133(3):237-245.

[21] Wahlin BE, Yri OE, Kimby E, Holte H, Delabie J, Smeland EB, et al. *Clinical significance of the WHO grades of follicular lymphoma in a population-based cohort of 505 patients with long follow-up times.* Br J Haematol 2012;156(2):225-23.

[22] Federico M, Bellei M, Marcheselli L, et al. *Follicular lymphoma international prognostic index 2: a new prognostic index for follicular lymphoma developed by the international follicular lymphoma prognostic factor project.* J Clin Oncol. 2009 Sep 20;27(27):4555-62.

[23] Brice P, Bastion Y, Lepage E, Brousse N, Haïoun C, Moreau P, et al. *Comparison in low-tumor-burden follicular lymphomas between an initial no-treatment policy, prednimustine, or interferon alfa: a randomized study from the Groupe d'Etude des Lymphomes Folliculaires.* Groupe d'Etude des Lymphomes de l'Adulte. J Clin Oncol 1997;15(3):1110-7.

[24] Guadagnolo BA, Li S, Neuberg D, Ng A, Hua L, Silver B, et al. *Long-term outcome and mortality trends in early-stage, Grade 1-2 follicular lymphoma treated with radiation therapy*. Int J Radiat Oncol Biol Phys 2006;64(3):928-34.

[25] Hoskin PJ, Kirkwood AA, Popova B, Smith P, Robinson M, Gallop-Evans E, et al. *4 Gy versus 24 Gy radiotherapy for patients with indolent lymphoma (FORT): a randomised phase 3 non-inferiority trial*. Lancet Oncology 2014;15(4):457-63.

[26] Ardeshna KM, Smith P, Norton A, Hancock BW, Hoskin PJ, MacLennan KA, et al. *Long-term effect of a watch and wait policy versus immediate systemic treatment for asymptomatic advanced-stage non-Hodgkin lymphoma: a randomised controlled trial*. Lancet 2003;362(9383):516-22.

[27] Ardeshna KM, Qian W, Smith P, Braganca N, Lowry L, Patrick P, et al. *Rituximab versus a watch-and-wait approach in patients with advanced-stage, asymptomatic, non-bulky follicular lymphoma: an open-label randomised phase 3 trial*. Lancet Oncol 2014;15(4):424-35.

[28] Kahl BS, Hong F, Williams ME, Gascoyne RD, Wagner LI, Krauss JC, et al. *Rituximab extended schedule or re-treatment trial for low-tumor burden follicular lymphoma: eastern cooperative oncology group protocol e4402*. J Clin Oncol 2014;32(28):3096-102.

[29] Marcus R, Imrie K, Solal-Celigny P, Catalano JV, Dmoszynska A, Raposo JC, et al. *Phase III study of R-CvP compared with cyclophosphamide, vincristine, and prednisone alone in patients with previously untreated advanced follicular lymphoma*. J Clin Oncol 2008;26(28):4579-86.

[30] Rumme MJ, Niederle N, Maschmeyer G, Banat GA, von Grünhagen U, Losem C, et al. *Bendamustine plus rituximab versus CHOP plus rituximab as first-line treatment for patients with indolent and mantle-cell lymphomas: an open-label, multicentre, randomised, phase 3 non-inferiority trial.* Lancet 2013;381 (9873): 1203-10.

[31] Flinn IW, van der Jagt R, Kahl BS, Wood P, Hawkins TE, Macdonald D, et al. *Randomized trial of bendamustine-rituximab or R-CHOP/ R-CVP in first-line treatment of indolent NHL or MCL: the BRIGHT study*. Blood 2014;123(19): 2944-52.

[32] Casulo C, Burack WR, Friedberg JW. *Transformed follicular non-Hodgkin lymphoma.* Blood. 2015;125(1):40-7.

[33] Hari P, Carreras J, Zhang MJ, Gale RP, Bolwell BJ, Bredeson CN, et al. *Allogeneic transplants in follicular lymphoma: Higher risk of disease progression after reduced-intensity compared to myeloablative conditioning*. Biol Blood Marrow Transplant 2008;14(2):236-45.

[34] Van Besien K, Ha CS, Murphy S, McLaughlin P, Rodriguez A, Amin K, et al. *Risk factors, treatment, and outcome of central nervous system recurrence in adults with intermediate-grade and immunoblastic lymphoma.* Blood 1998;91(4):1178-84.

[35] Coiffier B, Thieblemont C, Van Den Neste E, Lepeu G, Plantier I, Castaigne S, et al. *Long-term outcome of patients in the LNH-98.5 trial, the first randomized study comparing rituximab-CHOP to standard CHOP chemotherapy in DLBCL patients: a study by the Groupe d'Etudes des Lymphomes de l'Adulte.* Blood 2010;116 (12):2040-5.

[36] Schmitz N, Zeynalova S, Glass B, Kaiser U, Cavallin-Stahl E, Wolf M, et al. *CNS disease in younger patients with aggressive B-cell lymphoma: an analysis of patients treated on the Mabthera International Trial and trials of the German High-Grade Non-Hodgkin Lymphoma Study Group*. Ann Oncol 2012;23(5):1267-73.

[37] Miller TP, Dahlberg S, Cassady JR, Adelstein DJ, Spier CM, Grogan TM, et al. *Chemotherapy alone compared with chemotherapy plus radiotherapy for localized intermediate- and highgrade non-Hodgkin's lymphoma.* N Engl J Med 1998;339(2):21-6.

[38] Pfreundschuh M, Trumper L, Osterborg A, Pettengell R, Trneny M, Imrie K, et al. *CHOP-like chemotherapy plus rituximab versus CHOP-like chemotherapy alone in young patients with good-prognosis diffuse large-B-cell lymphoma: a randomised controlled trial by the MabThera International Trial (MInT) Group*. Lancet Oncol 2006;7(5):379-91.

[39] Ruan J, Martin P, Furman RR, Lee SM, Cheung K, Vose JM, et al. *Bortezomib plus CHOP-rituximab for previously untreated diffuse large B-cell lymphoma and mantle cell lymphoma.* J Clin Oncol 2011;29(6):690-7.

[40] Vitolo U, Chiappella A, Ferreri AJ, Martelli M, Baldi I, Balzarotti M, et al. *First-line treatment for primary testicular diffuse large B-cell lymphoma with rituximab-CHOP, CNS prophylaxis, and contralateral testis irradiation: Final results of an international phase II trial*. J Clin Oncol 2011;29(20):2766-72.

[41] Sehn LH, Berry B, Chhanabhai M, Fitzgerald C, Gill K, Hoskins P, et al. *The revised International Prognostic Index (R-IPI) is a better predictor of outcome than the standard IPI for patients with diffuse large B-cell lymphoma treated with R-CHOP*. Blood 2007;109(5):1857-61.

[42] Meignan M, Gallamini A, Meignan M, Gallamini A, Haioun C A. *Report on the First International Workshop on interim-PET scan in lymphoma.* Leuk Lymphoma 2009;50(8):1257-60.

[43] Haioun C, Itti E, Rahmouni A, Brice P, Rain JD, Belhadj K, et al. *[18F]fluoro-2-deoxy-D-glucose positron emission tomography (FDG-PET)in aggressive lymphoma: na early prognostic tool for predicting patient outcome*. Blood 2005;106(4):1376-81.

[44] Juweid ME, Wiseman GA, Vose JM, Ritchie JM, Menda Y, Wooldridge JE, et al. *Response assessment of aggressivenon-Hodgkin's lymphoma by integrated International Workshop Criteria and fluorine-18-fluorodeoxyglucose positron emission tomography.* J Clin Oncol 2005;23(21):4652-61.

[45] Ferreri AJ, Bruno-Ventre M, Donadoni G, Ponzoni M, Citterio G, Foppoli M, et al. *Risk-tailored CNS prophylaxis in a monoinstitutional series of 200 patients with diffuse large B-cell lymphoma treated in the rituximab era.* Br J Haematol 2015;168(5):654-62.

[46] Ferreri AJ, Reni M, Foppoli M, Martelli M, Pangalis GA, Frezzato M, et al. *High-dose cytarabine plus high-dose methotrexate versus high-dose methotrexate alone in patients with primary CNS lymphoma: a randomised phase 2 trial.* Lancet 2009;374(9700):1512-20.

[47] Aukema SM, Siebert R, Schuuring E, van Imhoff GW, Kluin-Nelemans HC, Boerma EJ, et al. *Double-hit B-cell lymphomas.* Blood 2011;117(8):2319-31.

[48] Petrich AM, Gandhi M, Jovanovic B, Castillo JJ, Rajguru S, Yang DT, et al. *Impact of induction regimen and stem cell transplantation on outcomes in double-hit lymphoma: a multicenter retrospective analysis.* Blood 2014;124(15):2354-61.

[49] Gisselbrecht C, Glass B, Mounier N, Singh Gill D, Linch DC, Trneny M, et al. *Salvage regimens with autologous transplantation for relapsed large B-cell lymphoma in the rituximab era.* J Clin Oncol. 2010;28(27):4184-90.

[50] Baron F, Maris MB, Sandmaier BM, Storer BE, Sorror M, Diaconescu R, et al. *Graft-versus-tumor effects after allogeneic hematopoietic cell transplantation with nonmyeloablative conditioning.* J Clin Oncol 2005;23(9):1993-2003.

[51] Oliansky DM, Czuczman M, Fisher RI, Irwin FD, Lazarus HM, Omel J, et al. *The role of cytotoxic therapy with hematopoietic stem cell transplantation in the treatment of diffuse large B cell lymphoma: update of the 2001 evidence-based review.* Biol Blood Marrow Transplant 2011;17(1):20-47.

[52] Cavalli F, Ceriani L, Zucca E. *Functional imaging using 18-fluorodeoxyglucose PET in the management of primary mediastinal large b-cell lymphoma: the contributions of the international extranodal lymphoma study group.* Am Soc Clin Oncol Educ Book. 2016;35:e368-75.

[53] Peyrade F, Jardin F, Thieblemont C, Thyss A, Emile JF, Castaigne S, et al. *Attenuated immunochemotherapy regimen (R-miniCHOP) in elderly patients older than 80 years with diffuse large B-cell lymphoma: a multicentre, single-arm, phase 2 trial.* Lancet Oncol 2011;12(5):460-8.

[54] Vose JM. *Mantle cell lymphoma: 2017 update on diagnosis, risk-stratification, and clinical management.* Am J Hematol 2017;92(8):806-13.

[55] Hsi ED, Martin P. *Indolent mantle cell lymphoma.* Leuk Lymphoma 2014;55(4):761-7.

[56] Tiemann M, Schrader C, Klapper W, Dreyling MH, Campo E, Norton A, et al. *Histopathology, cell proliferation indices and clinical outcome in 304 patients with mantle cell lymphoma (MCL): a clinicopathological study from the European MCL Network.* Br J Haematol 2005;131(1):29-36.

[57] Hoster E, Dreyling M, Klapper W, Gisselbrecht C, van Hoof A, Kluin-Nelemans HC, et al. *A new prognostic index (MIPI) for patients with advanced-stage mantle cell lymphoma.* Blood 2008;111(12):558-65.

[58] Martin P, Chadburn A, Christos P, Weil K, Furman RR, Ruan J, et al. *Outcome of deferred initial therapy in mantle-cell lymphoma.* J Clin Oncol 2009;27(8):1209-13.

[59] Delarue R, Haioun C, Ribrag V, Brice P, Delmer A, Tilly H. *CHOP and DHAP plus rituximab followed by autologous stem cell transplantation in mantle cell lymphoma: a phase 2 study from the Groupe d'Etude des Lymphomes de l'Adulte.* Blood 2013;121(1):48-53.

[60] Kluin-Nelemans HC, Hoster E, Hermine O, Walewski J, Trneny M, Geisler CH, et al. *Treatment of older patients with mantle-cell lymphoma.* N Engl J Med 2012;367(6):520-31

[61] Leitch HA, Gascoyne RD, Chhanabhai M, Voss NJ, Klasa R, Connors JM. *Limited-stage mantle-cell lymphoma.* Ann Oncol 2003;14(10):1555-61.

[62] Rosenbluth BD, Yahalom J. *Highly effective local control and palliation of mantle cell lymphoma with involved-field radiation therapy (IFRT).* Int J Radiat Oncol Biol Phys 2006;65(4):1185-91.

[63] Witzig TE, Vose JM, Zinzani PL, Reeder CB, Buckstein R, Polikoff JA, et al. *An international phase II trial of single-agent lenalidomide for relapsed or refractory aggressive B-cell nonHodgkin's lymphoma.* Ann Oncol 2011;22:1622-27.

[64] Wang ML, Rule S, Martin P, Goy A, Auer R, Kahl BS, et al. *Targeting BTK with ibrutinib in relapsed or refractory mantle-cell lymphoma.* N Engl J Med 2013;369(6):507-16.

[65] Redaelli A, Laskin BL, Stephens JM, Botteman MF, Pashos CL. *The clinical and epidemiological burden of chronic lymphocytic leukaemia.* Eur J Cancer Care 2004;13(3):279-87.

[66] Campo E, Swerdlow SH, Harris NL, Pileri S, Stein H, Jaffe ES, et al. *The 2008 WHO classification of lymphoid neoplasms and beyond: evolving concepts and practical applications.* Blood 2011;117(19):5019-32.

[67] Bruzzi JF, Macapinlac H, Tsimberidou AM, Truong MT, Keating MJ, Marom EM, et al. *Detection of Richter's transformation of chronic lymphocytic leukemia by PET/CT.* J Nucl Med 2006;47(8):1267-73.

[68] Hallek M, Cheson BD, Catovsky D, Caligaris-Cappio F, Dighiero G, Döhner H, et al. *Guidelines for the diagnosis and treatment of chronic lymphocytic leukemia: a report from the International Workshop on Chronic Lymphocytic Leukemia updating the National Cancer Institute-Working Group 1996 guidelines.* Blood 2008;111(12):5446-56.

[69] Rai KR, Sawitsky A, Cronkite EP, Chanana AD, Levy RN, Pasternack BS. *Clinical staging of chronic lymphocytic leukemia.* Blood 1975;46(2):219-34.

[70] Haas RL, Poortmans P, de Jong D, Aleman BM, Dewit LG, Verheij M, et al. *High response rates and lasting remissions after low-dose involved field radiotherapy in indolent lymphomas.* J Clin Oncol 2003;21(13):2474-80.

[71] Khalil MO, Morton LM, Devesa SS, Check DP, Curtis RE, Weisenburger DD. *Incidence of marginal zone lymphoma in the United States*, 2001-2009 with a focus on primary anatomic site. Br J Haematol 2014;165(1):67-77.

[72] Isaacson P, Wright DH. Malignant lymphoma of mucosa-associated lymphoid tissue. *A distinctive type of B-cell lymphoma.* Cancer 1983;52(8):1410-6.

[73] Farinha P, Gascoyne RD. Molecular pathogenesis of mucosa-associated lymphoid tissue lymphoma. J Clin Oncol 2005;23(26):6370-8.

[74] Hamoudi RA, Appert A, Ye H, Ruskone-Fourmestraux A, Streubel B, Chott A, et al. *Differential expression of NF-kappaB target genes in MALT lymphoma with and without chromosome translocation: insights into molecular mechanism.* Leukemia 2010;24(8):1487-97.

[75] Liu H, Ye H, Ruskone-Fourmestraux A, De Jong D, Pileri S, Thiede C, et al. *T(11;18) is a marker for all stage gastric MALT lymphomas that will not respond to eradication.* Gastroenterology 2002;122(5):1286-94.

[76] Sretenovic M., Colovic M., Jankovic G, Suvajdzic N, Mihaljevic B, Colovic N, et al. *More than a third of non-gastric malt lymphomas are disseminated at diagnosis: A single center survey.* European Journal of Haematology 2009;82(5):373-80.

[77] Akoum R, Serhal W, Farhat H. Disseminated Gastric MALT Lymphoma with Monoclonal Gammopathy, t(11;18)(q21;q21), and subsequent development of T-large granular lymphocytic leukemia: A case report and review of the literature. Case Rep Med 2015;2015:953297.

[78] Wotherspoon AC, Ortiz-Hidalgo C, Falzon MR, Pan L, Moschini A, de Boni M, et al. *Helicobacter pyloriassociated gastritis and primary B-cell gastric lymphoma.* Lancet 1991;338(8776):1175-6.

[79] Dreyling M, Thieblemont C, Gallamini A, Arcaini L, Campo E, Hermine O, Kluin-Nelemans JC, et al. *ESMO Consensus conferences: guidelines on malignant lymphoma. part 2: marginal zone lymphoma, mantle cell lymphoma, peripheral T-cell lymphoma.* Ann Oncol 2013;24(4):857-77.

[80] Salcedo JA, Al-Kawas F. *Treatment of Helicobacter pylori infection.* Arch Intern Med 1998;158(8):842-51.

[81] Wundisch T, Thiede C, Morgner A, Dempfle A, Günther A, Liu H, et al. *Long-term follow-up of gastric MALT lymphoma after helicobacter pylori eradication.* J Clin Oncol 2005;23(31):8018-24.

[82] Tsang RW, Gospodarowicz MK, Pintilie M, Wells W, Hodgson DC, Sun A, et al. *Localized mucosa-associated lymphoid tissue lymphoma treated with radiation therapy has excellent clinical outcome.* J Clin Oncol 2003;21(22):4157-64.

[83] Goda JS, Gospodarowicz M, Pintilie M, Wells W, Hodgson DC, Sun A, et al. *Long-term outcome in localized extranodal mucosa-associated lymphoid tissue lymphomas treated with radiotherapy.* Cancer 2010;116(16):3815-24.

[84] Tsai HK, Li S, Ng AK, Silver B, Stevenson MA, Mauch PM. *Role of radiation therapy in the treatment of stage I/II mucosa-associated lymphoid tissue lymphoma.* Ann Oncol 2007;18(4):672-8.

[85] Conconi A, Martinelli G, Thieblemont C, Ferreri AJ, Devizzi L, Peccatori F, et al. *Clinical activity of rituximab in extranodal marginal zone B-cell lymphoma of MALT type.* Blood 2003;102(8):2741-5.

[86] Hammel P, Haioun C, Chaumette MT, Gaulard P, Divine M, Reyes F, Delchier JC. *Efficacy of single-agent chemotherapy in low-grade B-cell mucosa-associated lymphoid tissue lymphoma with prominent gastric expression.* J Clin Oncol 1995;13(10):2524-9.

[87] Younes, A. *Marginal zone lymphoma.* Handbook of lymphoma. Switzerland: Springer International Publishing, 2016.

[88] Thieblemont C, Bernard S, Molina T. *Management of aggressive lymphoma in very elderly patients.* Hematol Oncol 2017;35(Suppl 1):49-53.

[89] Scadden DT. Epstein-Barr virus, the CNS, and AIDS-related lymphomas: as close as flame to smoke. J Clin Oncol 2000;18(19):3323-4.

[90] Coulon A, Lafitte F, Hoang-Xuan K, Martin-Duverneuil N, Mokhtari K, Blustajn J, et al. *Radiographic findings in 37 cases of primary CNS lymphoma in immunocompetent patients.* Eur Radiol 2002;12(2):329-40.

[91] Batchelor T, Loeffler JS. *Primary CNS lymphoma.* J Clin Oncol 2006;24(8):1281-8.

[92] Maher EA, Fine HA. *Primary CNS lymphoma.* Semin Oncol 1999;26(3):346-56.

[93] Abrey L, Ben-Porat L, Panageas K, Yahalom J, Berkey B, Curran W, et al. *Primary central nervous system lymphoma: the Memorial Sloan-Kettering Cancer Center prognostic model.* J Clin Oncol 2006;24:5711-5.

[94] Laperriere NJ, Cerezo L, Milosevic MF, Wong CS, Patterson B, Panzarella T. *Primary lymphoma of brain: results of management of a modern cohort with radiation therapy.* Radiother Oncol 1997;43(3):247-52.

[95] Nelson DF, Martz KL, Bonner H, Nelson JS, Newall J, Kerman HD, et al. *Non-Hodgkin's lymphoma of the brain: can high dose, large volume radiation therapy improve survival?* Report on a prospective trial by the Radiation Therapy Oncology Group (RTOG): RTOG 8315. Int J Radiat Oncol Biol Phys 1992;23(1): 9-17.

[96] Mead GM, Bleehen NM, Gregor A, Bullimore J, Shirley D, Rampling RP, et al. *A medical research council randomized trial in patients with primary cerebral non-Hodgkin lymphoma: cerebral radiotherapy with and without cyclophosphamide, doxorubicin, vincristine, and prednisone chemotherapy.* Cancer 2000;89(6):1359-70.

[97] Ferreri A. *How I treat primary CNS lymphoma.* Blood 2011;118(3):510-22.

[98] Morris PG, Correa DD, Yahalom J, Raizer JJ, Schiff D, Grant B, et al. *Rituximab, methotrexate, procarbazine, and vincristine followed by consolidation reduced-dose wholebrain radiotherapy and cytarabine in newly diagnosed primary CNS lymphoma: final results and long-term outcome.* J Clin Oncol 2013;31(31):3971-397.

[99] Thieblemont C, Grossoeuvre A, Houot R, Broussais-Guillaumont F, Traullé GSC, et al. *Non-Hodgkin's lymphoma in very elderly patients over 80 years.* A descriptive analysis of clinical presentation and outcome. Ann Oncol 2008;19(4):774-9.

[100] Dixon D, Neilan B, Jones SE, Lipschitz DA, Miller TP, Grozea PN, et al. *Effect of age on therapeutic outcome in advanced diffuse histyocitic lymphoma: The Southwest Group Experience.* J Clin Oncol 1986;4(3):295-305.

[101] van der Poel M, Mulder W, Ossenkoppele G, Maartense E, Wijermans P, Hoogendoorn M, et al. *Comorbidity and treatment decision-making in elderly non-Hodgkin's lymphoma patients: a survey among haematologists.* J Medicine 2014;72(3):165-9.

[102] Peyrade F, Jardin F, Thieblemont C, Thyss A, Emile JF, Castaigne S, et al. *Attenuated immunochemotherapy regimen (R-miniCHOP) in elderly patients older than 80 years with diffuse large B-cell lymphoma: a multicentre, single-arm, phase 2 trial.* Lancet Oncol 2011;12(5):460-8.

[103] Weisenburger D, Savage K, Harris N, Gascoyne RD, Jaffe ES, MacLennan KA, et al. *Peripheral T-cell lymphoma, not otherwise specified: a report of 340 cases from the International Peripheral T-cell Lymphoma Project.* Blood 2011;117(12):3402-8.

In: Cancer Management in Latin America II
Editors: Maurício F Silva et al.
ISBN: 978-1-53616-735-1

Chapter 9

MANAGEMENT OF BONE METASTASES

Pedro R León[1,*], MD, Gustavo Ferraris[2], MD, PhD, Marjorie Monteiro Rodrigues[3], MD, Gustavo Nader Marta[4,5], MD, PhD, Fiona Lim[6], MBBS, Bo Angela Wan[7], MD(C) and Mauricio F Silva[8,9,10], MD, PhD

[1]Department of Clinical Oncology and Radiation Oncology, Centro Médico Nacional del Noreste UMAE 25 IMSS, Monterrey, Nuevo León, México,
[2]Centro Médico Deán Funes, Catholic University of Córdoba, Córdoba, Argentina,
[3]Department of Radiation Oncology, Hospital Dilson de Quadros Godinho, Montes Claros, Brazil,
[4]Department of Radiology and Oncology, Faculty of Medicine, University of São Paulo, Brazil,
[5]Hospital Sírio-Libanês, São Paulo, Brazil,
[6]Instituto Brasileiro de Controle do Câncer, São Paulo, Brazil,
[4]Department of Oncology, Princess Margaret Hospital, Hong Kong, PR China,
[7]Odette Cancer Centre, Sunnybrook Health Sciences Centre, Toronto, Ontario, Canada,
[8]Radiation Oncology Unit, Santa Maria Federal University, Santa Maria, Brazil,
[9]Hospital de Caridade Astrogildo de Azevedo, Santa Maria, Brazil
[10]Latin America Cooperative Oncology Group, Porto Aegre, Brazil

[*] Corresponding Author's Email: rubenleonmx@yahoo.com.

Abstract

Bone is a frequent site of metastases and typically indicates a short-term prognosis in cancer patients. This narrative review summarizes local and systemic management strategies for bone metastases from the fields of radiation oncology, medical oncology and orthopedic surgery in Latin America countries. Local management strategies are organized according to different clinical scenarios. Despite improvement in surgical techniques and advances in systemic therapies, management of patients with bone metastatic disease remains a powerful cornerstone for the radiation oncologist. The primary goal of radiotherapy is to provide pain relief, preserving patient's quality of life. Multidisciplinary approach to treat patients with bone metastases is normally needed. In this chapter we review the clinical approach and treatment of bone metastases.

Introduction

Metastasis is a process that involves loss of intercellular cohesion, cell migration, angiogenesis, access to systemic circulation, survival in circulation, evasion of local immune responses, and growth at distant organs. The reason bone is a favorite site of metastasis from many types of cancer is not yet fully understood. One possible reason is that the microenvironment of the bone marrow is appropriate for the growth of cancer cells (1).

Metastases from carcinomas are the most common malignant tumors affecting bone. Carcinomas with the greatest tendency to metastasize to this site include breast and prostate (65–75% of cases), thyroid (60% of cases), lung (30–40% of cases) and kidney (20–25% of cases) (1).

Bone metastases can be lytic, blastic or mixed depending on the type of cancer. Osteoblastic metastases are typical in prostate cancer and are sometimes detected in breast and undifferentiated type stomach cancer. Osteolytic metastases are detected in many types of cancers, such as breast, lung, thyroid, and stomach cancers. The frequency of serious complications depends on the site and type of lesion.

The overall incidence of bone metastases is not known. The cases of cancer detected in Latin American countries are smaller than in Europe and in the United States, but the mortality is higher because they are detected in advanced stages. In recent decades, Latin America and the Caribbean have been undergoing political, economic, and social transformations that have caused changes in the morbidity and mortality profile of the population. The ratio between mortality and incidence in Latin America is 0.59 higher than the European Union (0.43) and the United States (0.35), which reflects better support of cancer treatment in developed countries (2).

The bone is the third most common site of metastases after the lungs and the liver (3, 4). On the other hand, bone metastases are the most frequent malignancy of the bone and typically occurs via hematogenous dissemination (3, 5). The most frequent sites of metastases in the bone are the lumbar vertebrae, followed by the thoracic vertebrae, cervical vertebrae and sacrum, whereas metastases in the appendicular skeleton are rare (6). The treatment strategy for bone metastases (BM) from variable primary cancers should be planned comprehensively, taking into consideration if bone disease is localized or widespread, if there is evidence of extra skeletal metastases, the kind of cancer, symptoms and the general performance status of the patient. Treatments can often shrink or slow the growth of bone metastases and can help with symptoms, but they are not curative.

To achieve the best approach a multidisciplinary team is necessary with interdisciplinary meetings and strong focus on prevention of complications and reduction in the morbidity, hospitalization and overall costs associated with management of advanced-stage cancers (see Figure 1).

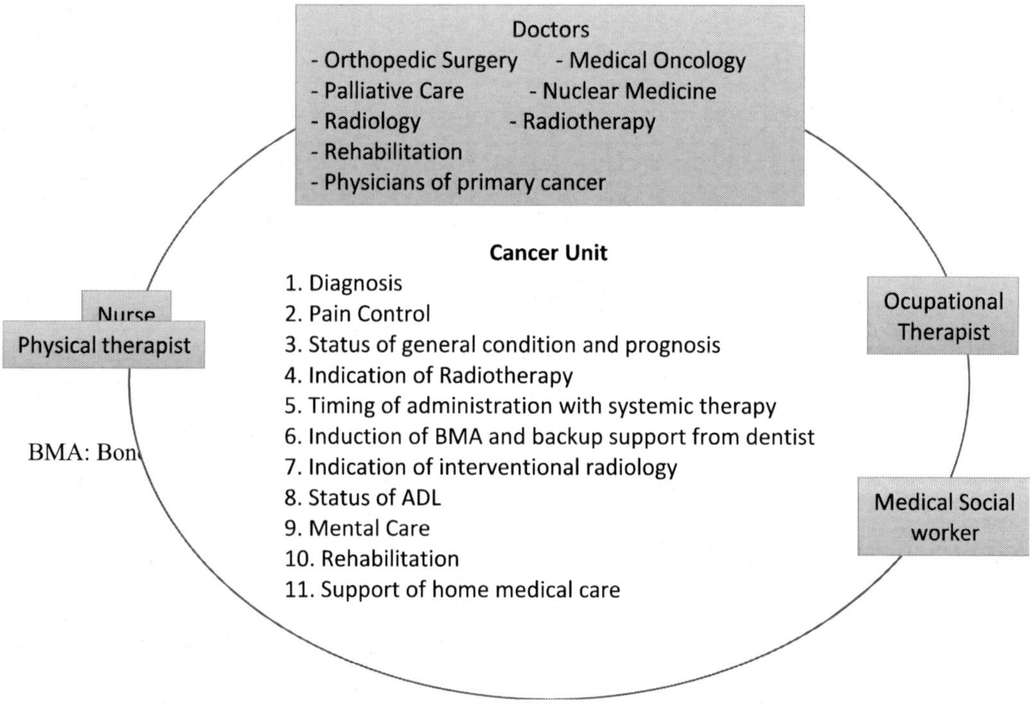

Figure 1. Cancer Unit for the management of bone metastases.

OUR LITERATURE REVIEW

This chapter contains opinions based on a narrative literature review of the publications including books and peer-reviewed journal articles. The authors summarize the most relevant historical aspects and current concepts on approach of patient with bone metastatic disease.

Table 1. Management of skeletal related events

Skeletal Related Event	Management	Effects
Bone pain	NSAIDs, Opioids	Analgesic effects
	Bisphosphonates	Inhibition of pathological bone resorption Analgesic effects
	Denosumab	Inhibition of pathological bone resorption Analgesic effects
	Radiotherapy	Analgesic effects Tumor shrinkage
Pathological bone fracture	Surgery	Stabilization of fracture
	Radiotherapy	Supportive therapy to prevent local recurrence
	Bisphosphonates	Prophylaxis
	Denosumab	Prophylaxis
Spinal cord compression	Steroids	Stabilization of vascular membranes Reduction of inflammation and edema
	Radiotherapy	Tumor shrinkage effects
	Surgery	Relief for the compression
	Bisphosphonates	Prophylaxis
	Denosumab	Prophylaxis
Hypercalcemia	Hydration	Promotion of renal calciuresis
	Loop diuretics	Promotion of renal calciuresis
	Bisphosphonates	Inhibition of pathological bone resorption
	Denosumab	Inhibition of pathological bone resorption

Note: NSAID = nonsteroidal anti-inflammatory drug.

GENERAL ASPECTS

Morbidities, such as pathological fractures and spinal paralysis, cause impairment in activities of daily life (ADLs) and quality of life (QOL) and affect prognosis because of deterioration of the affected patient's general condition and discontinuation of treatment for the primary disease (7–11).

Skeletal complications associated with bone metastases include cancer-induced bone pain, hypercalcemia, pathological bone fractures and spinal cord compression (12). Pain is one of the most frequent skeletal complications in patients with metastatic disease occurring in approximately 68% of patients (13). Other serious skeletal complications, such as pathological fractures, spinal cord compression and hypercalcemia, worsen patients' QOL and reduce survival rates (7-10, 14, 15). Information on the management of BM is shown in table 1.

Nine to 29% of patients with bone metastases develop pathological fractures (16, 17). Pathological fractures not only reduce QOL, but also impair on survival of patients (18, 19). Pathological fractures are mainly treated with surgery to stabilize the fractured bones to improve QOL via pain relief and restoration of function and mobility (20).

Radiotherapy is administered as a supportive therapy to prevent local recurrence by eliminating residual disease and relief pain (21).

Table 2. Analgesic management

NSAIDs + adjuvants (steroids)
NSAIDs + Weak opioids + adjuvant
NSAIDs + Strong opioids + adjuvant
Adjuvants
Tricyclic antidepressants: Amitriptyline, Nortriptyline
Antiseizure drugs: Carbamazepine, Gabapentin

Note: NSAIDs = Non-steroidal anti-inflammatory drugs.

PHARMACOLOGICAL MANAGEMENT OF BONE PAIN

Steroids are used in case of mixed type pain due to soft tissue involvement and neuropathic pain. Dexamethasone and methylprednisolone are of choice in doses that must be individualized and evaluating risks vs. benefits. The medical analgesic management of bone metastases is based on the World Health Organization and should be done as Table 2.

RADIOTHERAPY

Indications for radiotherapy for bone metastases include pain, risk for pathologic fracture and neurological complications arising from spinal cord compression. For most patients, external beam radiotherapy (EBRT) provides excellent palliation for localized metastatic bone pain. In most clinical situations, the clinical benefit can be achieved with a short treatment schedule. Moreover, EBRT leads an improvement in QOL with little toxicity (22, 23). The mechanism of pain relief after radiotherapy is poorly understood. The median time to onset of pain relief is around three weeks. Overall pain relief is obtained in 60% to 80% of patients and 25% of patients achieve complete response after conventional EBRT (24, 25).

Numerous randomized trials have been conducted on dose-fractionation schedules of palliative radiotherapy. One of the first randomized trials was conducted by the Radiation Therapy Oncology Group (RTOG 74-02) where patients were randomly assigned to 8 Gy in one treatment fraction or 30 Gy in 10 treatment fractions. Ninety percent of patients experienced some pain relief and 54% achieved complete pain relief. Both regimens were equivalent in terms of pain and narcotic relief at 3 months and were ell tolerated with few adverse effects. The 8 Gy arm had higher rate of re-treatment but had less acute toxicity (26).

The Dutch Bone Metastases Study found no difference in pain relief or QOL following single 8 Gy or 24 Gy in 6 daily treatment fractions. However, the re-irradiation rates were 25% in the single arm and 7% in the multiple treatment arm (27).

A meta-analysis by Wu et al. included 3,260 patients from 8 randomized trials and compared single 8-Gy fraction with several multifractionation regimens. They found equivalent complete pain relief in about 33% of patients and a similar overall pain response rate of approximately 60% in both the 8 Gy regimen and the multifractionation regimens (28). Another meta-analysis of 11 trials by Sze et al. (29) reported similar findings. Fewer treatment visits and patient convenience are advantages of single-fraction therapy. However, the need for retreatment may be higher for those who receive shortfractionation treatment (29).

A recent published update of palliative radiotherapy fractionation schedules for painful uncomplicated bone metastases compared single fraction to multiple fractions and showed that the overall response rate was similar in patients for single fraction treatments (61%) and those for multiple fraction treatments (62%). Similarly, complete response rates were nearly identical in both groups (23% vs 24%, respectively). Re-treatment was significantly more frequent in the single fraction treatment arm, with 20% receiving additional treatment to the same site versus 8% in the multiple fraction treatment arm. No significant difference was seen in the risk of pathological fracture at the treatment site, rate of spinal cord compression at the index site, or in the rate of acute toxicity (30).

Patients initially treated with single fraction of 8 Gy are 2.6 times more likely to require re-treatment than those who received multiple fractions. Interestingly, radiation oncologists seem more likely to offer re-treatment after initial 8 Gy RT versus initial multiple fractions schedule, may be due to the limits of radiation tolerance (30).

The choice of palliative radioteraphy regime depends on a large number of factors, including, primary site, histology, performance status, type of lesion (osteolytic vs. osteoblastic), location of the metastases, weight-bearing vs. non–weight-bearing site, extent of disease, number of painful sites and level of pain prior to treatment. The effectiveness of the treatment also depends on the goal: palliation of pain, prevention of pathologic fracture, avoidance of future treatments or local control of the disease. The doses required and volumes treated may be quite different for each of these goals. In addition to pain relief, other symptoms may be relieved by radiotherapy. Patients who have improvement in pain after radiotherapy may also have improvement in emotional functioning, decreased insomnia and decreased constipation, and overall improvement in QOL scores. Radiotherapy should be an integral part of palliative treatment for bone metastases for treatment of pain and prevention of other symptoms (23).

Stereotactic radiosurgery is a modern treatment modality that delivers high doses to metastatic bone with a great accuracy, minimizing the dose to the adjacent critical structures. It has emerged as a new treatment option for the multidisciplinary management of metastases. The goals of stereotactic radiosurgery parallel those of brain radiosurgery, that is to improve local control over conventional fractionated radiotherapy and to be effective for the treatment of previously irradiated lesions with an acceptable safety profile (31).

Stereotactic radiosurgery offers several theoretical advantages for spinal tumors: early treatment of these lesions before a patient becomes symptomatic and the stability of the spine, it avoids the need to irradiate large segments of the spinal cord, the early treatment of spinal lesions may obviate the need for extensive spinal surgery for decompression and fixation in these already debilitated patients and may also avoid the need to irradiate large segments of the spinal column, which is known to have a deleterious effect on bone marrow reserve in these patients. The avoidance of open surgery and the preservation of bone-marrow function facilitate continuous chemotherapy in this patient population. Other advantage is the shorter overall treatment time. Practically speaking, a shorter treatment course is also much more convenient for patients, especially those with limited mobility. However, patients do need to be able to tolerate a longer treatment time per fraction than with conventional treatment. As always, treatment decision-making needs to be multifactorial and individualized to the situation when considering SBRT (32, 33).

Dose and fractionation schedules are different in each institution. Single-fraction SRS doses range from 16 to 24 Gy, while hypofractionated regimens consist of 6 Gy×5 fractions, 8 Gy×3 fractions, or 9 Gy×3 fractions (34).

The efficacy of spinal radiosurgery in local disease control was assessed clinically and radiologically in some studies. Chang et al. (35) reported radiological control of spinal metastases in 90% of the patients at 6 months and in 80% at 12 months, like Garg et al. (36), who obtained an imaging control rate of 88% of the patients after 18 months of follow-up.

In a series of 103 metastases with a variety of histopathologies treated with 18-24 Gy (median, 24 Gy) single-fraction spinal SRS, Yamada, et al. demonstrated an actuarial local control rate of 90% overall at a median follow-up of 15 months, with improved LC with 24 Gy vs. 18-23 Gy dosing. The median time to local failure was 9 months (range, 2-15 months) from the time of treatment and morbidity was limited to grade 1-2 toxicities (37).

An RTOG phase II/III study was initiated comparing 16 or 18 Gy with 8 Gy, of which the phase II feasibility results are available, but the phase III results are still pending (38).

RE-IRRADIATION

Re-irradiation should be considered after initial palliative radiotherapy for no response/parcial response in previously irradiated area or pain relapse after initial satisfactory response. Patients requiring re-irradiation represent a substantial group, considering that up to 40% of patients do not obtain any pain relief after initial radiotherapy and pain relapse occurs in approximately 50% of initial responders within one year after radiotherapy (39).

The International Bone Metastases Consensus Working Party recommends a 4-week interval for re-treatment in those patients who do not achieve a response to initial RT (40). The best available evidence on re-treated patients was presented by van der Linden et al. (41). They reanalyzed the database of the Dutch Bone Metastasis Study that compared 8 Gy single fraction versus 24 Gy in multiple fractions for painful bone metastases and found that the mean time to re-treatment was 13 weeks in single fraction patients and 21 weeks in multiple fractions patients. Response was recorded in 66% initial 8 Gy patients and 46% initial multi fractions patients ($p = 0.12$), with longer mean duration of remission in initial single fraction patients (16 weeks versus 8 weeks) (41).

The preferred dose schedule for re-irradiation must be determined. This question iniciated the phase III international randomised trial that compared single 8 Gy with 20 Gy in multiple fractions for re-irradiation of painful bone metastases (NCIC CTG SC20) whose results have recently been published by Chow et al. (42) and showed that re-irradiation is efficacious and a sigle dose of 8 Gy is non-inferior (45% of patients responded to the single fraction while 51% of patients responded to the multiple fractions) and less toxic tan multiple fractions of 20 Gy. The most frequent toxicities were lack of appetite (56% and 66% of patients treated with 8Gy and 20Gy respectively) and diarrea (23% and 31% of patients treated with 8 Gy and 20 Gy, respectively). (42, 43).

At present careful patient selection in terms of performance status, number of metastases, primary tumor type and loco-regional anatomy should be considered.

SYSTEMIC THERAPY

The rationale for using systemic therapy in the management of bone metastasis is compelling. In selecting systemic antitumor treatment for metastatic bone disease, the pathological type of the tumor is most important. Chemotherapy, targeted therapies and hormone therapy may contribute to pain relief by reducing tumor bulk and/or by modulating pain signaling pathways. However, primary tumor type, disease extent, and treatment-related toxicity are important considerations. (44).

In advanced hormonally driven tumors such as prostate and breast, the first line treatment is hormone deprivation to cut off the proliferative signaling in the cancers. While chemotherapy is an integral part of systemic treatment, the role of endocrine therapy is particularly important in bone-only or bone-predominant metastases from breast cancer (45).

Among patients with recurrent breast cancer, those with estrogen receptor (ER)-positive tumors are twice as likely to develop bone metastases as those with ER-negative tumors (46). Current guidelines recommend endocrine therapy in preference to chemotherapy for women with ER-positive advanced breast cancer, except in the presence of rapidly progressive visceral disease. (47).

Development and approval of immunotherapy for cancers in general has made considerable progress and attracted interest in recent years. In the advanced prostate cancer field, Sipuleucel-T has been approved after showing a survival benefit in castration-resistant prostate cancer patients who are asymptomatic or minimally symptomatic. As the field of immune oncology continues to expand, specific bone directed therapies may materialize (48).

Effective systemic anti-cancer therapy is paramount in the management of bone metastases. Novel mechanistic insights into the complex multistep process of bone metastases will, undoubtably, lead to improved detection of micrometastases and a significant expansion of new and better treatment options.

Spinal cord compression

Spinal cord compression is an oncological emergency that can reduce survival and QOL if the treatment is not performed (49). The spinal cord is damaged by compression or by vascular compromising due to tumor growth. The damage can be irreversible if the arterial flow to the spinal cord is disturbed. The symptoms are pain; motor weakness; sensory deficits; gait disturbance; and urinary, bowel, and sexual dysfunction. Immediate diagnosis must be done with computed tomography or magnetic resonance imaging to determine compression site and rule out multifocality. Early initiation of corticosteroids is also necessary to stabilize vascular membranes and reduce inflammation and edema (50).

Even though the efficacy of radiotherapy is promising, surgery was shown to be effective to relieve compression. In a randomized, multi-institutional trial, patients with spinal cord compression caused by metastatic cancer were assigned to either surgery followed by radiotherapy or radiotherapy alone. The primary endpoint was the ability to walk. More patients in the surgery group (84%) than in the radiotherapy group (57%) were able to walk after treatment ($p = 0.001$) (51).

Prompt decision-making is very important to reduce damage to the spinal cord. The optimum dose and treatment regimen of radiotherapy for spinal cord compression is still controversial. The short course radiotherapy is preferable because the survival prognosis of most patients with metastatic epidural spinal cord compression is only a few months (52). However, the high daily doses might be more toxic and less effective for the treatment of acute compression and prevention of recurrence. Only a randomized trial showed the non-inferiority of short course radiotherapy to the longer course (53). In this trial, a total of 203 patients with metastatic epidural spinal cord compression and poor to intermediate expected survival were randomly assigned to either 4 Gy × 5 in 1 week (n = 101) or 3 Gy × 10 in 2 weeks (n = 102). The primary endpoint was overall response regarding motor deficits at 1 month after radiotherapy, defined as improvement or no further progression. The overall response rates regarding motor function were not significantly different, 87.2% after 4 Gy × 5 and 89.6% after 3 Gy × 10. However, both regimens were still non-standard short schedules.

Further randomized trials are required to compare them with a standard, more protracted schedule.

Surgery

Surgery is indicated for fractures of long bones and hip joints, in spinal cord involvement or peripheral nerve compression. The goals of surgical management are palliation of pain and functional preservation and restoration. Most patients without fracture do not require surgery for bone metastases. If a pathological fracture of a long bone is present, it is often best treated with internal fixation and instrumentation. Other goals of surgical intervention include immediate weight-bearing and return to activity. The surgical strategy will depend on both the prognostic factors and the biological and mechanical features of metastatic disease. There have been reports indicating that surgical intervention for patients with cancer with impending pathologic fractures lead better outcomes than that for patients with cancer with completed pathologic fractures (54, 55).

The morbidity and mortality from a completed fracture are greater than that of a properly managed impending fracture; however, the true risk of pathologic fracture can be difficult to determine. Accurate prediction of pathologic fractures in various clinical situations remains an active area of investigation. Those bones that bear weight and experience torsional forces are at the highest risk, though any bone sufficiently weakened by tumor may fracture with the slightest force (56).

An understanding of the risk of pathological fractures in patients with bone metastases is an unmet need for prompt prevention, detection, and treatment. Mirels proposed a scoring system to quantify the risk of sustaining a pathologic fracture through a metastatic lesion in a long bone (57). The scoring system is based on characteristics and all the features were assigned progressive scores ranging from 1 to 3 (see Table 3). A score of > 8 suggests prophylactic fixation should be considered.

Table 3. Mirels' scoring system for diagnosing impending pathologic fractures in a long bone

Score	Site of Lesion	Size of Lesion	Nature of Lesion	Pain
1	Upper limb	<1/3 of cortex	Blastic	Mild
2	Lower limb	1/3–2/3 of cortex	Mixed	Moderate
3	Trochanteric region	>2/3 of cortex	Lytic	Functional

In developing a care plan, the merits of prophylactic surgery should be considered for patients with bone metastases. With early diagnosis, timely intervention is essential to prevent pathologic fractures.

Bisphosphonates and Inhibitors of NF-KB Activating Receptor Ligand (RANKL) in Bone Metastases

Bisphosphonates are analogues of pyrophosphate, a natural inhibitor of bone demineralization. They bind avidly to exposed bone mineral around resorbing osteoclast and this leads to very high local concentrations of product in the resoption lacunae. Then, bisphosphonates are internalized by the osteoclast causing disruption of the chemical process involved in bone resorption (58, 59).

In oncology, bisphosphonates are the standard treatment for tumor induced hypercalcaemia and a new form of therapy for bone metastases (60). The most common adverse events include flu-like symptoms, anemia, nausea, bone pain, dyspnea and peripheral edema. These events are mostly limited and mild to moderate (58). A rare but very serious side effect is osteonecrosis of the jaw (61).

Denosumab is a human monoclonal antibody that inhibits the RANKL, preventing the development of osteoclasts. It can help prevent or delay problems like fractures in patients with bone metastases. It also can be helpful when zoledronate is no longer working. Side effects are like bisphosphonates, including nausea, diarrhea, weakness and can cause osteonecrosis of the jaw too (62).

The duration of treatment with denosumab or zoledronate remains undefined. Since many patients with bone metastases survive beyond two years, the decision to maintain treatment for a period longer than 24 months depends on a risk-benefit balance. All bisphosphonates undergo renal clearance so, patients with renal impairment should not receive the treatment. Patients doing these treatments should take a supplement containing calcium and vitamin D (61).

Radiotherapy is the treatment of choice for localized bone pain, but in presence of poorly localized bone pain or recurrence of pain in previously irradiated skeletal sites, the bisphosphonates are an alternative treatment approach (63).

RADIOISOTOPES

Radiopharmaceuticals such as strontium-89, rhenium-186 or samarium-153, have been shown to be effective in palliation of metastatic bone pain. They are preferentially taken up at sites for bone formation, so they probably are most effective for osteoblastic metastases. The principal side effects are myelosuppression and pain flare (63, 64).

There are also available radium-223, calcium mimetic and alpha emitter that selectively binds to areas of increased bone turnover in bone metastases. It bounds into newly formed bone stroma and the radiation induces mainly double-stranded DNA breaks that result in a potent and highly localized cytotoxic effect. Toxic effects on adjacent tissues and particularly the bone marrow is minimal due to the short path of the alpha particles. Radium-223 significantly prolonged overall survival in patients who had castration-resistant prostate cancer and bone metastases, with a 30% reduction in the risk of death (65).

DISCUSSION

Cancer is a major public health issue in Latin America and the Caribbean. It is estimated that by 2030, approximately 1.7 million people will have been diagnosed with cancer in the region and that more than 1 million people per year will die from the disease. Consequently, major difficulties will arise when addressing the increasing morbidity and mortality associated with the disease, especially in advanced stages (66), in a region characterized by major population growth under unfavorable conditions, such as widespread poverty, persistent and severe social inequality, scarce institutional development and poor social security (67).

Opioid consumption in Latin America and the Caribbean is variable. According to international standards, moderate levels of consumption are reported in Argentina, Chile, Brazil, Colombia, Cuba, Mexico, Costa Rica and Uruguay, as well as in Guatemala, Honduras and Bolivia, where particularly low levels have been recorded. Nevertheless, average consumption remains far below international levels, suggesting that pain management is inadequate for much of the Latin American population (68).

The presence of bone metastases is a sign of disseminated disease and foretells a short-term prognosis in cancer patients. The bone metastases have an important impact on patient's QOL thus, new strategies are necessary to prevent skeletal disease and palliate established skeletal events. Palliative care is needed to provide physical and psychosocial relief and to improve the quality of life of patients and their families (69).

Palliative-care services have progressed in recent years in Latin America; however, there remains limited access to care and medications for patients with advanced cancer.

Palliative care must be a priority for health-care policy makers. Education and training in palliative care must be supported and valued and it must be approached by a multidisciplinary team and at the same time interdisciplinary that allows a better approach and communication both within the treating medical team and between the patient and his family in order to provide better alternatives of treatment, autonomy and above all QOL.

Bone metastases present a variety of challenges. Innovative combined modality approaches are required in order to improve survival with acceptable toxicity. This treatment may include combinations of external beam irradiation plus surgery, hormone therapy, radioisotopes, bisphosphonates and chemotherapy but the treatment should be individualized according to the patient's clinical condition and life expectancy.

Latin America has had to overcome a situation with more limited resources compared to North America and Europe, however, it has been compensated with the regulation of resources based on local consensus, while the challenge being to stay ahead on the integral management of bone metastases in the future.

REFERENCES

[1] Coleman RE. *Metastatic bone disease: clinical features, pathophysiology and treatment strategies.* Cancer Treat Rev 2001;27(3):165-76.

[2] Goss PE, Lee BL, Badovinac-Crnjevic T, Strasser-Weippl K, Chavarri-Guerra Y, St Louis J et al. *Planning cancer control in Latin America and the Caribbean.* Lancet Oncol 2013;14(5):391-436.

[3] Hage WD, Aboulafia AJ, Aboulafia DM. *Incidence, location, and diagnostic evaluation of metastatic bone disease.* Orthop Clin North Am 2000;31(4),515-28.

[4] Hosono N, Yonenobu K, Fuji T, Ebara S, Yamashita K, Ono K. *Orthopaedic management of spinal metastases.* Clin Orthop Relat Res 1995;(312):148-59.

[5] Karr JP, Yamanaka H. Prostate Cancer and Bone Metastasis, 1st ed. New York: Springer, 1992.

[6] Moriwaki S. *Histopathology and statistical analysis of spinal metastases of carcinomas in autopsy cases.* Orthop Surg Traumatol 1993; 36:233-41.

[7] Coleman RE. Skeletal complications of malignancy. Cancer 1997;80 (8 Suppl):158 8-94.

[8] Plunkett TA, Rubens RD. *The biology and management of bone metastases.* Crit Rev Oncol Hematol 1999,31(1):89-96.

[9] Nørgaard M, Jensen AØ, Jacobsen JB, Cetin K, Fryzek JP, Sørensen HT. *Skeletal related events, bone metastasis and survival of prostate cancer: A population-based cohort study in Denmark (1999 to 2007).* J Urol 2010;184(1):162-7.

[10] Yong M, Jensen AÖ, Jacobsen JB, Nørgaard M, Fryzek JP, Sørensen HT. *Survival in breast cancer patients with bone metastases and skeletal-related events: A population-based cohort study in Denmark (1999–2007).* Breast Cancer Res Treat 2011;129(2):495-503.

[11] Sathiakumar N, Delzell E, Morrisey MA, Falkson C, Yong M, Chia V, et al. *Mortality following bone metastasis and skeletal-related events among men with prostate cancer: A population-based analysis of us medicare beneficiaries,* 1999–2006. Prostate Cancer Prostatic Dis 2011;14(2):177-83.

[12] Tsuzuki S, Park SH, Eber MR, Peters CM, Shiozawa Y. *Skeletal complications in cancer patients with bone metastases.* Int J Urol 2016;23(10):825-32.

[13] van den Beuken-van Everdingen MHJ, de Rijke JM, Kessels AG, Schouten HC, van Kleef M, Patijn J. *Prevalence of pain in patients with cancer: A systematic review of the past 40 years.* Ann Oncol Off J Eur Soc Med Oncol England; 2007;18(9):1437-49.

[14] McKay R, Haider B, Duh MS, Valderrama A, Nakabayashi M, Fiorillo M, et al. *Impact of symptomatic skeletal events on health-care resource utilization and quality of life among patients with castration-resistant prostate cancer and bone metastases.* Prostate Cancer Prostatic Dis England; 2017;20(3):276-82.

[15] Howard LE, De Hoedt AM, Aronson WJ, Kane CJ, Amling CL, Cooperberg MR, et al. *Do skeletal-related events predict overall survival in men with metastatic castration-resistant prostate cancer?* Prostate Cancer Prostatic Dis England 2016;19(4):380-4.

[16] Aaron AD. *Treatment of metastatic adenocarcinoma of the pelvis and the extremities. J Bone Joint Surg Am United States*; 1997 Jun;79(6):917-32.

[17] Bohm P, Huber J. *The surgical treatment of bony metastases of the spine and limbs.* J Bone Joint Surg Br 2002;84(4);521-9.

[18] Hansen BH, Keller J, Laitinen M, Berg P, Skjeldal S, Trovik C. *The scandinavian sarcoma group skeletal metastasis register. Survival after surgery for bone metastases in the pelvis and extremities.* Acta Orthop Scand Suppl 2004;75(311): 11-5.

[19] Mavrogenis AF, Pala E, Romagnoli C, Romantini M, Calabro T, Ruggieri P. *Survival analysis of patients with femoral metastases.* J Surg Oncol 2012;105(2): 135-41.

[20] Bryson DJ, Wicks L, Ashford RU. *The investigation and management of suspected malignant pathological fractures: A review for the general orthopaedic surgeon.* Injury 2015;46(10):1891-9.

[21] Frassica DA. *General principles of external beam radiation therapy for skeletal metastases.* Clin Orthop Relat Res 2003;415(Suppl): S158-64.

[22] Zeng L, Chow E, Bedard G, Zhang L, Fairchild A, Vassiliou V, et al. *Quality of life after palliative radiation therapy for patients with painful bone metastases: results of an international study validating the EORTC QLQ-BM22.* Int Radiat Oncol Biol Phys 2012;84(3): e337-42.

[23] Lutz S, Berk L, Chang E, Chow E, Hahn C, Hoskin P, et al. *Palliative radiotherapy for bone metastases: an ASTRO evidence-based guideline.* Int J Radiat Oncol Biol Phys 2011;79(4):965-76.

[24] Steenland E, Leer JW, Van Houwelingen H, Post WJ, van den Hout WB, Kievit J, et al. *The effect of a single fraction compared with multiple fraction on painful bone metastases: a global analysis of the Dutch Bone Metastases Study.* Radiother Oncol 1999;52(2):101-9.

[25] Chow E, Hoskin P, Mitera G, Zeng L, Lutz S, Roos D, et al. *Update of the international consensus on palliative radiotherapy endpoints for future clinical trials in bone metastases.* Int Radiat Oncol Biol Phys 2012;82(5):1730-7.

[26] Hartsell WF, Scott CB, Bruner DW, Scarantino CW, Ivker RA, Roach M 3rd, et al. *Randomized Trial of Short- Versus Long-Course Radiotherapy for Palliation of Painful Bone Metastases.* J Natl Cancer Inst 2005;97(11):798-804.

[27] Meeuse JJ, van der Linden YM, van Tienhoven G, Gans RO, Leer JW, *Reyners AK, et al. Efficacy of radiotherapy for painful bone metastases during the last 12 weeks of life: results from the Dutch Bone Metastasis Study Cancer* 2010;116(11):2716-25.

[28] Wu JS, Wong R, Johnston M, Bezjak A, Whelan T. *Meta-analysis of dose-fractionation radiotherapy trials for the palliation of painful bone metastases.* Int J Radiat Oncol Biol Phys 2003;55(3):594-605.

[29] Sze WM, Shelley M, Held I, Mason M. *Palliation of metastatic bone pain: single fraction versus multifraction radiotherapy: A systematic review of the randomised trials.* Cochrane Database Syst Rev. 2004(2):CD004721.

[30] Chow E, Zeng L, Salvo N, Dennis K, Tsao M, Lutz S. *Update on the systematic review of palliative radiotherapy trials for bone metastases.* Clin Oncol (R Coll Radiol) 2012;24(2):112-24.

[31] Seil Sohn, Chun Kee Chung. *Role of Stereotactic Radiosurgery in Metastasis to the Spine.* J Korean Neurosurg Soc 2012;51(1):1-7.

[32] Jhaveri P, Teh B, Bloch C, Amato R, Butler EB, Paulino AC. *Stereotactic body radiotherapy in the management of painful bone metastases.* Oncology 2008;22(7):782-8.

[33] Sohn S, Chung C. *The role of stereotactic radiosurgery in metastasis to the spine.* J Korean Neurosurg Soc 2012;51(1):1-7.

[34] Gagnon GJ, Nasr NM, Liao JJ, Molzahn I, Marsh D, McRae D, Henderson FC. *Treatment of spinal tumors using cyberknife fractionated stereotactic radiosurgery: pain and quality-of-life assessment after treatment in 200 patients.* Sr Neurosurgery 2009;64(2):297-306.

[35] Chang UK, Cho WI, Kim MS, Cho CK, Lee DH, Rhee CH. *Local tumor control after retreatment of spinal metastasis using stereotactic body radiotherapy; comparison with initial treatment group.* Acta Oncol 2012;51(5):589-95.

[36] Garg AK, Shiu AS, Yang J, Wang XS, Allen P, Brown BW, et al. *Phase 1/2 trial of single-session stereotactic body radiotherapy for previously unirradiated spinal metastases.* Cancer 2012;118(20):5069-77.

[37] Yamada Y, Bilsky MH, Lovelock DM, Venkatraman ES, Toner S, Johnson J, et al. *High-Dose, Single-Fraction Image-Guided Intensity-Modulated Radiotherapy for Metastatic Spinal Lesions.* Int J Radiat Oncol Biol Phys 2008;71(2):484-490.

[38] Ryu S, Pugh SL, Gerszten PC, Yin FF, Timmerman RD, Hitchcock YJ, et al. *RTOG 0631 phase 2/3 study of image guided stereotactic radiosurgery for localized (1-3) spine metastases: phase 2 results.* Pract Radiat Oncol 2014;4(2):76-81.

[39] Huisman M, van den Bosch MA, Wijlemans JW, van Vulpen M, van der Linden YM, Verkooijen HM. *Effectiveness of reirradiation for painful bone metastases: a systematic review and meta-analysis.* Int J Radiat Oncol Biol Phys 2012;84(1):8-14.

[40] Chow E, Hoskin P, Mitera G, Zeng L, Lutz S, Roos D, et al. International Bone Metastases Consensus Working Party. *Update of the international consensus on palliative radiotherapy endpoints for future clinical trials in bone metastases.* Int J Radiat Oncol Biol Phys 2012;82(5):1730-7.

[41] van der Linden YM, Lok JJ, Steenland E, Martijn H, van Houwelingen H, Marijnen CA, et al. *Dutch Bone Metastasis Study Group. Single fraction radiotherapy is efficacious: a further analysis of the Dutch Bone Metastasis Study controlling for the influence of retreatment.* Int J Radiat Oncol Biol Phys 2004;59(2):528-37.

[42] Chow E, Hoskin PJ, Wu J, Roos D, van der Linden Y, Hartsell W, et al. *A phase III international randomised trial comparing single with multiple fractions for re-irradiation of painful bone metastases: National Cancer Institute of Canada Clinical Trials Group (NCIC CTG) SC 20.* Clin Oncol 2006;18(2):125-8.

[43] Chow E, van der Linden YM, Roos D, Hartsell WF, Hoskin P, Wu JS, et al. *Single versus multiple fractions of repeat radiation for painful bone metastases: a randomized, controlled, noninferiority trial.* Lancet Oncol 2014;15(2):164-71.

[44] Gough N, Miah AB, Linch M. *Nonsurgical oncological management of cancer pain. Curr Opin Support Palliat Care 2014*;8(2):102-11.

[45] Wong MH, Pavlakis N. *Optimal management of bone metastases in breast cancer patients.* Breast Cancer Targets Ther 2011; 3:35-60.

[46] Hess KR1, Pusztai L, Buzdar AU, Hortobagyi GN. *Estrogen receptors and distinct patterns of breast cancer relapse.* Breast Cancer Res Treat 2003;78(1):105-18.

[47] Beslija S, Bonneterre J, Burstein HJ, Cocquyt V, Gnant M, Heinemann V. *Third consensus on medical treatment of metastatic breast cancer.* Ann Oncol 2009;20(11):1771-85.

[48] Kantoff PW, Higano CS, Shore ND, Berger ER, Small EJ, Penson DF. *Sipuleucel-T immunotherapy for castration-resistant prostate cancer.* N Engl J Med 2010;363(5):411-22.

[49] Prasad D, Schiff D. *Malignant spinal-cord compression.* Lancet Oncol 2005; 6(1):15-24.

[50] Cole JS, Patchell RA. *Metastatic epidural spinal cord compression.* Lancet Neurol 2008;7(5):459-66.

[51] Patchell RA, Tibbs PA, Regine WF, Payne R, Saris S, Kryscio RJ. *Direct decompressive surgical resection in the treatment of spinal cord compression caused by metastatic cancer: A randomised trial.* Lancet 2005;366(9486):643-8.

[52] Rades D, Abrahm JL. *The role of radiotherapy for metastatic epidural spinal cord compression.* Nat Rev Clin Oncol 2010;7(10):590-8.

[53] Rades D, Segedin B, Conde-Moreno AJ, Garcia R, Perpar A, Metz M, et al. *Radiotherapy with 4 gy x 5 versus 3 gy x 10 for metastatic epidural spinal cord compression: Final results of the score-2 trial (aro 2009/01).* J Clin Oncol 2016;34(6):597-60.

[54] Johnson SK, Knobf MT. *Surgical interventions for cancer patients with impending or actual pathologic fractures.* Orthop Nurs 2008,27(3):160-71.

[55] Ward WG, Holsenbeck S, Dorey FJ, Spang J, Howe D. *Metastatic disease of the femur: Surgical treatment.* Clin Orthop Relat Res 2003;415(Suppl): S230-44.

[56] Nielsen OS, Munro AJ, Tannock IF. *Bone metastases: pathophysiology and management policy.* J Clin Oncol 1991;9(3):509-24.

[57] Mirels H. *Metastatic disease in long bones: A proposed scoring system for diagnosing impending pathologic fractures.* Clin Orthop Relat Res 1989;(249):256-64.

[58] Selvaggi G, Scagliotti G. *Management of bone metastases in cancer: A review.* Crit Rev Oncol Hematol 2005;56(3):365-78.

[59] Rogers M, Xiong X, Ji X, Ebetino FH, Mönkkönen J, Russell RG, Williamson MP, et al. *Inhibition of growth of Dictyostelium discoideum amoebae by bispho-sphonates is dependent on cellular uptake.* Pharmacol Res 1997;14(5):625-30.

[60] Body J, Coleman R, Piccart M. Use of bisphosphonates in cancer patients. Cancer Treat Rev 1996;22(4):265-87.

[61] Steger G, Bartsch R. *Denosumab for the treatment of bone metastases in breast cancer: evidence and opinion.* Ther Adv Med Oncol 2011;3(5):233-43.

[62] Green JR, Rogers MJ. *Pharmacologic profile of zoledronic acid: a highly potent inhibitor of bone resorption.* Drug Dev Res 2002; 55:210-24.

[63] Maisano R, Pergolizzi S, Cascinu S. *Novel therapeutic approaches to cancer patients with bone metastasis.* Crit Rev Oncol Hematol 2001;40(3):239-50.

[64] Robinson R, Preston D, Baxter K, Dusing RW, Spicer JA. *Clinical experience with strontium89 in prostatic and breast cancer patients.* Semin Oncol 1993;20 (3 suppl 2):44-8.

[65] Parker C, Nilsson S, Heinrich D, Helle SI, O'Sullivan JM, FOssa SD. *Alpha emitter Radium-223 and survival in metastatic prostate cancer.* N Engl J Med 2013;369(3):213-23.

[66] Goss PE, Lee BL, Badovinac-Crnjevic T, Strasser-Weippl K, Chavarri-Guerra Y, St Louis J, et al. *Planning cancer control in Latin America and the Caribbean.* Lancet Oncol 2013;14(5):391-436.

[67] UN. *Older Persons in Latin America and the Caribbean: Situation and Policies.* ECLAC Population Division – Latin American and Caribbean Demographic Centre (CELADE). Santiago: UN, 2003.

[68] Cleary J, De Lima L, Eisenchlas J, Radbruch L, Torode J, Chermy NI. *Formulary availability and regulatory barriers to accessibility of opioids for cancer pain in Latin America and the Caribbean: a report from the Global Opioid Policy Initiative (GOPI).* Ann Oncol 2013;24(11): xi4150.

Macedo F, Ladeira K, Pinho F, Saraiva N, Bonito N, Pinto L, et al. *Bone Metastases: An Overview.* Oncol Rev 2017;11(1):321.

In: Cancer Management in Latin America II
Editors: Maurício F Silva et al.
ISBN: 978-1-53616-735-1

Chapter 10

MANAGEMENT OF BRAIN METASTASES

Fernando Mariano Obst[1,*], MD, MSc, Karine Campagnolo[1], MD, Tiago Pereira de Leão[2], MD, Fiona Lim[3], MBBS, Bo Angela Wan[4], MD(C) and Mauricio F Silva[5,6,7], MD, PhD

[1]Radiation Oncology Unit, São Lucas Hospital of Pontifical Catholic University, Porto Alegre, Brazil
[2]Radiation Oncology Unit, General Hospital of Caxias do Sul, Brazil
[3]Department of Oncology, Princess Margaret Hospital, Hong Kong, PR China
[4]Odette Cancer Centre, Sunnybrook Health Sciences Centre, University of Toronto, Toronto, Ontario, Canada
[5]Radiation Oncology Unit, Santa Maria Federal University, Santa Maria, Brazil
[6]Hospital de Caridade Astrogildo de Azevedo, Santa Maria, Brazil
[7]Latin America Cooperative Oncology Group, Porto Alegre, Brazil

ABSTRACT

This chapter is an overview of the most relevant topics on management of brain metastases in the literature. Brain metastases are common and often be present in patients whose systemic cancer is asymptomatic. When brain metastases occur, they considerably decrease the quality of life in patients who otherwise might be functional. The goal of this chapter is to review important prognostic factors that may guide treatment selection, discuss the roles of surgery, radiation, and systemic therapy in the treatment of patients with brain metastases, and present new directions in brain metastasis therapy under active investigation. An early diagnosis and effective treatment of the brain metastasis, may lead

* Corresponding Author's Email: fmobst@gmail.com.

to a useful remission of the brain symptoms and may prolong survival, preserving neurologic and neurocognitive function, and maximize life quality.

INTRODUCTION

Brain metastases are the most common intracranial malignancy, causing significant morbidity and mortality in oncology patients. The current treatment for brain metastasis depends on the patient's overall health status, the primary tumor pathology, and the number and location of brain lesions. The modern management options for these tumors including surgical resection, radiotherapy, and chemotherapy. With an increased understanding of the pathophysiology of brain metastasis come increased future therapeutic options. Therapy targeted to specific tumor molecular pathways, such as those involved in blood-brain barrier transgression, cell-cell adhesion, and angiogenesis, are also reviewed. A personalized plan for each patient, based on molecular characterizations of the tumor that are used to better target radiotherapy and chemotherapy, is undoubtedly the future of brain metastasis treatment.

CLINICAL PRESENTATION

Epidemiology

Intracranial or brain metastases (BM) are the most commonly diagnosed central nervous system (CNS) tumor in the United States, these tumors are estimated to occur as much as 10 times more frequently than primary malignant brain tumors (1-8). Estimates for the frequency of these tumors vary significantly, but previous studies have reported that they occur in 9-10% of all cancer diagnoses (9, 10). Early studies that attempted to estimate the frequency of BM were based on autopsy data collected at single centers. These studies estimated the overall frequency of BM in persons who die of cancer to be approximately 25% (11, 12). These estimates varied significantly by cancer histology, with the highest reported frequencies in melanoma and lung cancer. There are many limitations to autopsy studies for estimating frequency of BM. These studies are often conducted at a single institution, and thus largely reflect the experience of a single large tertiary referral center only. Most of these studies are over 20 years old, and since this time period, the proportion of individuals receiving autopsy after death has declined significantly. Precise incidence or prevalence of BM is difficult to calculate, as it is not possible to use the same methodologies that are most often used for primary cancers. There have been a few attempts to estimate incidence of BM from population-based samples, but incidence estimated by these studies has varied. The proportion of cancers that present with BM increases with increasing age, peaking at approximately 60 years old. This pattern is largely due to the increasing risk of cancer with increasing age, as well as the low frequency of BM in cancers more common in younger persons. Lung cancer is the strongest example of this, though this pattern is also present in other cancer histologies.

Diagnosis

The majority of patients present with neurologic signs and symptoms (13-17). Although differential diagnoses such as an abscess or a stroke must be considered, new-onset neurologic symptoms in a known cancer patient should always be presumed to be from BM until proven otherwise. Patients presenting with acute neurologic signs and symptoms will likely undergo an initial noncontrast CT because of its ease of completion and ability to rule out life-threatening etiologies. However, contrast-enhanced MRI represents the most sensitive imaging modality to detect brain metastases, especially for identifying small lesions, which can have a significant effect on the patient's prognosis and treatment course. The majority of brain metastases will be located in the cerebral hemisphere (80%) at the junction of gray-white matter. Although there is no pathognomonic MRI characteristics of BM, they generally tend to be T1 iso- or hypointense, T2 hyperintense and enhance with contrast administration (18, 19). Full systemic workup (e.g., positron emission tomography [PET] and CT) should be promptly initiated if BM is the presenting event. Performance status and extracranial disease status have consistently been shown to impact prognosis. Contemporary series have further refined the class division by incorporating disease-specific prognostic factors, thereby creating and validating a diagnosis-specific graded prognostic assessment (DS-GPA) index to estimate survival outcomes with BM (20).

TREATMENT

Initial therapy for suspected or confirmed BM should instantly start with corticosteroids (e.g., dexamethasone or methylprednisolone), which effectively improve edema and neurologic deficits in approximately two-thirds of patients within 24 to 48 hours (21). Patients may present to the radiation oncologist already started on prophylactic anticonvulsants. This represents one of the most preventable causes of neurocognitive decline in brain tumor patients given the known negative impact on quality of life and neurocognition with anticonvulsants. Based on four negative randomized trials, the American Academy of Neurology in 2000 recommended that prophylactic anticonvulsants not be initiated in newly diagnosed brain tumor patients who have not experienced a seizure (22).

The decision-making for BM care are driving by patient factors and tumor factors. Patient factors include the patient's overall age, condition, and systemic disease burden, summarized as life expectancy independent of central nervous system (CNS) disease. Tumor factors include histological type, number, and location of lesions, and, more recently, the biology of the tumor based on molecular and genetic testing. Patients with poor life expectancy independent of CNS disease may reasonably be offered palliative care or no treatment for the CNS disease, regardless of the nature of the brain involvement. Patients in good medical condition with a low systemic disease burden, and hence a good survival chance independent of the brain metastases, may warrant aggressive treatment. Certain histological types of tumors (small cell lung cancer, breast cancer) are more likely to respond to adjuvant treatment with irradiation or chemotherapy, which can make their use beneficial even for numerous or poorly located lesions. Lesions in eloquent parts of the brain (those that subserve a discrete function, such as speech or movement) or in parts of the brain less accessible via open neurosurgery also connote a poorer prognosis. Neurosurgical resection of individual symptomatic brain metastases remains the standard of care. Lesions causing deficits due to local mass effect and cerebral edema should almost always undergo surgical extirpation once diagnosed, particularly if the lesion is a new diagnosis and tissue is required for pathology.

Surgical resection

Surgical resection can aid in obtaining a pathologic diagnosis of intracranial lesions, provide immediate relief of tumor mass effect, and may cure a small percentage of patient with single or solitary lesions. Given that up to 50% of brain metastases can present as a single lesion, there has been historical interest in evaluating the role of surgery in the management of brain metastases (23). There have now been three phase III trials testing the hypothesis that surgical resection to single brain metastasis is potentially beneficial. All three trials included patients with either a single lesion, defined as the presence of only one intracranial lesion regardless of the extracranial disease status, or a solitary lesion, defined as the intracranial lesion being the only site of metastatic disease (24-26). The studies by Patchell et al. (24) and Noordijk et al. (25) included better performance status patients compared with the Mintz et al. (26) study, which may have contributed to the differences in the outcomes between these studies. Additionally, 45% of patients in the study by Mintz et al. (26) had extracranial metastases, as compared to 37.5% and 31.7% in the studies by Patchell et al. (24) and Noordijk et al. (25), respectively. Similarly, as highlighted by Noordijk et al. the survival benefit to the addition of surgery to WBRT was most pronounced in the patient with inactive or stable extracranial disease, with no survival benefit present for patients with active or progressive extracranial disease. The results of these studies suggest that surgical resection should be reserved for lesions causing life-threatening complications, requiring pathologic confirmation or in patients with good performance status (KPS $\geq$ 70) with controlled extracranial disease burden.

Whole brain radiotherapy (WBRT)

The standard of care in select patients with diffuse brain metastasis ($\geq$5 brain metastases) continues to be WBRT. WBRT is well known to provide improvement in neurologic symptoms with overall response rates of 70% to 93% (27). The optimal dose and fractionation schedule for WBRT are not defined, despite numerous studies are designed to determine the optimal delivery. A dose of 30 Gy in 10 fractions or 37.5 Gy in 15 fractions continue to remain the standards for a vast majority of patients receiving WBRT: the radiographic overall response rate with this fractionation scheme is 59% (24% CR and 35% PR) (28). For patients with poor performance status, and/or uncontrolled extracranial disease burden, there an option of shorter fractionation scheme (e.g., 20 Gy in 5 fractions), though a supportive care-alone strategy may also be considered. A phase III randomized, non-inferiority study, the QUARTZ (Quality of Life after Treatment of Brain Metastases) trial, compared the Quality Adjusted Life Years (QALY) between optimal supportive care (OSC) alone and OSC + WBRT (20 Gy in 5 daily fractions) for NSCLC patients with brain metastases unsuitable for resection or stereotactic radiotherapy. OSC consisted of dexamethasone on patient's symptoms as well as patient access to palliative care clinicians and nurses. Results revealed a difference in mean QALY of 4.7 days (46.4 QALY days for OSC + WBRT vs. 41.7 QALY days for OSC), which was within the prespecified non-inferiority margin of 7 days. Overall survival was not significantly different between randomization arms (OSC + WBRT: 9.2 weeks vs. OSC alone: 8.5 weeks). Subgroup analysis suggested a survival benefit in favor of OSC + WBRT for patients younger than 60, KPS $\geq$ 70, and controlled extracranial primary (29-31).

WBRT has been frequently cited as a cause of neurocognitive decline in cancer patients on the literature, the Memorial Sloan-Kettering Cancer Center experience reported by DeAngelis et al. shows an 11% risk of radiation-induced dementia in patients undergoing WBRT for brain metastasis (32). The 11% figure is very misleading: of the 47 patients who survived 1 year after WBRT, 5 patients (11%) developed severe dementia. When these 5 patients were examined, all were treated in a fashion that would significantly increase the risk of late radiation toxicity, with large daily fractions and concurrent radiosensitizer. No patient who received the standard 30 Gy in 10 fractions

WBRT alone experienced dementia. RTOG 0933 and 0614 evaluating the role of hippocampal avoidance WBRT (HA-WBRT) and use of WBRT + memantine, respectively, in an effort to preserve memory-related dysfunction as was identified by Li et al. (33). RTOG 0933 was a phase II trial comparing the 4- month decline in HVLT-delayed recall scores with HA-WBRT (30 Gy in 10 fractions) relative to a historical control group receiving standard WBRT (30 Gy in 10 fractions). HA-WBRT resulted in a mean decline of 7% in HVLT-DR scores from baseline to 4 months, which was significantly lower than the mean decline of 30% for historical controls (34). RTOG 0614 was a phase III placebo controlled trial randomizing patients to WBRT (37.5 Gy in 15 fractions) with or without 24 weeks of memantine administration. The primary end point was the effect of memantine use on delayed recall at 24 weeks, which trended in favor of memantine use, though was not statistically significant (p = 0.059). Use of memantine resulted in superior results in delayed recognition, executive function, and processing speed (35).

Radiosurgery

Radiosurgery bring a satisfactory alternative to conventional surgery. The three above-mentioned randomized trials of surgical resection were all performed before the large scale availability of stereotactic radiosurgery (SRS). Although no randomized trials have been performed comparing surgery with SRS, SRS boost appears to provide at least comparable, if not improved, local control rates (80% to 90% when combined with WBRT). Thus, in the setting of limited intracranial disease burden, unless emergent surgery is warranted, SRS alone or as a boost can serve as a noninvasive alternative. There is an ample evidence that assessed the efficacy of SRS boost in the treatment of multiple metastases (36, 37). The study RTOG-95-08, the inclusion criteria was limited to 1 to 3 metastases, with maximum diameter of 4 cm for the largest lesion with additional lesions not exceeding 3 cm. WBRT dose was 37.5 Gy in 15 fractions, whereas SRS boost dose was lesion size based in accordance with the results of RTOG 90-05. The primary end point was overall survival, which was not statistically different between the WBRT plus SRS and WBRT-alone arms (6.5 and 5.7 months, respectively; P = .1356), although the SRS boost improved the survival in the subgroup (planned analysis) of patients with single metastasis (38). For secondary end points, the local control and performance measures were higher in the SRS boost arm, but this did not translate into a lower death rate from neurologic progression. Based on the major end points for multiple metastases, this study should be considered a negative trial. More recently, a secondary analysis of RTOG 95- 08 to determine the efficacy of SRS boost with patients re-stratified by DS-GPA scores. Their secondary analysis predominantly included lung cancer primaries (84%). Results revealed an overall survival benefit to SRS boost in patients with DS-GPA score of 3.5 to 4, irrespective of number of metastases (WBRT alone:10.3 months vs. WBRT + SRS: 21 months, $p = 0.05$). No survival benefit for SRS boost was observed with DS-GPA scores <3.5. These results should be interpreted with caution, however, given the small sample size and potential nonrandom selection of patients in the secondary analysis (39). In conclusion, although SRS boost is indicated (from RTOG-95-08 and from the extrapolation of surgical resection data) in patients with a single metastasis, it is difficult to justify its routine use in patients with multiple metastases in light of the equivocal phase III SRS boost trials.

An ongoing controversy in the treatment of brain metastasis is the role of WBRT postoperatively or post-SRS. In an earlier study by Sneed et al. patients who were initially treated with SRS alone without WBRT experienced worse freedom from new brain metastasis and overall brain freedom from progression despite the imbalance of the prognostic factors that favored the SRS-alone group, although the overall survival was not different (40). Because of the equivalency of overall survival, many have advocated withholding upfront WBRT with salvage therapies including repeat SRS or delayed WBRT for failures (41). The omission of upfront WBRT may have even more serious consequences for patients with more radioresistant tumors such as renal-cell carcinoma (RCC). The SRS dose given is typically limited by tumor size and volume, not by whether the patient received additional dose with WBRT, a patient treated with WBRT plus SRS receives much higher tumor dose than SRS alone (42,43). Given the long-term cognitive impact attributed to WBRT, however, contemporary series have evaluated the efficacy of postoperative SRS as an alternative to upfront WBRT. No phase III trials have been published to date, though two prospective trials have recently completed and reported in presentation form. Mahajan et al. (44) prospectively evaluated local tumor control rates of resected metastases receiving postoperative cavity SRS vs. observation in 1 to 3 brain metastases. All lesions not resected received definitive SRS. Secondary objectives included distant brain control and overall survival. Results revealed 1-year local control rates for observation and postoperative SRS of 45% and 72%, respectively ($p = 0.01$). One-year freedom from distant brain failure with observation and postoperative SRS was 33% and 43%, respectively ($p = 0.29$). Similarly, overall survival did not differ with use of postoperative cavity SRS (observation: 17 months vs. postoperative SRS: 17 months, $p = 0.37$). Have now been four phase III trials that have evaluated the role of SRS alone versus the addition of WBRT. In the Japanese Radiation Oncology Study Group JROSG-99-1 phase III trial of one to four lesions, the SRS-only arm experienced increased 1-year total brain recurrence rate ($p < 0.001$), increased 1-year rate of distant brain relapse ($p = 0.003$), and increased 1-year local tumor failure ($p = 0.002$). This resulted in more frequent use of salvage therapy ($p < 0.001$) in the SRS-alone arm (49). Furthermore, the average time until Mini-Mental State Examination (MMSE) deterioration was significantly longer for the WBRT plus SRS arm (16.5

months vs. 7.6 months; p = 0.05), in large part due to increased recurrence in the SRS group (45).

Median overall survival did not differ between groups (WBRT + SRS: 7.5 months vs. SRS alone: 8 months, p = 0.42). Despite, no overall survival benefit for the entire group, this study demonstrates the importance of WBRT in decreasing brain failure. Subsequently, this group has performed a secondary analysis evaluating the outcomes of post-SRS WBRT in non-small-cell lung primaries restratified by DS-GPA. Significantly increased median overall survival was observed with DSGPA score of 2.5 to 4 (WBRT + SRS: 16.7 months vs. SRS alone: 10.6 months, p = 0.04), whereas no survival differential was observed with DS-GPA scores <2.5. No significant difference in neurocognitive function, as assessed by the MMSE, was observed at baseline or during follow-up for WBRT + SRS or SRS alone arms for either DS-GPA scores <2.5 or >2.5 (56). The results of the secondary analyses of the RTOG 95-08 and JROSG-99-1 trials therefore indicate that patients with brain metastases from NSCLC primary with favorable DS-GPA scores may benefit more from combined treatment (WBRT + SRS) than either treatment alone. Future prospective examination of this conclusion is warranted. Muacevic et al. randomized single brain metastasis patients (KPS ≥ 70, size ≤ 3 cm, stable systemic disease) to SRS alone versus resection plus WBRT (46). Although this trial is not exactly an SRS ± WBRT trial, it addresses the benefit of WBRT to local therapies. Those randomized to SRS alone experienced worse distant (p = 0.04) recurrences, but there were no differences in neurologic death rates or overall survival.

The results of EORTC-22952-26001 have been reported with the primary end point of evaluating duration of functional independence (47). In this study, patients with one to three brain metastases underwent local therapy with either surgery or SRS and were then randomized to the addition of WBRT versus observation. WBRT did not improve duration of functional independence or overall survival but was associated with a significant decrease in 2-year local and distant brain relapse rate versus observation with either surgery or SRS. This resulted in a 16% decrease in the risk of neurologic death. Although there was no difference in duration of functional independence between the two arms, the authors conclude that this is likely because of a variety of factors, including the subjective definition of functional independence, the routine use of MRI imaging rendering the majority of recurrences as asymptomatic, and the potential impact of systemic progression on performance status.

Chang et al. (48) reported on a series of 58 patients with one to three brain metastases randomized to SRS with or without WBRT. The primary end point of the study was neurocognitive function, which was assessed using the Hopkins Verbal Learning Test-Revised at 4 months after therapy. They found that patients receiving combined therapy were more likely to have a decline in learning and memory function at 4 months compared with patients who did not receive WBRT. The median survival was 15.2 months for the SRS-alone group and 5.7 months for the WBRT/SRS group (p = 0.003).

However, the local (100% vs. 67%; p = 0.012) and distant (73% vs. 45%; p = 0.02) brain control rates were worse in the SRS-alone group compared with the WBRT/SRS group.

There are multiple criticisms of this study worth noting (49). First, because the primary end point was neurocognitive function, the authors did not stratify by baseline neurocognitive function or other factors known to impact neurocognition. Second, the authors chose a single test at a single time point. Ideally, a whole battery of tests should be performed at multiple time points to adequately assess the trend of something as complex as neurocognition. Most importantly, the combined arm inexplicably had a shorter survival, contrary to the four previously mentioned trials that demonstrated equivalent survivals. The median survival of 5.7 months was within two months of the primary end point mark, which classically falls within the time point of progressively worsening cognition seen in terminally ill patients (50, 51). The superior survival in spite of inferior local and distant brain control is unprecedented and can possibly be explained by an improper randomization, which is possible in a small study.

In summary, four of the five phase III local with or without WBRT trials unequivocally show a meaningful benefit of WBRT in terms of preventing neurologic deaths or brain failure. It is difficult to ignore the level I evidence provided by these phase III trials. Adjuvant WBRT, therefore, should be strongly considered after local therapy with surgical resection or SRS. However, this has become very controversial. Therefore, it is critical for radiation oncologists to help patients navigate through the risks and benefits of additional WBRT.

Given the success of SRS in treating patients with 1-4 brain metastases and the ability of modern machines and techniques that allow the delivery high doses of radiation in a more efficient manner, more centers are using SRS for patients with multiple (> 4) brain metastases. In addition, some centers have become particularly concerned about the impact of WBRT on neurocognitive function and have favored SRS alone as primary treatment option.

One potential concern of treating multiple lesions with SRS is the cumulative whole brain dose. Yamamoto and his colleagues reviewed the median cumulative dose to the whole brain for patients with at least 10 lesions who were treated by gamma knife (GK) radiosurgery (52). For this study, the median number of lesions treated with SRS was 17 (range 10-43). The median volume for all tumors was 8.02 cc (range: 0.46-81.41 cc). The median prescribed dose was 20 Gy (range 12-25 Gy). The median cumulative dose to the whole brain was 4.71 Gy (range 2.16-8.51 Gy). The median brain volumes receiving >10 Gy, 15 Gy, and 20 Gy were 64 cc, 24 cc, and 8 cc, respectively.

Another study from Yang (53) reported that 50% of the brain received less than 5 Gy when a maximum tumor dose of 40 Gy was used when treating 25 metastatic intracranial tumors. Hunter (54) reported the Cleveland Clinic experience for patients with 5 or more brain metastases treated with linac or GK radiosurgery. Patients were treated using the RTOG 9005 dosing regimen. The median survival after SRS was 7.5 months. Minimum

KPS of 80 significantly influenced overall survival (4.8 months for KPS 70 or lower versus 8.8 months for KPS of 80 or higher; $p = 0.0097$). The number of lesions (8 or fewer versus 9 or more) and primary site did not affect survival. On multivariate analysis, KPS and prior WBRT significantly predicted for better survival.

Yamamoto reported on 456 consecutive patients with brain metastases from non-lung cancers treated with GK from 1991 to 2004 (55). The mean and median tumor numbers were 6 and 2, respectively (range 1-55). Median cumulative treatment volume was 7.3 cc (range 0.041 to 122 cc). A dose of 20 Gy or more was used in 70% of patients. If the brain had already been irradiated or the cumulative tumor volume was relatively large, the dose was reduced by 30%. The median survival was 7 months after GK. Significant predictors for survival included number of lesions, maximum and cumulative tumor volumes, well controlled primary tumors, no extracranial metastases, KPS > 80, prior surgeries and minimum of two GK procedures.

The University of Pittsburgh evaluated their outcomes after single GK radiosurgery session for 205 patients with 4 or more intracranial metastases (56). Median number of lesions was 5 (range 4-18) with a median total tumor volume of 6.8 cc (range 0.6 51 cc). The median SRS dose was 16 Gy (range 12-20). The median survival after SRS was 8 months. One year local control rate was 71%. The median time to progressive/new brain metastases was 9 months. The median overall survival for RTOG RPA class 1, 2, and 3 was 18, 9 and 3 months, respectively($p < 0.00001$). On multivariate analysis, the number of brain metastases was not statistically significant. Total treatment volume, age, RPA classification and marginal dose were significant prognostic factors.

Serizawa reported on 2,390 consecutive patients with brain metastases who underwent GK radiosurgery from 1998 to 2005 at the Gamma House, Chiba Cardiovascular Center (Chiba) and Mito GammaHouse Katsuta Hospital (Mito) (57). The number of lesions treated ranged from 1 to 25+ brain metastases, with 204 patients (17.3%) at Chiba and 210 patients (17.3%) at Mito having 11 or more metastases. Whole brain radiation therapy was not used as initial management. Median survival was 7.7 months at Chiba and 7 months at Mito.

A Japanese multi-institutional prospective study (JLGK0901) prospectively evaluated patients with 1-10 brain metastases treated by GK SRS alone (58). The study evaluated 778 consecutive patients who met the following inclusion criteria: newly diagnosed brain metastases, 1-10 lesions, largest tumor < 10 cc, total tumor volume < 15 cc, no MRI evidence of CSF spread, and no impairment of daily activity secondary to extracranial disease. Whole brain radiation therapy was not used as initial treatment. Repeat SRS or WBRT was used when distant brain lesions occurred. Patients were stratified based on number of lesions: 1, 2, 3-4, 5-6, and 10. The number of lesions did not influence overall survival (0.83 years for 1, 0.69 years for 2, 0.69 years for 3-4, 0.59 years for 5-6, and 0.62 years for 7-10 lesions). On multivariate analysis, survival was significantly influenced by active systemic disease, KPS < 70, and male gender.

Table 1.

	N	Number of lesions	12-month local control	12-month recurrence	median survival (months)
Radiation Therapy Group 95-08 (N = 331)					
WBRT+SRS	164	1-3	82%	25%	6.5
WBRT	167	1-3	71%	30%	5.7
Japanese Radiation Oncology Study Group 99-1 (N = 132)					
SRS + WBRT	65	1-4	88,7%	47%	7.5
SRS	67	1-4	72,5%	76%	8.0
MD Anderson Cancer Center (N = 58)					
SRS + WBRT	28	1-3	100%	27%	5.7
SRS	30	1-3	67%	73%	15.2
NCCTG (Alliance) N0574 (N = 213)					
SRS+ WBRT	102	1-3	84.9%	-	7.4
SRS	111	1-3	50.5%	-	10.4

WBRT: whole brain radiotherapy; SRS: stereotactic radiotherapy.

Table 2.

	N	Treatment	Selection	Brain RR	OS	PFS
Porta et al. (63)	17	Erlotinib	EGFR mutated	82%	12.9 months	11.7 months
Park et al. (64)	28	Gefitinib or Erlotinib	EGFR mutated	83%	15.9 months	6.6 months
Li (65)	9	Gefitinib	EGFR mutated	89%	NS	NS
Kim et al. (66)	23	Gefitinib or Erlotinib	Asian non-smokers	74%	18.8 months	7.1 months
Welsh et al. (67)	40	Erlotinib	Unselected	86%	11.8 months	8 months
Iuchi et al. (68)	41	Gefitinib	EGFR mutated	88%	21.9 months	14.5 months
Hofknecht et al. (69)	32	Afatinib	EGFR mutated/ TKI pretreated	35%	9.8 months	3.6 months
Costa et al. (70)	40	Crizotinib	ALK-rearranged	25%	NS	7 months
Kim et al. (71)	124	Ceritinib	ALK-rearranged	69%	NS	6.9 months
Shaw et al. (72)	64	Ceritinib	ALK-rearranged	NS	20.3 months	6.9 months
Gadgeel et al. (73)	21	Alectinib	ALK-rearranged	52.%	NS	31.1 months
Ou et al. (74)	34	Alectinib	ALK-rearranged	55.9%	NS	10.3 months
Gandhi et al. (75)	48	Alectinib	ALK-rearranged	68.8%	NS	NS

RR: response rate; OS: overall survival; PFS: progression-free survival.

Targeted agents

The majority of traditional chemotherapies have shown limited activity in the central nervous system, which has been attributed to the blood-brain barrier and the molecular structure of the used agents. The discovery of driver mutations and drugs targeting these mutations has changed the treatment landscape. Several of these targeted small-molecule tyrosine kinase inhibitors do cross the blood-brain barrier and/or have shown activity in the central nervous system. Another major advance in the care of brain metastases has been the advent of new immunotherapeutic agents, for which initial studies have shown intracranial activity. Epidermal growth factor receptor (EGFR) mutations as well as anaplastic lymphoma kinase (ALK) rearrangements, which occur in 15% to 20% of advanced NSCLC cases represent two commonly targeted mutations (31).

Zimmerman et al. (59) identified a brain metastasis response rate of 74% to 89% with the use of EGFR tyrosine kinase inhibitors (TKIs). Similarly, Rusthoven et al. (60) noted response rates of 36% to 67% with next-generation TKI's, such as alectinib, in ALK-positive NSCLC brain metastases. Magnuson et al. (61) have reported the largest pooled multi-institutional analysis to date evaluating the optimal sequencing of EGFR-TKI's and radiation therapy in patients with EGFR-mutant NSCLC brain metastases. TKI naive patients who had developed brain metastases underwent one of three treatment regimens: SRS followed by EGFRTKI, WBRT followed by EGFR-TKI, or EGFR-TKI followed by SRS or WBRT at a time of intracranial progression. Patients receiving upfront EGFR-TKI had smaller (<1 cm) and less symptomatic intracranial disease. Median OS for the upfront SRS, WBRT, and EGFR-TKI arms was 46, 30, and 25 months, respectively ($p < 0.001$). Both upfront SRS and WBRT use were independently associated with improved OS relative to upfront EGFR-TKI. Use of upfront SRS or WBRT was also associated with a trend toward lower risk of intracranial progression, highlighting the potential for inferior outcomes with deferral of early radiotherapy (61). On the contrary, Gerber et al. (62) found equivalent survival outcomes with use of upfront EGFR-TKI or WBRT in patients with EGFR mutant brain metastases. Prospective trials remain assured at this time to address the role of targeted agents.

Conclusion

Brain metastasis is the most common intracranial tumor and the incidence is increasing due to advancements in systemic therapy (improved extracranial control) with limited penetration of the blood-brain barrier in conjunction with increased utilization of MRI/surveillance imaging. Steroids reduce leakage from tumor vessels, therefore decreasing edema and mass effect in patients with symptomatic brain metastasis. Surgery should be considered for patients with single lesion amenable to resection, controlled or absent extracranial disease, KPS >70, age <60 years old, life expectancy >2 months, need for immediate relief of neurologic surgery secondary to mass effect or need to establish a tissue diagnosis. The standard of care in select patients with diffuse brain metastasis (≥5 brain metastases) continues to be WBRT. The most commonly utilized WBRT dose is 30 Gy/10 and 25% of patients have a complete response to WBRT for brain metastases. Adjuvant WBRT reduced the 2-year relapse rate both at initial sites and new sites, with decreased rates of death secondary to intracranial progression without improvement in the duration of functional independence or OS. The criteria for SRS includes: spherical/pseudospherical target, generally noninfiltrative lesions (<3-4 cm) located along the gray-white junction (non-eloquent regions), ability to deliver a higher dose than can be achieved with WBRT alone (improved LC), treatment of unresectable lesions, and reduced risk of neurocognitive decline depending on location of lesion(s). The SRS boost after WBRT dose was dependent on size in accordance: 24 Gy if <2-cm diameter, 18 Gy if 2-3 cm, and 15 Gy if 3-4 cm. The addition of SRS improved the median survival for patients with a single brain metastasis. The omission of WBRT after SRS for 1-4 brain metastases does not affect survival but increases the risk of intracranial relapse and thus increases the need for salvage therapy. The SRS dose was based on size lesions ≤2 cm to 22-25 Gy and lesions >2 cm to 18-20 Gy. There are a recommendation for initial treatment of 1-3 newly diagnosed brain metastasis with SRS alone with close observation (MRI is generally recommended every 2-4 months) in order to preserve cognitive function. The new immunotherapeutic agents, for which initial studies have shown intracranial activity, was also associated with a trend toward lower risk of CNS progression

References

[1] Gavrilovic IT, Posner JB. *Brain metastases: epidemiology and pathophysiology*. J Neurooncol 2005;75(1):5-14.

[2] Kaal EC, Niel CG, Vecht CJ. *Therapeutic management of brain metastasis*. Lancet Neurol 2005;4:289-98.

[3] Nathoo N, Chahlavi A, Barnett GH, Toms SA. *Pathobiology of brain metastases*. J Clin Pathol 2005;58(3):237-42.

[4] Fox BD, Cheung VJ, Patel AJ, Suki D, Rao G. *Epidemiology of metastatic brain tumors*. Neurosurg Clin North Am 2011;22(1):1-6,v.

[5] Davis FG, Dolecek TA, McCarthy BJ, Villano JL. *Toward determining the lifetime occurrence of metastatic brain tumors estimated from 2007 United States cancer incidence data*. Neuro Oncol 2012;14(9):1171-7.

[6] Nayak L, Lee EQ, Wen PY. *Epidemiology of brain metastases*. Curr Oncol Rep 2002;14(1):48-54.

[7] Feng W, Zhang P, Zheng X, Chen M, Mao WM. *Incidence and treatment of brain metastasis in patients with esophageal carcinoma*. World J Gastroenterol 2015;21(19):5805-12.

[8] Villano JL, Durbin EB, Normandeau C, Thakkar JP, Moiranguthem V, Davis FG. *Incidence of brain metastasis at initial presentation of lung cancer*. Neuro Oncol 2015;17(1):122-8.

[9] Schouten LJ, Rutten J, Huveneers, Twijnstra A, et al. *Incidence of brain metastases in a cohort of patients with carcinoma of the breast, colon, kidney, and lung and melanoma*. Cancer 2002;94(10):2698-705.

[10] Barnholtz-Sloan JS, Sloan AE, Davis FG, Vigneau FD, Lai P, Sawaya RE. *Incidence proportions of brain metastases in patients diagnosed (1973 to 2001) in the Metropolitan Detroit Cancer Surveillance System*. J Clin Oncol 2004;22(14): 2865-72.

[11] Posner JB, Chernik NL. *Intracranial metastases from systemic cancer*. Adv Neurol 1978;19:579-92.

[12] Takakura K. *Metastatic tumors of the central nervous system*. Tokyo: Igaku-Shoin, 1982.

[13] Lagerwaard FJ, Levendag PC, Nowak PJ, Eijkenboom VM, Hanssens PE, Schmitz PI. *Identification of prognosticfactors in patients with brain metastases: a review of 1292 patients*. Int J Radiat Oncol Biol Phys 1999;43(4):795-803.

[14] DeVita VT, Lawrence TS, Rosenberg SA. *DeVita, Hellman, and Rosenberg's Cancer: Principles & Practice of Oncology*. 10th ed. Philadelphia: Wolters Kluwer, 2015.

[15] Nussbaum ES, Djalilian HR, Cho KH, Hall WA. *Brain metastases. Histology, multiplicity, surgery, and survival*. Cancer 1996;78(8):1781-8.

[16] Barnholtz-Sloan JS, Sloan AE, Davis FG, Vigneau FD, Lai P, Sawaya RE. *Incidence proportions of brain metastases in patients diagnosed (1973 to 2001) in the Metropolitan Detroit Cancer Surveillance System*. J Clin Oncol 2004;22(14):28 65-72.

[17] Posner JB. *Brain metastases: 1995. A brief review*. J Neurooncol 1996;27(3):287-93.

[18] Fink KR, Fink JR. *Imaging of brain metastases*. Surg Neurol Int 2013;4(Suppl 4):S209-19.

[19] Soffietti R, Cornu P, Delattre JY, Grant R, Graus F, Grisold W, et al. *EFNS Guidelines on diagnosis and treatment of brain metastases: report of an EFNS Task Force*. Eur J Neurol 2006;13(7):674-81.

[20] Sperduto PW, Kased N, Roberge D, Xu Z, Stanley R, Luo X, et al. *Summary report on the graded prognostic assessment: an accurate and facile diagnosis-specific tool to estimate survival for patients with brain metastases*. J Clin Oncol 2012;30(4):419-25.

[21] Ruderman NB, Hall TC. *Use of glucocorticoids in the palliative treatment of metastatic brain tumors*. Cancer 1965;18:298-306.

[22] Glantz MJ, Cole BF, Forsyth PA, Recht LD, Wen PY, Chamberlain MC, et al. *Practice parameter: anticonvulsant prophylaxis in patients with newly diagnosed brain tumors*. Report of the Quality Standards Subcommittee of the American Academy of Neurology. Neurology 2000;54(10):1886-93.

[23] Delattre JY, Krol G, Thaler HT, Posner JB. *Distribution of brain metastases*. Arch Neurol 1988;45(7):741-4.

[24] Patchell RA, Tibbs PA, Walsh JW, Dempsey RJ, Maruyama Y, Kryscio RJ, et al. *A randomized trial of surgery in thetreatment of single metastases to the brain*. N Engl J Med 1990;322(8):494-500.

[25] Noordijk EM, Vecht CJ, Haaxma-Reiche H, Padberg GW, Voormolen JH, Hoekstra FH, et al. *The choice of treatment of single brain metastasis should be based on extracranial tumor activity and age*. Int J Radiat Oncol Biol Phys 1994;29(4):711-7.

[26] Mintz AH, Kestle J, Rathbone MP, Gaspar L, Hugenholtz H, Fisher B, et al. *A randomized trial to assess the efficacy of surgery in addition to radiotherapy in patients with a single cerebral metastasis*. Cancer 1996;78(7):1470-6.

[27] Coia LR. *The role of radiation therapy in the treatment of brain metastases*. Int J Radiat Oncol Biol Phys 1992;23(1):229-38.

[28] Nieder C, Berberich W, Schnabel K. *Tumor-related prognostic factors for remission of brain metastases after radiotherapy*. Int J Radiat Oncol Biol Phys 1997;39(1):25-30.

[29] Mulvenna P, Nankivell M, Barton R, Faivre-Finn C, Wilson P, McColl E, et al. *Dexamethasone and supportive care with or without whole brain radiotherapy in treating patients with nonsmall cell lung cancer with brain metastases unsuitable for resection or stereotactic radiotherapy (QUARTZ): results from a phase 3, noninferiority, randomised trial*. Lancet 2016;388(10055):2004-14.

[30] Cagney DN, Alexander BM, Aizer AA. Whole brain radiotherapy for nonsmall cell lung cancer. Lancet 2017;389(10077):1394-5.

[31] Zhu J, Kang M, Fan X. *Whole brain radiotherapy for non-small cell lung cancer.* Lancet 2017;389(10077):1395.

[32] DeAngelis LM, Mandell LR, Thaler HT, Kimmell DW, Galicich JH, Fuks Z, et al. *The role of postoperative radiotherapy after resection of single brain metastases.* Neurosurgery 1989;24(6):798-805.

[33] Li J, Bentzen SM, Renschler M, Mehta MP. *Regression after whole-brain iradiation therapy for brain metastases correlates with survival and improved neurocognitive function.* J Clin Oncol 2007;25(10):1260-66.

[34] Gondi V, Pugh SL, Tome WA, Caine C, Corn B, Kanner A, et al. *Preservation of memory with conformal avoidance of the hippocampal neural stem-cell compartment during whole-brain radiotherapy for brain metastases (RTOG 0933): aphase II multi-institutional trial.* J Clin Oncol 2014;32(34):3810-6.

[35] Brown PD, Pugh S, Laack NN, Wefel JS, Khuntia D, Meyers C, et al. *Memantine for the prevention ofcognitive dysfunction in patients receiving whole-brain radiotherapy: arandomized, double-blind, placebo-controlled trial.* Neuro Oncol 2013;15(10):1429-37.

[36] Kondziolka D, Patel A, Lunsford LD, Kassam A, Flickinger JC. *Stereotactic radiosurgery pluswhole brain radiotherapy versus radiotherapy alone for patients with multiple brain metastases.* Int J Radiat Oncol Biol Phys 1999;45(2):427-34.

[37] Chougule P, Burton-Williams M, Saris S, Zheng Z, Ponte B, Noren G, et al. Randomized treatment of brain metastasis with gamma knife radiosurgery, whole brain radiotherapy or both. Int J Radiat Oncol Biol Phys 2000;3(48):114.

[38] Sperduto PW, Shanley R, Luo X, Andrews D, Werner-Wasik M, Valicenti R, et al. *Secondary analysis of RTOG 9508, a phase 3 randomized trial of whole-brain radiation therapy versus WBRT plus stereotactic radiosurgery in patients with 1-3 brain metastases; poststratified by the graded prognostic assessment (GPA).* Int J Radiat Oncol Biol Phys 2014;90(3):526-31.

[39] Sneed PK, Suh JH, Goetsch SJ, Sanghavi SN, Chappell R, Buatti JM, et al. *A multi-institutional review of radiosurgery alone vs. radiosurgery with whole brain radiotherapy as the initial management of brain metastases.* Int J Radiat Oncol Biol Phys 2002;53(3):519-26.

[40] Sneed PK, Lamborn KR, Forstner JM, McDermott MW, Chang S, Park E, et al. *Radiosurgery for brain metastases: is whole brain radiotherapy necessary?* Int J Radiat Oncol Biol Phys 1999;43(3):549-58.

[41] Regine WF, Huhn JL, Patchell RA, St Clair WH, Strottmann J, Meigooni A, et al. *Risk of symptomatic brain tumor recurrence and neurologic deficit after radiosurgery alone in patients with newly diagnosed brain metastases: Results and implications.* Int J Radiat Oncol Biol Phys 2002;52(2):333-8.

[42] Manon R, O'Neill A, Knisely J, Werner-Wasik M, Lazarus HM, Wagner H, et al. *Phase II trial of radiosurgery for one to three newly diagnosed brain metastases from renal cell carcinoma, melanoma, and sarcoma: an Eastern Cooperative Oncology Group study (E6397).* J Clin Oncol 2005;23(34):8870-76.

[43] Patchell RA, Tibbs PA, Regine WF, Dempsey RJ, Mohiuddin M, Kryscio RJ, et al. *Postoperative radiotherapy in thetreatment of single metastases to the brain: A randomized trial.* JAMA1998;280(17):1485-9.

[44] Mahajan A, Ahmed S, Li J, McAleer MF, Weinberg J, Brown PD, et al. *Postoperative stereotactic radiosurgery versus observation for completely resected brain metastases: results of a prospective randomized study.* Int J Radiat Oncol Biol Phys 2016;96(2S):S2.

[45] Aoyama H, Tago M, Kato N, Toyoda T, Kenjyo M, hirota S, et al. *Neurocognitive function of patients with brain metastasis who received either whole brain radiotherapy plus stereotactic radiosurgery or radiosurgery alone.* Int J Radiat Oncol Biol Phys 2007;68(5):1388-95.

[46] Muacevic A, Wowra B, Siefert A, Tonn JC, Steiger HC, Kreth FW, et al. *Microsurgery plus whole brain irradiation versus Gamma Knife surgery alone for treatment of single metastases to the brain: a randomized controlled multicentre phase III trial.* J Neurooncol 2008;87(3):299-307.

[47] Kocher M, Soffietti R, Abacioglu U, Villa S, Fauchon F, Baumert BG, et al. *Adjuvant whole-brain radiotherapy versus observation after radiosurgery or surgical resection of one to three cerebral metastases: results of the EORTC 22952-26001 study.* J Clin Oncol 2011;29(2):134-41.

[48] Chang EL, Wefel JS, Hess KR, Allen PK, Lang FF, Kornguth DG, et al. *Neurocognition in patients with brain metastases treated with radiosurgery or radiosurgery plus whole-brain irradiation: a randomised controlled trial.* Lancet Oncol 2009;10(11):1037-44.

[49] Mahmood U, Kwok Y, Regine WF, Patchell RA. *Whole-brain irradiation for patients with brain metastases: still the standard of care.* Lancet Oncol 2010;11(3):221-222; author reply 223.

[50] Lawlor PG, Gagnon B, Mancini IL, Pereira JL, Hanson J, Suarez-Almazor ME, et al. *Occurrence, causes, and outcome of delirium in patients with advanced cancer: a prospective study.* Arch Intern Med 2000;160(6):786-94.

[51] Pereira J, Hanson J, Bruera E. *The frequency and clinical course of cognitive impairment in patients with terminal cancer.* Cancer 1997;79(4):835-42.

[52] Yamamoto M, Ide M, Nishio S, Urakawa Y. *Gamma knife radiosurgery for numerous brain metastases: is this a safe treatment.* Int J Radiat Oncol Biol Phys 2002;53(5):1279-83.

[53] Yang CC, Ting J, Wu X, Markoe A. *Dose volume histogram analysis of the gamma knife radiosurgery treating twenty-five metastatic intracranial tumors.* Stereotact Funct Neurosurg 1998;70(Suppl 1):41-9.

[54] Suzuki S, Omagari J, Nishio S, Nishiye E, Fukui M. *Gamma knife radiosurgery for simultaneous multiple metastatic brain tumors.* J Neurosurg 2000;93(Suppl 3):30-1.

[55] Hunter G, Suh J, Reuther AM, Vogelbaum M, Barnett GH, Angelov L, et al. *Treatment of five or more brain metastases with stereotactic radiosurgery.* Int J Radiat Oncol Biol Phys 2012;83(5):1394-8.

[56] Yamamoto M, Barfod BE, Urakawa Y. *Gamma knife radiosurgery for brain metastases of non-lung cancer origin: focusing on multiple brain lesions.* Prog Neurol Surg 2009;22:154-69.

[57] Serizawa T, Yamamoto M, Nagano O, Higuchi Y, Matsuda S, Ono J, et al. *Gamma knife surgery for metastatic brain tumors.* J Neurosurg 2008;109 (Suppl 1):118-21.

[58] Serizawa T, Hirai T, Nagano O, Higuchi Y, Matsuda S, Ono H, et al. *Gamma knife radiosurgery for 1-10 brain metastases without prophylactic whole-brain radiation therapy: analysis of cases meeting the Japanese prospective multi-institute study (JLG0901) inclusion criteria.* J Neurooncol 2010;98(2):163-7.

[59] Zimmermann S, Dziadziuszko R, Peters S. *Indications and limitations of chemotherapy and targeted agents in non-small cell lung cancer brain metastases.* Cancer Treat Rev 2014;40(6):716-22.

[60] Rusthoven CG, Doebele RC. *Management of brain metastases in ALK positive non-small-cell lung cancer.* J Clin Oncol 2016;34(24):2814-9.

[61] Magnuson WJ, Lester-Coll NH, Wu AJ, Yang TJ, Lockney NA, Gerber NK, et al. *Management of brain metastases in tyrosine kinase inhibitor-naive epidermal growth factor receptor-mutant non-small-cell lung cancer: a retrospective multi-institutional analysis.* J Clin Oncol 2017;35(10):1070-7.

[62] Gerber DE, Ghandi L, Costa DB. *Management and future directions in non-small cell lung cancer with known activating mutations.* Am Soc Clin Oncol Educ Book 2014:e353-65.

[63] Porta R, Sanchez-Torres JM, Paz-Ares L, Massuti B, Reguart N, Mayo C, et al. *Brain metastases from lung cancer responding to erlotinib: the importance of EGFR mutation.* Eur Respir J 2011;37(3):624-31.

[64] Park SJ, Kim HT, Lee DH, Kim KP, Kim SW, Suh C, et al. *Efficacy of epidermal growth factor receptor tyrosine kinase inhibitors for brain metastases in non-small-cell lung cancer harbouring either exon 19 or 21 mutation.* Lung Cancer 2012;77(3):556-60.

[65] Li Z. *The retrospective analysis of the frequency of EGFR mutations and the efficacy of gefitinib in NSCLC patients with brain metastases.* J Clin Oncol 2011;29(Suppl):e18065.

[66] Kim JE, Lee DH, Choi Y, Yoon DH, Kim SW, Suh C et al. *Epidermal growth factor receptor tyrosine kinase inhibitors as a first-line therapy for never-smokers with adenocarcinoma of the lung having asymptomatic synchronous brain metastasis.* Lung Cancer 2008;65(3):351-4.

[67] Welsh JW, Komaki R, Amini A, Munsell MF, Unger W, Allen PK, et al. *Phase II trial of erlotinib plus concurrent whole-brain radiation therapy for patients with brain metastases from non-small-cell lung cancer.* J Clin Oncol 2013;31(7):895-902.

[68] Iuchi T, Shingyoji M, Sakaida T, Hatano K, Nagano O, Itakura M, et al. *Phase II trial of gefitinib alone without radiation therapy for Japanese patients with brain metastases from EGFR-mutant lung adenocarcinoma.* Lung Cancer 2013;82(2): 282-7.

[69] Hoffknecht P, Tufman A, Wehler T, Pelzer T, Wierodt R, Schütz M, et al. *Efficacy of the irreversible ErbB family blocker afatinib in epidermal growth factor receptor (EGFR) tyrosine kinase inhinbitor (TKI)-pretreated non-small-cell lung cancer patients with brain metastases or brain metastases or leptomeningeal disease.* J Thorac Oncol 2015;10(1):156-63.

[70] Costa DB, Kobayashi S and Pandya SS. *CSF concentration of the anaplastic lymphoma kinase inhibitor crizotinib.* J Clin Oncol 2011;29(15):e443-5.

[71] Kim DW, Mehra R, Tan DSW, Felip E, Chow LQM, Camidge DR, et al. *Ceritinib in advanced anaplastic lymphoma kinase (ALK)-rearranged (ALK+) non-small cell lung cancer (NSCLC): Results of the ASCEND-1 trial.* J Clin Oncol 2014;32(5s): 422s.

[72] Shaw AT, Kim DW, Nakagawa K, Seto T, Crinó L, Ahn MJ, et al. *Crizotinib versus chemotherapy in advanced ALK-positive lung cancer.* N Engl J Med 2013;368(25):2385-94.

[73] Gadgeel SM, Gandhi L, Riely GJ, Chiappori AA, West HL, Azada MC, et al. *Safety and activity of alectinib against systemic disease and brain metastases in patients with crizotinib-resistant ALK-rearranged non-small-cell lung cancer (AF-002JG): results from the dosefinding portion of a phase 1/2 study.* Lancet Oncol 2014;15(10):1119-28.

[74] Ou SHI, Ahn JS, Petris DE, Gowindan R, Yang JCH, Hughes BGH, et al. *Efficacy and safety of the ALK inhibitor alectinib in ALK+ non-small-cell lung cancer (NSCLC) patients who have failed prior crizotinib: an open-label, single-arm, global phase 2 study (NP28673).* J Clin Oncol 2015;33(Suppl 15s):424s.

[75] Gandhi L, Shaw A, Gadgeel SM, Riely G, Cetnar J, West HJ, et al. *A phase II, open-label, multicentre study of the ALK inhibitor alectinib in an ALK+ non-small-cell lung cancer (NSCLC) U.S./Canadian population who had progressed on crizotinib (NP28761).* J Clin Oncol 2015;33(Suppl 15s):426s.

In: Cancer Management in Latin America II
Editors: Maurício F Silva et al.
ISBN: 978-1-53616-735-1

Chapter 11

MANAGEMENT OF CANCER EMERGENCIES

Jorge Henrique Leal[1,*], MD, MSc, Heather L McArthur[2], MD, MPH, Fiona Lim[3], MBBS, Bo Angela Wan[4], MD(C), Beatriz Amendola[5], MD and Mauricio F Silva[6,7,8], MD, PhD

[1]CLION – CAM Group, Salvador, Bahia, Brazil,
[2]Cedars-Sinai Medical Center, Los Angeles, California, United States of America,
[3]Princess Margaret Hospital, Hong Kong, PR China,
[4]Odette Cancer Centre, Sunnybrook Health Sciences Centre, Toronto, Ontario, Canada,
[5]Innovative Cancer Institute, South Miami, Florida, United States of America,
[6]Radiation Oncology Unit, Santa Maria Federal University, Santa Maria, Brazil,
[7]Radiation Oncology Unit, Hospital de Caridade Astrogildo de Azevedo, Santa Maria, Brazil
[8]Latin America Cooperative Oncology Group, Porto Alegre, Brazil

ABSTRACT

Cancer emergencies comprise a group of medical conditions presented by patients with an underlying malignant neoplasm and demands high clinical suspicion. Proper management depends on a fast and precise diagnosis, and the outcomes may impact patient survival and quality of life. In countries where early detection programs are not adequately implemented, a significant proportion of patients present with emergency symptoms as their first sign of disease. This chapter will give an overview of diagnosis and treatment of hypercalcemia, tumor lysis syndrome, cardiac tamponade, metastatic spinal cord compression and superior vena cava syndrome.

* Corresponding Author's Email: jorge.leal@clion.com.org.

INTRODUCTION

Cancer is a major cause of morbidity and mortality, with approximately 14 million new cases and 8 million cancer-related deaths in 2012, affecting populations in all countries and all regions, with 60% occurring in Africa, Asia, Central and South America (1). Despite worldwide efforts to promote early detection, some patients still present with emergency symptoms as the first sign of disease (2). Thus, medical education regarding diagnosis and treatment of major cancer related emergencies remains critically important. This chapter will review some of the practical aspects of the five most common oncological emergencies diagnosed in emergency departments.

HYPERCALCEMIA

Hypercalcemia of malignancy (HM) is one of the most common types of paraneoplastic syndromes, with various incidences reported depending on study populations and designs. In hematological malignancies, the incidence of HM in multiple myeloma and acute T-cell lymphocytic leukemia (ATLL) is 30% and 70%, respectively (3). In adults with non-hematological cancers, hypercalcemia may occur in up to 30% of patients during the course of their disease (4). Furthermore, it is considered an important cancer emergency, since it conveys a poor prognostic factor for hospitalized patients, with a 30-day mortality incidence of 50% (5). The degree of hypercalcemia can be classified by total or ionized serum calcium level as mild (10.5–11.9 mg/dL or 5.6-8.0 mg/dL), moderate (12.0–13.9 mg/dL or 8.0-10.0 mg/dL), or severe (≥14.0 mg/dL or 10-12 mg/dL), but since half of serum calcium is protein-bound and formulas to correct for hypoalbuminemia are imprecise, the use of ionized calcium as the standard of care for evaluating hypercalcemia is recommended (6).

Maintaining calcium balance involves a complex homeostatic interplay involving parathyroid glands, bone, kidney and gut, orchestrated by parathyroid hormone (PTH) and active vitamin D [1,25(O)2D]. The calcium ion (Ca^{2+}) is intimately involved in its own short-term regulation through a calcium-sensing receptor (CaSR) found in parathyroid glands (as well as other tissues). A change in Ca^{2+} concentration from the physiologic range of 1.10 to 1.35mmol/l results in an appropriate compensatory change in PTH release and formation (7).

Depending on the etiology and pathogenesis, HM can be classified in four different types: humoral hypercalcemia of malignancy (80%), local osteolytic hypercalcemia (20%), followed by rare cases of 1,25 $(OH)_2D$-secreting lymphomas (1%) and ectopic hyperparathyroidism (1%) (8). Except for the osteolytic hypercalcemia, all others are considered as paraneoplastic syndromes, with no alterations in parathyroid gland nor presence of bone metastasis. More than 80% of the cases results from secretion of parathyroid hormone-related protein (PTHrP) by cancer cells. Composed of 139-173 amino acids, PTHrP shares 13 N-terminal homologies with PTH, and stimulates osteoclastic bone resorption and renal tubular calcium reabsorption (9). It occurs most commonly in squamous cell tumors (lung, head and neck, esophagus and cervix cancers) but it is also seen in other cancer types such as renal cell, ovarian, endometrial, breast, HTLV-associated lymphoma and neuroendocrine gastrointestinal cancers (GI-NETs) (10). Rarely, hypercalcemia may result from ectopic 1,25-dihydroxy (OH)2 vitamin D secretion, particularly in association with certain hematological malignancies (lymphomas) and NETs, or from ectopic PTH secretion (11). The second most common cause of MH is the local osteolytic hypercalcemia, mostly related to marked increase in osteoclastic bone resorption in areas surrounding the malignant cells within the bone marrow space due to cytokines as IL-1, IL-6 and IL-8. It can be a consequence of metastatic bone disease from epithelial tumors (breast cancer) or from hematological malignancies directly involving the marrow (multiple myeloma and lymphoma) (12).

Hypercalcemia as a syndrome has a myriad of symptoms such as lethargy, mental confusion, constipation, nausea, vomiting, cardiac dysrhythmias, but can also present as only a laboratory abnormality. In patients with high risk for cancer related hypercalcemia, any suspicion should be followed by a laboratory panel with complete blood count, ionized serum calcium levels, electrolyte panel, renal function and albumin level and electrocardiogram (13). In cases where patients are in cancer remission, a PTH test level should be obtained in order to rule out primary hyperparathyroidism (14).

After a diagnosis of HM has been stablished, the goal is to treat the underlying malignant condition contributing for the hypercalcemia associated with adequate supportive measures, patient hydration and use of some specific medications. General supportive measures: removal of any source of calcium intake (parenteral, enteral or oral); discontinuation of medications that may independently lead to hypercalcemia (e.g., lithium, calcitriol, vitamin D, and thiazides); treat hypophosphatemia (e.g., keep the calcium-phosphorus product below 40 with adequate renal function) (8). Restoring adequate intravascular volume is fundamental to improving glomerular filtration rate and decreasing passive sodium–calcium reabsorption from the proximal tubule. Normal saline infusion is recommended at 200–500 mL/hr and adjusted for a urine output of 100–150 mL/hour, in the absence of any contraindications. This will increase the glomerular filtration rate (inhibiting calcium reabsorption in proximal nephron) and allow safe use of loop diuretics to inhibit calcium reabsorption in the ascending loop of Henle (15). Hemodialysis is generally indicated for congestive heart failure, severe kidney injury (glomerular filtration rate <10–20 mL/min), clinically significant neurological findings, or calcium concentration >18 mg/dL (16). The most effective and safest specific medications used in the treatment of MH are intravenous bisphosphonates. These drugs work by blocking osteoclastic bone resorption. Because they are poorly absorbed when given orally (approximately 1 to 2 percent of an oral dose is absorbed), only intravenously administered bisphosphonates are used for this indication (17). Bisphosphonate therapy should be initiated as soon as hypercalcemia is discovered, because a response requires two to four days, and the nadir in serum calcium generally occurs within four to seven days after therapy is initiated (18). Zoledronic acid was shown to have greater efficacy than pamidronate in the treatment of hypercalcaemia of malignancy in a pooled analysis of two randomised, double-blind, phase 3 trials involving 275 patients with moderate-to-severe hypercalcaemia of malignancy. Treatment with zoledronic acid resulted in a significantly higher proportion of complete responses by day 10 (88.4 versus 69.7%; $p = 0.002$), more rapid calcium normalization, and more durable responses than treatment with pamidronate (19). Both drugs have been reported to cause or exacerbate renal failure, but this effect has generally occurred in patients receiving multiple doses (20). Since hypercalcemia is a frequent cause of renal dysfunction in patients with MH, effective treatment of the hypercalcemia associated with cancer often improves renal function, although in patients with CrCl < 30mL/min their use it is not recommended (21). Ibandronate, also a nitrogen-containing bisphosphonate, has been successfully used, notably in patients with myeloma and renal failure (22). Although not currently indicated for the treatment of hypercalcemia of malignancy, ibandronate may offer an alternative therapy for patients with renal failure (23).

More than 90% of patients with hypercalcaemia of malignancy can be successfully treated with rehydration and bisphosphonates; however, some patients do not respond to or experience relapse on bisphosphonate therapy. Persistent or relapsed hypercalcaemia of malignancy remains a difficult complication to manage (24). The receptor activator of nuclear factor K ligand (RANKL) system is the molecular pathway that leads to osteoclast recruitment and differentiation and bone resorption in hypercalcemia associated with cancer. Denosumab, a fully-human IgG2 monoclonal antibody against RANKL that disrupts signaling through RANK and prevents tumour-mediated activation of osteoclasts (25), has been shown to be effective for the treatment of patients with bisphosphonate-refractory hypercalcaemia. In a single-arm, open-label study, 33 patients with hypercalcaemia of malignancy despite recent bisphosphonate treatment received denosumab 120 mg on days 1, 8, 15, and 29, and then every 4 weeks. In total, 64% of patients responded to denosumab treatment by day 10, with 36% of patients experiencing a complete response (26). The results of this study formed the basis of the approval of denosumab for the treatment of bisphosphonate-refractory hypercalcaemia of malignancy in the USA, Australia, Canada, and Russia (27-30). Denosumab, therefore, offers a new treatment option for patients with persistent hypercalcaemia that does not respond to bisphosphonates or hypercalcaemia that relapses following bisphosphonate treatment.

Several agents commonly used before the advent of bisphosphonates are now used infrequently, usually when bisphosphonates are ineffective or contraindicated. Some examples are the use of calcitonin, glucocorticoids (31), mithramycin (32), and gallium nitrate (33). Table 1 summarizes the physiopathology of malignant hypercalcemia and suggested treatment interventions mentioned above.

Table 1. Physiopathology of malignant hypercalcemia (MH) and suggested sequence interventions

<table>
<tr><th>Type of MH (Frequency)</th><th>Physiopathology</th><th>Common tumors</th><th>Suggested intervention sequence</th></tr>
<tr><td>Humoral hypercalcemia (80%)</td><td>Secretion of PTHrP by cancer cells</td><td>squamous cell tumors (lung cancer, head and neck, esophagus and cervix cancers), renal cell, ovarian, endometrial, breast, lymphomas and NETs</td><td rowspan="4">Direct cancer therapy (systemic or surgery)

IV bisphosphonates

Intravenous Saline (200-500mL/hr)

Furosemide (calciuresis)

Correct serum phosphorus (repletion)

Denosumab*

Glucocorticoids**</td></tr>
<tr><td>Local osteolytic hypercalcemia (20%)</td><td>Induction of osteoclastic bone resorption by cytokines and growth factors, RANKL, PTHrP</td><td>Breast, multiple myeloma, lymphoma, leukemias</td></tr>
<tr><td>1.25(OH)$_2$D-secreting lymphomas (<1%)</td><td>Ectopic 1,25-dihydroxy(OH)2 vitamin D secretion</td><td>Lymphomas</td></tr>
<tr><td>Ectopic hyperparathyroidism (<1%)</td><td>Ectopic PTH secretion</td><td>Primary parathyroid carcinoma</td></tr>
</table>

1,25(OH)2D, 1,25-dihydroxyvitamin D; PTHrP, parathyroid hormone-related protein; PTH, parathyroid hormone; RANKL, receptor activator of nuclear factor kB ligand; NET, neuroendocrine tumors; IV, intra venous.
* For bisphosphonate refractory hypercalcemia ** Should be part of initial treatment in lymphomas.

TUMOUR LYSIS SYNDROME

Acute tumor lysis syndrome (TLS) is a potentially life-threatening emergency characterized by metabolic derangements as consequence of tumor cells releasing their contents in the bloodstream, spontaneously or in response to cancer treatment (34). The hallmark of this syndrome is the presence of at least two of the following laboratory abnormalities: hyperuricemia, hyperkalemia, hypocalcemia, and hyperphosphatemia. These metabolic disturbances can progress to clinical toxic effects including end organ damage such as renal insufficiency, cardiac arrhythmias, seizures, and finally death (35). Patients at highest risk for TLS are those with treatment-sensitive malignancy with a high proliferation rate and/or a large tumor burden. Other factors such as pre-existing kidney disease, elevated pretreatment uric acid, and volume depletion may also predict a higher risk for TLS. If undiagnosed or diagnosed too late, TLS can lead to death in 20%–50% of cases (36). The incidence of this important medical emergency depends on several factors, such as type of cancer (hematological vs. solid malignancies), disease volume (low volume vs. bulky disease), patient characteristics (pre-existing renal disease vs. healthy individual) and treatment strategies (high vs. low response rate regimens). In patients diagnosed with leukemia and non-Hodgkin's lymphoma, a retrospective analysis within four European countries revealed a TLS incidence of 28% (37). Others have reported incidences varying from 9.8% to 41% after treatment of hematological malignancies (38, 39). TLS is rare in patients with solid malignancies; if present, it is usually a post treatment complication, with case reports in colon cancers after Cetuximab (40), non-small cell lung cancer after radiation therapy (41), endometrial cancer after a taxane-platinum combination therapy (42), hepatocellular carcinoma after sorafenib treatment (43) and breast cancer after treatment with trastuzumab and pertuzumab based therapy (44).

When cancer cells lyse, they release potassium, phosphorus, and nucleic acids, which are metabolized into hypoxanthine, then xanthine, and finally uric acid. The tumor lysis syndrome occurs when more potassium, phosphorus, nucleic acids, and cytokines are released during cell lysis than the body's homeostatic mechanisms can deal with (45). Renal excretion is the primary means of clearing urate, xanthine, and phosphate, which can precipitate in any part of the renal collecting system. Crystal-induced tissue injury occurs in the tumor lysis syndrome when calcium phosphate, uric acid, and xanthine precipitate in renal tubules and cause inflammation and obstruction (46). High levels of both uric acid and phosphate render patients with the tumor lysis syndrome at particularly high risk for crystal-associated acute kidney injury, because uric acid precipitates readily in the presence of calcium phosphate, and calcium phosphate precipitates readily in the presence of uric acid (47).

In patients with known malignancy with recently initiated therapy presenting to an emergency department with any laboratory abnormality that could possibly be related to TLS, immediate measures should take place. The laboratory definition of tumor lysis syndrome is the sum of two or more of the following blood test results, as follows: potassium $\geq$ 6.0 mmol/L or 6 mEq/dL; phosphorus $\geq$ 2.1 mmol/L for children or $\geq$ 1.45 mmol/L for adults; uric acid $\geq$ 476 mmol/L or 8 mg/dL and calcium $\leq$ 1.75mmol/L. Renal function test could be normal or with signs of acute renal injury. Patients could be asymptomatic or present with muscle cramps, paresthesias, nausea, vomiting, diarrhea, lethargy, seizures, or hypotension. Electrocardiography could demonstrate dysrhythmias (48).

Management of acute TLS consists of prophylactic measures to reduce the risk of renal impairment and treatment of metabolic abnormalities. For that, it is imperative to stratify patients according to their risk of developing TLS, otherwise prophylactic measures will not take place. Cairo et al. published an international expert consensus panel with recommendations regarding risk stratification for TLS, subdividing patients in three risk groups: low risk, intermediate risk and high-risk patients (49). Low risk patients comprise those with solid tumors (non-bulky disease, low chemotherapy sensitivity), multiple myeloma, chronic myeloid leukemia (CML), chronic lymphocytic leukemia (CLL) not in biological therapies and acute myeloid leukemia (AML) with LDH < 2 times upper limit normal (ULN). Intermediate risk patients are those diagnosed with AML with LDH ≥ 2 times ULN or white blood count (WBC) ≥ 25.000, acute lymphoblastic leukemia with WBC < 100.000 and LDH < 2 times ULN and bulky solid tumors highly sensitive to chemotherapy (neuroblastoma, germ-cell tumours and small-cell lung cancers). The high-risk patients are those with AML and WBC ≥ 100.000, ALL with high LDH (> 2xULN) or WBC ≥ 100.000, Burkitt lymphoma, and other high-grade lymphomas (49).

The British Committee for Standards in Hematology published their guideline in 2015 summarising their recommendation with respective levels of evidence. For prophylactic measures, the primary intervention for high- risk patients are volume loading with intravenous hydration to increase glomerular filtration rate, urine flow, and minimize acidosis, preventing precipitation of uric acid crystals (Grade 1B). The exact fluid volume required is not known but it seems reasonable to aim for 3 litres per 24 hours in adults. The practice of alkalinizing urine is no longer supported because it increases the risk of xanthine nephropathy (Grade 1C). The use of allopurinol, a xanthine oxidase inhibitor, or rasburicase, a recombinant urate oxidase, is strongly recommended. For patients with high risk for TLS, rasburicase is recommended (Grade 1B) (50). The only two randomized trials comparing rasburicase and allopurinol for prophylaxis of TLS in high risk patients showed a significant reduction in puric acid levels, serum phosphorus and creatinine levels, but no impact in mortality. The standard recommended dose of rasburicase is 0.2 mg/kg/day given as a 30-min infusion. The duration of treatment should be determined by the clinical response, but it is usually recommended from 3-7 days (51). For patients with low risk of TLS, intravenous fluids and allopurinol is usually enough, with close monitoring of laboratory tests (Grade 2C). The intermediate risk patients also should receive fluid over load and up to seven days of allopurinol after chemotherapy initiation (Grade 2C).

For patients with stablished TLS, a multidisciplinary approach is mandatory, including hematology, oncology, nephrology and intensive care specialists, for the patient condition can deteriorate very quickly (Grade 1C). Once again, the need for vigorous hydration and careful monitoring of fluid balance is imperative to maintain a high urine output, that should be measured every 6 hours, together with laboratory tests (Grade 1A). The aim is to prevent uric acid crystallization and calcium phosphate deposition in the renal tubules. The build-up of these products in the renal tubules creates a vicious circle of deteriorating renal function leading to worsening hyperuricaemia, hyperkalaemia, hyperphosphataemia and hypocalcaemia. These biochemical abnormalities in turn drive further tubular deposition of uric acid and calcium phosphate (52). Since allopurinol is a xanthine oxidase inhibitor, it acts by preventing the development of uric acid crystals in the renal tubules but it does not influence the breakdown of uric acid that has already been deposited; therefore, it should not be used in this setting (Grade 1B) (53). As for rasburicase, a recombinant urate oxidase that metabolizes urate directly to the more soluble compound allantoin, it is recommended with the purpose of braking down deposits of uric acid and reduce urate levels quickly (Grade 1B). The only exceptions are patients with previous allergic reactions to rasburicase or have G6PD deficiency, since hydrogen peroxide, a breakdown product from uric acid, can cause methemoglobinemia and hemolytic anemia (54). Patients with intractable fluid overload, hyperkalaemia, hyperuricaemia, hyperphosphatemia or hypocalcaemia are indications for renal dialysis (Grade 1A) (50).

A summary of the suggested interventions for prophylaxis and treatment of TLS and metabolic abnormalities is compiled in Table 2.

Table 2. Suggested management of tumor lysis syndrome (TLS)

TLS Risk Stratification	Low Risk	Intermediate Risk	High Risk	Stablished TLS
Management	Intravenous fluids[1] Allopurinol[2] Daily laboratory tests	Intravenous fluids[1] Allopurinol[2] Inpatient monitoring Laboratory tests every 6 hours	Intravenous fluids[1] Rasburicase[3] Cardiac monitoring Laboratory tests every 6 hours	Intravenous fluids[1] Rasburicase[3] Cardiac monitoring Intensive care unit Laboratory tests every 4-6 hours Treat laboratory abnormalities

Intravenous fluids: 3000mL/day adults, or 2500-3000mL/m^2/day.
Allopurinol: 200-400mg/m2/day divided in1-3 doses maximum 800mg/day. Monitor renal function.
Rasburicase: 0.2mg/Kg/day recommended.

CARDIAC TAMPONADE

Pericardial tamponade is a life-threatening disorder caused by excessive fluid accumulation in the pericardial space leading to extracardiac compression and hemodynamic instability (54). In the Western world, cancer is the most common cause of pericardial tamponade, comprising up to 43% of the cases presenting to a general hospital (55). In Northern India, up to 33% of patients presenting to an emergency department with cardiac tamponade had cancer as their cause of pericardial effusion, the second most common etiology after tuberculosis (56). But the pericardial effusion that occurs in patients with malignancy could be secondary to malignancy itself or could be an inflammatory process like benign idiopathic pericarditis and radiation-induced pericarditis (57). Most malignant pericardial disease is due to metastases from sites of disease outside of the heart and pericardium, primarily from lung, breast, and hematologic sources (58). Primary neoplasms of the pericardium are exceedingly rare, up to 0.02% of cases from autopsy series in the United States, and these include malignant mesotheliomas, malignant pericardial tumors, cardiac sarcomas and lymphomas (59).

Patients with malignancies most commonly develop pericardial effusion either by direct local extension (60), metastatic spread via blood or lymphatic vessels (60) or obstruction to the lymphatic drainage (61). The pericardium is composed of a visceral layer formed by a single layer of mesothelial cells adhered to the surface of the heart and a fibrous parietal layer formed by the pericardium reflecting back on itself. The space between these two layers contains up to 50 mL of fluid serving as a lubricant. Fluid filling the pericardial sac initially has a flat pressure response until reaching the pericardial reserve volume, i.e., the volume that begins to distend the pericardium. Pressure then begins to rise abruptly due to the relative inextensibility of the parietal pericardium (54). The steep rise in pressure with minimal increment in pericardial fluid volume eventually leads to a critical intrapericardial pressure, which in turn results in impaired filling of the cardiac chambers and hemodynamic compromise (62).

Patients with pericardial tamponade can present with symptoms such as exertional dyspnea, syncope, chest pain, palpitations, nonspecific chest discomfort, and simple fatigue. Beck's triad of hypotension increased jugular venous pressure, and muffled heart tones is usually present (63). Although cardiac tamponade is a clinical diagnosis, Doppler echocardiography play major roles in the identification of pericardial effusion, evaluating hemodynamic significance and assessing percutaneous treatment relieve. The 2015 European Society of Cardiology (ESC) Guidelines recommend echocardiography as the initial imaging technique to assess the hemodynamic impact of a pericardial effusion and a judicious clinical evaluation that includes echocardiographic findings to guide the timing of pericardiocentesis (64). Pericardiocentesis and the cytology of pericardial fluid or pericardial biopsy are essential for the definitive diagnosis of malignant pericardial disease. Additional tests such as culture, adenosine deaminase and polymerase chain reaction of the pericardial fluid is indicated in cases where the diagnosis of malignant pericardial infusion is not stablished (65).

The treatment of malignant pericardial effusions and tamponade is a combination of symptoms control and cancer treatment to prevent recurrences. Percutaneous drainage is the mainstay for symptomatic relief and hemodynamical stability, but it usually does not resolve the problem, for the risk of recurrence is high (66). In order to prevent fluid from reaccumulating, a number of palliative percutaneous techniques have been tested (67). The most frequently used procedures are prolonged catheter drainage (68), pericardial chemical sclerosis with doxycycline or bleomycin (69, 70), balloon pericardiotomy and surgical decompression (71).

A systematic review assessing the safety and efficacy of various percutaneous interventions for malignant pericardial effusion with primary endpoint of recurrence of pericardial effusion evaluated trials using pericardiocentesis alone or followed by extended catheter drainage, pericardial instillation of sclerosing agents or percutaneous balloon pericardiotomy (72). The most effective procedure was percutaneous balloon pericardiotomy, with pooled recurrence rates of 10.3%, very similar to extended catheter drainage (12.1%) and pericardial sclerosis (10.8%). Patients in the isolated pericardiocentesis studies experienced recurrences of up to 38.3%. Another percutaneous treatment strategy for malignant pericardial effusion is intrapericardial chemotherapy. Several chemotherapy agents have been tested in this scenario, with no randomized controlled trials published to date, only retrospective analysis or single centers prospective cohorts (73-76). In a prospective cohort study from European Institute of Oncology, Milan, 33 patients with malignant pericardial effusion confirmed by cytology where submitted to intrapericardial treatment with thiotepa, an alkylating agent, 15 mg total dose on days 1, 3 and 5 via the pericardiocentesis catheter. Most of the patients had metastatic breast or lung cancer. No procedure related complications were observed, only three recurrences occurred, receiving additional intrapericardial treatment. The median survival was 115 days (77).

Surgical decompression of the pericardium, also known as pericardiotomy, is another treatment modality for malignant pericardial effusion. The procedure can be accomplished using different surgical technics (open surgery, video assisted surgery), with series of retrospective trials demonstrating acceptable local control (78, 79). While there are no randomized controlled trials comparing surgical pericardiectomy with other procedures, a systematic review with data from 59 retrospective studies looking at success rates of surgical and non-surgical malignant pericardial effusions treatments demonstrated a superior success rate with surgical modality (93-100% vs 55-90%), although no conclusions can be drawn because of bias related to the trials retrospective natures (80). Malignant pericardial effusions with consequent pericardial tamponade confers a very dismal prognosis, with median survival of 4 months (range 0 to 39 months), with some variation depending of the cancer type. Usually, patients present with disseminated disease and not amenable to curative treatment (80).

METASTATIC SPINAL CORD COMPRESSION

Metastatic spinal cord compression (MSCC), also known as neoplastic epidural spinal cord compression, is a devastating oncological emergency, with a time dependent outcome associated with serious morbidity. It occurs in 3-5% of all cancer patients and is more common in patients between the ages of 40-60 years and in cases of prostate cancer (17%), multiple myeloma (15%) and breast cancer (7%) (81). In a population-based study of over 15,000 cases of hospitalizations due to spinal cord compression, the three most common cancers responsible for the event were lung cancer (25%), prostate cancer (16.2%) and multiple myeloma (11%) (82). The definition of spinal cord compression is based on any radiologic evidence of indentation of the thecal sac, but it varies in the literature (83). In approximately 20% of the cases, the MSCC is the initial presentation of malignancy (84). Approximately 60% of the cases occurs in the thoracic spine, 30% in the lumbar spine and 10% in the cervical spine (85).

MSCC was first described in 1925 by Spiller, defined as cancer metastasis to the spine or epidural space with consequent spinal cord compression (86). There are two possible mechanisms involved in this process: growth of a paravertebral tumor directly into the spinal canal (15% cases) or haematogenous metastasis to the vertebral body with consequent spread to the epidural space (85% cases) (87). Damage caused in the spinal cord occurs both by direct compression, causing demyelination and axonal damage, and by vascular compromise and vasogenic edema (88). The beneficial actions of corticosteroids in MSCC may be related to resolution of vasogenic edema and reduction in local levels of prostaglandins and serotonin (89).

Pain is the most frequent symptom from MSCC, and it usually present for a prolong period of time, with a median of 2 months before the diagnosis of cord compression (90). Localized pain that is confined to the region of the spine affected by the metastases is usually the first symptom; typically, the pain progressively increases in intensity over time. Radicular pain due to compression or invasion of the nerve roots is commonly present, frequently unilateral, with cervical or lumbosacral spine involvement, or bilateral, with thoracic spine involvement (91). Weakness is the second most common symptom at diagnosis, most of the time referred as heaviness or clumsiness that, on examination, is weakness (92). There is a strong association between weakness and the ability to walk; about 50-68% of patients are unable to walk when they are first diagnosed with MSCC93.

Other symptoms are less common and variable, like sensory deficits, ataxia, bowel or bladder dysfunctions (93). In patients with bone metastases, it is very important for the treating physician to be aware of the following red flags: limb weakness, difficulty walking, sensory loss, bladder or bowel dysfunctions and thoracic or cervical pain (94). Patients with red flags should prompt an assessment to rule out MSCC. Magnetic resonance imaging (MRI) is the method of choice for the diagnosis of MSCC, overall accuracy is 95% (sensitivity 93%, specificity 97%) (95). It has advantages over CT, adding new information regarding nerves and soft tissue and, for 40% of patients, the MRI information changes the radiation fields used. Furthermore, the entire spine can be imaged in one sitting, which is important because up to a third of patients have more than one site of spinal cord compression (96).

Once the patient has a confirmed diagnosis of MSCC, the main treatment goals include pain control, avoidance of neurological complications preserving neurological function. If the patient is at high risk of MSCC (metastatic tumor with bone lesions, recent pain, neurological symptoms), initial treatment with corticosteroids is mandatory for edema reduction. The rational for this strategy is based on a randomized trial with patients from solid tumors (97). The experimental treatment regimen comprised a 96 mg intravenous bolus of dexamethasone, then 96 mg per day oral dexamethasone for 3 days with a 10-day taper before radiotherapy. The control arm had radiation with no steroids. The investigators found 3-month and 6-month ambulatory rates of 81% versus 63% ($p<0{\cdot}05$) and 59% versus 33% ($p<0{\cdot}05$), respectively, in favor of the group who received dexamethasone. With the objective to reduce this fairly high loading dose, a small randomized trial compared a loading dose of 10mg and 100mg, with continued doses of 16mg a day. Both groups showed significant reductions in pain from baseline ($p<0{\cdot}001$ for both groups) but there were no differences between the two treatment arms with respect to pain reduction, ambulation or bladder function (98). Another small trial randomized 20 patients with MSCC to a bolus dose of 96 mg vs 16 mg and radiation therapy (99). The trial accrual was poor, only 20 patients randomized. No difference was observed regarding ambulation scores and symptom control. For patients with neurologic deficits and being treated with radiation therapy, the recommendation is a bolus of 8-10 mg of dexamethasone, followed by a 16 mg per day dosing schedule that should be tapered as symptoms improve (100).

Another treatment option for patients with MSCC is external beam radiotherapy. Considered the standard of care for this oncological emergency since 1950, the method has never been directly compared with best supportive care, so it is very important to select patients who can benefit the most based on tumor type (breast, prostate, lymphoma and myeloma), no visceral metastasis and good performance status (101). The standard dosing and schedule are 30Gy given in 10 fractions, based on a prospective study data (102). However, selection of optimal dose fraction and schedule is extremely important, especially for patients with poor prognosis. Maranzano and colleagues have reported two randomized control trials addressing the question of dose fractionation schedule. In the first trial, 300 patients with MSCC where randomized 1:1 to a split course of RT (15 Gy in three fractions, 4-day break, then 15 Gy in five fractions), or hypofractionated RT (8 Gy in two fractions 1 week apart) (103). All patients were given dexamethasone 16 mg daily during RT. Patients were assessed for ability to ambulate (with/without assistance), duration of ambulation, bladder function, overall survival, toxicity, and pain relief. With a median follow-up time was 33 months, no significant differences where observed in any of these outcomes. In the second randomized trial reported in 2009, the authors randomized 327 patients with MSCC and poor prognosis to 16 Gy in two fractions over 1 week vs. 8 Gy in one fraction (104). Dexamethasone was also administered in both groups. With a short median follow-up, no significant differences were reported between the treatment arms for ambulation, duration of ambulation, bladder control, pain response, and overall survival.

New methods to deliver more focused radiation are in development, with the potential to deliver higher radiation doses to the tumor with less exposure to the spinal cord and healthy tissue. One example is stereotactic body RT (SBRT). In the phase 2 trial RTOG 0631, patients with 1-3 spine metastasis with a Numerical Rating Pain Scale (NRPS) score ≥5 received 16 Gy single fraction SRS107. The primary endpoint was SRS feasibility: image guidance radiation therapy (IGRT) targeting accuracy ≤2 mm, target volume coverage >90% of prescription dose, maintaining spinal cord dose constraints (10 Gy to ≤10% of the cord volume from 5-6 mm above to 5-6 mm below the target or absolute spinal cord volume <0.35 cc) and other normal tissue dose constraints. A feasibility success rate <70% was considered unacceptable for continuation of the phase 3 component. With 46 patients accrued and 44 eligible, median NRPS was 7 at presentation. Final pretreatment rapid review was approved in 100%. Accuracy of image guided SRS targeting was in compliance with the protocol at 95%. The target coverage and spinal cord dose constraint were in accordance with the protocol requirements in 100% and 97%. Overall compliance for other normal tissue constraints was per protocol in 74%. There were no cases of grade 4-5 acute treatment-related toxicity (105). A phase 3 RTOG trial is underway to further confirm these findings.

For some very selected patients, surgery is an optional for treating MSCC. The strongest evidence comes from a randomized multi- institutional control trial by Patchell et al. In this trial, 101 patients with MESCC confirmed by MRI to receive decompressive surgical resection with RT 14 days later, or RT alone of 30 Gy in 10 fractions (106). All patients were directed to receive dexamethasone 100 mg bolus plus 96 mg daily (dose reduced for patients with contraindications to high-dose steroids). Patients in the combined therapy group were more likely to retain or maintain their ambulatory status longer than were patients receiving RT alone (84% vs. 57%, p = 0.001), experienced better ambulatory time (122 days vs. 13 days, p = 0.003), urinary continence (74% vs. 57%, p = 0.005), duration of continence (median 157 days vs. 17 days, p = 0.016), functional status (maintenance of Frankel and American Spinal Injury Association (ASIA) ASIA scores, p = 0.001). There was a difference in survival favoring the combined modality arm (median 126 days vs. 100 days, p = 0.033) (106). This trial established the effectiveness of radical surgery in this scenario. In a meta-analysis of conventional RT vs. surgery for the management of MSCC, authors concluded that surgery treated patients were more likely to recover ambulation and to better pain control, but no prognostic and predictive factors were adjusted for in this analysis (107). Given the data above, considering the trials limitations and patient selection, surgery can be an effective treatment option, but a multidisciplinary approach is the best options for the patients, taking in considerations tumor factors, patients prognosis, performance status and center expertise for performing such procedure. A suggested flow chart for diagnosis and treatment of metastatic spinal cord compression is outlined in Figure 1.

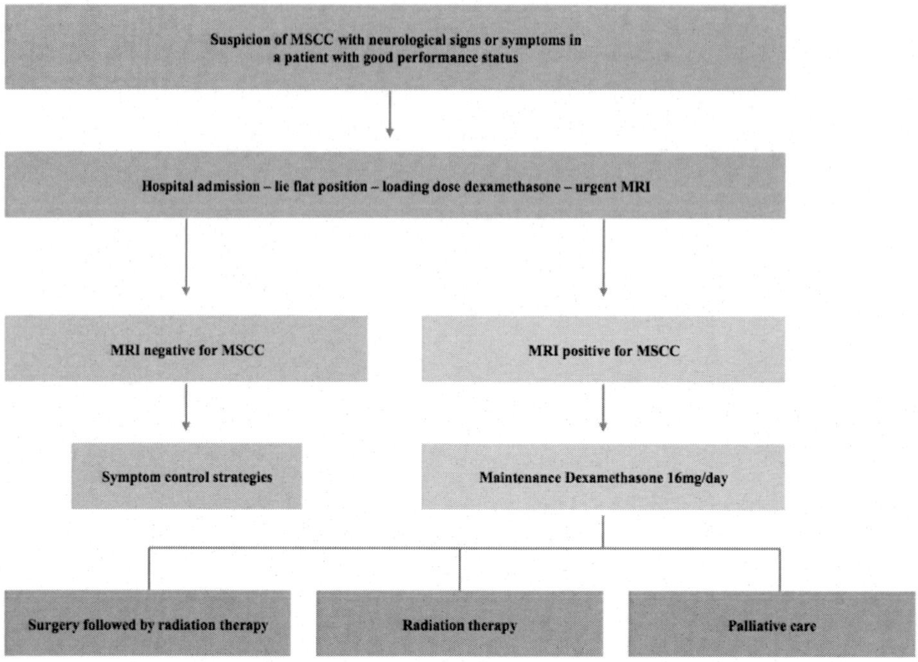

Figure 1. Flow chart for diagnosis and treatment of metastatic spinal cord compression.

SUPERIOR VENA CAVA SYNDROME

Superior vena cava syndrome (SVCS) is defined by compression of the vena cava impeding normal blood flow. The obstruction can be caused by invasion or external compression of the superior vena cava by a malignant process involving the right lung, lymph nodes, and other mediastinal structures, or by thrombosis of blood within the SVC (108). Other benign etiology can cause SVCS, but cancer is responsible for 60-90% of the cases according to a recently published series (109). Approximately 2% to 4% of all patients with lung cancer develop SVCS at some time during their disease course, been more frequent in small cell lung cancer (10%), given its predilection for mediastinal involvement and rapid growth (110). The second most prevalent malignancy is non-Hodgkin's lymphoma (NHL), representing 2-4% of all cases (111).

The superior vena cava (SVC) is the major vessel collecting venous return to the heart from the head, arms, and upper body. When a tumor growth produces compression of the SVC, there is increased resistance to venous blood flow, which is then diverted through collateral networks that may develop (112). Collateral vessels that are commonly found include the azygos, intercostal, mediastinal, paravertebral, hemiazygos, thoracoepigastric, internal mammary, thoracoacromioclavicular, and anterior chest wall veins. The severity of the obstruction is a component of anatomical site (more intense if bellow the azygos vein) and tumor biology (worse in rapidly growing tumors) (113).

When a patient with a confirmed cancer diagnosis presents with facial or neck edema, arm swelling, dyspnea, cough and dilated chest veins, it is mandatory to rule out SVCS (114). When stridor, confusion and obtundation are also present it means that major airway is obstructed by the tumor, the situation needs to be addressed more urgently as it may be more life threatening (115).

After clinical diagnosis, a chest CT with contrast (to evaluate the SVC) should be ordered. This method will allow the diagnosis and assessment of the level and extent of the blockade (116). Common findings on CT include enlarged paratracheal lymph nodes with or without additional lung or pleural abnormalities (117). Magnetic resonance venography is an alternative approach that may be useful for patients with a contrast dye allergy or for those in whom venous access cannot be obtained for contrast-enhanced studies (118). Superior vena cava venography should be used when a CT does not confirm the diagnosis, when a thrombotic obstruction is suspected, or when san interventional stent is planned (119).

Initial treatment should involve a multidisciplinary approach including medical oncology, radiation oncology, radiology, surgery and endovascular intervention. A balance between disease extension, severity of symptoms and patient's prognosis is crucial for a detailed treatment plan (120). The treatment options include supportive measures, radiation therapy (RT), chemotherapy, and stent insertion. Surgery is virtually never an option, as the presence of SVCS almost always signifies unresectable tumor within the mediastinum, but it may be possible after induction treatment (121). Initial supportive care measures are focused on symptom relief, usually considering head elevation, oxygen, pain relief and corticosteroids, which are used to reduce local edema and aid airway obstruction. No specific dosing or protocol exist; one suggestion is an initial dose of 4 mg 2-4 times a day, with tapering as soon as symptoms improve (122). Venous thrombosis usually accompanies SVCS, contributing to symptom severity and posing greater life risk to the patient. The incidence of thromboembolic events in patients with malignant SVCS has been reported as high as 38%, but there are no specific guidelines regarding prophylactic anticoagulation in these patients, which is currently administered only when a thrombus is evident in the radiological workup (123).

With the diagnosis confirmed and etiology determined, treatment options include: radiation therapy, chemotherapy, stent placement or a combination of these strategies. Radiotherapy (RT) is an effective modality in the treatment of SVCS due to malignancy, with complete relief of symptoms within two weeks in 78% and 63% of patients with SCLC and NSCLC, respectively (122). Treatment should be focused on tumor histology as well as the intent of treatment (curative or palliative). Using the example of NSCLC, a definitive course of radiation therapy can take 6 to 7 weeks to administer in daily fractions of 2 Gy (124). Palliative treatments are typically administered over a course of 1 to 2 weeks with larger fraction sizes of 3 Gy to 5 Gy (e.g., 20 Gy in 5 fractions, 30 Gy in 10 fractions), with the goal of achieving a more rapid response by using larger daily doses. Abbreviated treatments of two 6-Gy fractions (12 Gy/2 fractions) have been reported to be effective in older patients with poorer performance status (125).

Chemotherapy is often used as the initial treatment for SVCS from tumors with high-chemotherapy sensitivity, such as lymphomas, germ cell tumors and SCLC, conferring good response rates in up to 2 weeks (126). This strategy can relieve the symptoms of SVCS in up to 80% of patients with NHL and 77% with SCLS (110, 111). Combination chemotherapy and radiation may increase response rates and symptom relief, with special considerations for cases where a curative intent is considered, such as some lymphomas and SCLC (127, 128). The choice of drug and regimen will depend on tumor histology and patient performance status (120).

Stent placement can be especially useful in patients without a tissue diagnosis or who have previously been treated with RT or in those who have known chemotherapy and radiation-resistant tumors (129). In the very symptomatic patient with local assessment to endovascular procedures, stent placement can be considered a first choice for treatment, followed by cancer directed therapy (130).

Table 3. Advantages and disadvantages of treatment strategies for cancer related vena cava syndrome (VCS)

Radiation therapy		Endovascular stent		Chemotherapy	
Advantages	**Disadvantages**	**Advantages**	**Disadvantages**	**Advantages**	**Disadvantages**
Noninvasive procedure	No immediate symptom relief (usually 7-15 days)	Immediate symptom relief (24-72 hours)	Invasive procedure	Noninvasive procedure	No immediate symptom relief (usually 7-15 days)
Treats underlying malignancy	May cause tissue inflammation in the beginning	Allows option for further direct cancer treatment	Bleeding complications	Treats underlying malignancy	Needs a minimum performance status to tolerate treatment
-	Needs special equipment	Gives time to define disease etiology	Increased risk of thrombosis	Does not require special equipment	Important systemic toxicities
-	-	-	Does not treat underlying cancer	Can be administered in ICU	-

Adapted from Wan FJ et al. Superior Vena Cava Syndrome. Emerg Med Clin N Am 27 (2009) 243–255.
Abbreviation: ICU, intensive care unit.

There are no randomized, controlled trials comparing the efficacy of endovascular stenting with radiation or chemotherapy. That been said, the most extensive data come from a systemic review of the literature by Rowell and Gleeson in which 23 studies on stents were combined for a total of 159 patients with SVCS due to either SCLC or NSCLC (122). The results showed that 95% of the patients experienced complete or partial relief of their symptoms following stenting with a relapse rate of 11%. In comparison, relief rates in 487 patients with SCLC treated with chemotherapy alone, chemoradiotherapy, or RT were 77%, 83%, and 78% respectively; however, in NSCLC, relief rates in 243 patients treated with chemotherapy or RT were 59% and 63%, respectively.

A brief summary of the treatment strategies discussed here, with their advantages and disadvantages is outlined at Table 3.

REFERENCES

[1] Ferlay J, Soerjomataram I, Ervik M, Dikshit R, Eser S, Mathers C, et al. GLOBOCAN 2012 v1.0, *Cancer Incidence and Mortality Worldwide.* IARC Cancer Base 2013;11.

[2] Savage P, Sharkey R, Kua T, Papanastasopoulos P, McDonald-Burrows Z, Hassan S, et al. *Clinical characteristics and outcomes for patients with an initial emergency presentation of malignancy: a 15 month audit of patient level data.* Cancer Epidemiol 2015;39(1):86-90.

[3] Sargent JT, Smith OP. *Haematological emergencies managing hypercalcaemia in adults and children with haematological disorders.* Br J Haematol 2010;149(4):465-77.

[4] Esbrit P. *Hypercalcemia of malignancy-new insights into an old syndrome.* Clin Lab 2001;47:(1-2):67-71.

[5] Ralston SH, Gallacher SJ, Patel U, Campbell J, Boyle IT. *Cancer-associated hypercalcemia: morbidity and mortality.* Clinical experience in 126 treated patients. Ann Intern Med 1990;112(7):499-504.

[6] Endres D.B. *Investigation of hypercalcemia.* Clinical Biochemistry 2012;45(12):954-63.

[7] Peacock M. *Calcium metabolism in health and disease.* Clin J Am Soc Nephrol 2010;5(Suppl1):S23–30.

[8] Stewart AF. Clinical practice. *Hypercalcemia associated with cancer.* N Engl J Med 2005;352(4):373-9.

[9] Van den Eyden GG, Neyret A, Fumey G, Rizk-Rabin M, Vermeulen PB, Bouizar Z, et al. *PTHrP, calcitonin and calcitriol in a case of severe, protracted and refractory hypercalcemia due to a pancreatic neuroendocrine tumour.* Bone 2007;40(4):1166–1171.

[10] Donovan PJ, Achong N, Griffin K, Galligan J, Pretorius CJ, McLeod DS. *PTHrP-mediated hypercalcemia: causes and survival in 138 patients.* J Clin Endocrinol Metab 2015;100(5):2024-9.

[11] Dimitriadis GK, Angelousi A, Weickert MO, Randeva HS, Kaltsas G, Grossman A. *Paraneoplastic endocrine syndromes.* Endocr Relat Cancer 2017;24(6):R173-90.

[12] Roodman GD. *Mechanisms of bone metastasis.* N Engl J Med 2004;350(16):1655-64.

[13] Fallah-Rad N, Morton AR. *Managing hypercalcaemia and hypocalcaemia in cancer patients.* Curr Opin Support Palliat Care 2013;7(3):265-71.

[14] Bayne MC, Illidge TM. *Hypercalcaemia, parathyroid hormone-related protein and malignancy.* Clin Oncol 2001;13(5):372-7.

[15] McCurdy MT, Shanholtz CB. *Oncologic emergencies*. Crit Care Med 2012;40(7):2212-22.

[16] Koo WS(1), Jeon DS, Ahn SJ, Kim YS, Yoon YS, Bang BK. *Calcium-free hemodialysis for the management of hypercalcemia*. Nephron 1996;72(3):424-8.

[17] Fleisch H. *Bisphosphonates: mechanisms of action*. Endocr Rev 1998;19(1):80-100.

[18] Nussbaum SR, Younger J, Vandepol CJ, Gagel RF, Zubler MA, Chapman R, et al. *Single-dose intravenous therapy with pamidronate for the treatment of hypercalcemia of malignancy: comparison of 30-, 60-, and 90-mg dosages*. Am J Med 1993;95(3):297-304.

[19] Major P, Lortholary A, Hon J, Abdi E, Mills G, Menssen HD, et al. *Zoledronic acid is superior to pamidronate in the treatment of hypercalcemia of malignancy: a pooled analysis of two randomized, controlled clinical trials*. J Clin Oncol 2001;19(2):558-67.

[20] Markowitz GS, Fine PL, Stack JI, Kunis CL, Radhakrishnan J, Palecki W, et al. *Toxic acute tubular necrosis following treatment with zoledronate (Zometa)*. Kidney Int 2003;64(1):281-9.

[21] Machado CE, Flombaum CD. *Safety of pamidronate in patients with renal failure and hypercalcemia*. Clin Nephrol 1996;45(3):175-9.

[22] Henrich D, Hoffmann M, Uppenkamp M, Bergner R. *Ibandronate for the treatment of hypercalcemia or nephrocalcinosis in patients with multiple myeloma and acute renal failure: Case reports*. Acta Haematol 2006;116(3):165-72.

[23] Body JJ, Diel IJ, Tripathy D, Bergstrom B. *Intravenous ibandronate does not affect time to renal function deterioration in patients with skeletal metastases from breast cancer: phase III trial results*. Eur J Cancer Care 2006;15(3):299-302.

[24] Body JJ, Louviaux I, Dumon JC. *Decreased efficacy of bisphosphonates for recurrences of tumor-induced hypercalcemia*. Support Care Cancer 2000;8(5):398-404.

[25] Kostenuik PJ, Nguyen HQ, McCabe J, Warmington KS, Kurahara C, Sun N, et al. *Denosumab, a fully human monoclonal antibody to RANKL, inhibits bone resorption and increases BMD in knock-in mice that express chimeric (murine/human) RANKL*. J Bone Miner Res 2009;24(2):182-95.

[26] Hu MI, Glezerman IG, Leboulleux S, Insogna K, Gucalp R, Misiorowski W, et al. *Denosumab for treatment of hypercalcemia of malignancy*. J Clin Endocrinol Metab 2014;99(9):3144-52.

[27] Food and Drug Administration. XGEVA (denosumab) *Prescribing information*. Accessed 2012 October Oct 12. URL: http://www.accessdata.fda.gov/drugsa tfda_docs/label/2013/125320s094lb l.pdf.

[28] *Therapeutic Goods Administration Australia*. XGEVA (denosumab) Product Information. URL: https://www.ebs.tga.gov.au/ebs/picmi/picmirepository.nsf/ pdf? OpenAgent&id = CP-2012-PI-02073-3&d = 20160503161114622483.

[29] *Health Canada. XGEVA (denosumab) Product monograph*. Accessed 2016 May 03. URL: https://ww w.amgen.ca/Xgeva_PM.pdf.

[30] *Russian State register of medicines. Registration certificate*. URL: http://grls.ros minzdrav.ru /Grls_View_v2.aspx?idReg = 425821&t.

[31] Binstock ML, Mundy GR. *Effect of calcitonin and glucocorticoids in combination on the hypercalcemia of malignancy*. Ann Intern Med 1980;93(2):269-72.

[32] Perlia CP, Gubisch NJ, Wolter J, Edelberg D, Dederick MM, Taylor SG III. *Mithramycin treatment of hypercalcemia*. Cancer 1970;25(2):389-94.

[33] Leyland-Jones B. *Treatment of cancer related hypercalcemia: the role of gallium nitrate*. Semin Oncol 2003;30(Suppl 5):13-9.

[34] Shukla DK, Gupta D, Aggarwal A, Kumar D. *A case report of newly diagnosed epithelial ovarian carcinoma presenting with spontaneous tumor lysis syndrome and its successful management with rasburicase*. Indian J Med Paediatr Oncol. 2017;38(3):360-2.

[35] Cairo MS, Bishop M. *Tumour lysis syndrome: new therapeutic strategies and classification*. Br J Haematol 2004;127(1):3–11.

[36] Magrath IT, Semawere C, Nkwocha J. *Causes of death in patients with Burkitt's lymphoma — the role of supportive care in overall management.* East Afr Med J 1974;51(9):623-32.

[37] Annemans L, Moeremans K, Lamotte M, Garcia Conde J, van den Berg H, Myint H, et al. *Incidence, medical resource utilisation and costs of hyperuricemia and tumour lysis syndrome in patients with acute leukaemia and non-Hodgkin's lymphoma in four European countries.* Leuk Lymphoma 2003;44(1):77-83.

[38] Mato AR, Riccio BE, Qin L, Heitjan DF, Carroll M, Loren A, et al. *A predictive model for the detection of tumor lysis syndrome during AML induction therapy.* Leuk Lymphoma 2006;47(5):877-83.

[39] Cortes J, Moore JO, Maziarz RT et al. *Control of plasma uric acid in adults at risk for tumor Lysis syndrome: efficacy and safety of rasburicase alone and rasburicase followed by allopurinol compared with allopurinol alone-results of a multicenter phase III study.* J Clin Oncol 2010;28(27):4207-13.

[40] Krishnan G, D'Silva K, Al-Janadi A. *Cetuximab-related tumor lysis syndrome in metastatic colon carcinoma.* J Clin Oncol 2008;26(14):2406-8.

[41] Noh GY, Choe DH, Kim CH, Lee JC. *Fatal tumor lysis syndrome during radiotherapy for non-small-cell lung cancer.* J Clin Oncol 2008;26(36):6005-6.

[42] Godoy H, Kesterson JP, Lele S. *Tumor lysis syndrome associated with carboplatin and paclitaxel in a woman with recurrent endometrial cancer.* Int J Gynaecol Obstet 2010;109(3):254.

[43] Joshita S, Yoshizawa K, Sano K, Kobayashi S, Sekiguchi T, Morita S, et al. *A patient with advanced hepatocellular carcinoma treated with sorafenib tosylate showed massive tumor lysis with avoidance of tumor lysis syndrome.* Intern Med 2010;49(11):991-4.

[44] Baudon C, Duhoux FP, Sinapi I, Canon JL. *Tumor lysis syndrome following trastuzumab and pertuzumab for metastatic breast cancer: a case report.* J Med Case Rep 201616;10:178.

[45] Shimada M, Johnson RJ, May WS Jr, Lingegowda V, Sood P, Nakagawa T, et al. *A novel role for uric acid in acute kidney injury associated with tumour lysis syndrome.* Nephrol Dial Transplant 2009;24(10):2960-4.

[46] LaRosa C, McMullen L, Bakdash S, Ellis D, Krishnamurti L, Wu HY, et al. *Acute renal failure from xanthine nephropathy during management of acute leukemia.* Pediatr Nephrol 2007;22(1):132-5.

[47] Pais VM Jr, Lowe G, Lallas CD, Preminger GM, Assimos DG. *Xanthine urolithiasis.* Urology 2006;67(5):1084.

[48] Pession A, Masetti R, Gaidano G, Tosi P, Rosti G, Aglietta M, et al. *Risk evaluation, prophylaxis, and treatment of tumor lysis syndrome: consensus of an Italian expert panel.* Adv Ther 2011;28(8):684-97.

[49] Cairo MS, Coiffier B, Reiter A, Younes A. *Recommendations for the evaluation of risk and prophylaxis of tumour lysis syndrome (TLS) in adults and children with malignant diseases: an expert TLS panel consensus.* Br J Haematol 2010;149(4): 578-86

[50] Jones GL, Will A, Jackson GH, Webb NJ, Rule S; British Committee for Standards in Haematology. *Guidelines for the management of tumour lysis syndrome in adults and children with haematological malignancies on behalf of the British Committee for Standards in Haematology.* Br J Haematol 2015;169(5):661-71.

[51] Goldman SC, Holcenberg JS, Finklestein JZ, Hutchinson R, Kreissman S, Johnson FL et al. A randomized comparison between rasburicase and allopurinol in children with lymphoma or leukemia at high risk for tumor lysis. Blood 2001;97(10):2998-3003.

[52] Hagemeister F, Huen A. *The status of allopurinol in the management of tumor lysis syndrome: a clinical review.* Cancer J. 2005;11(Suppl 1):S1-10.

[53] Dinnel J, Moore BL, Skiver BM, Bose P. *Rasburicase in the management of tumor lysis: an evidence-based review of its place in therapy.* Core Evid 201510:23-38.

[54] Spodick DH. *Acute cardiac tamponade.* N Engl J Med 2003;349(7):684-90.

[55] Gornik HL, Gerhard Herman M, Beckman JA. *Abnormal cytology predicts poor prognosis in cancer patients with pericardial effusion*. J Clin Oncol 2005;23(22): 521-6.

[56] Jain S, Sharma N, Varma S, Rajwanshi A, Verma JS, Sharma BK. *Profile of cardiac tamponade in the medical emergency ward of a North Indian hospital*. Can J Cardiol 1999;15(6):671-5.

[57] Marwan M. Refaat, William E. Katz. *Neoplastic pericardial effusion*. Clin Cardiol 2011;34(10):593-8.

[58] Imazio M, Demichelis B, Parrini I, Favro E, Beqaraj F, Cecchi E, et al. *Relation of acute pericardial disease to malignancy*. Am J Cardiol 2005;95(11):1393-4.

[59] Burazor I, Aviel-Ronen S, Imazio M, Markel G, Grossman Y, Yosepovich A, et al. *Primary malignancies of the heart and pericardium*. Clin Cardiol 2014;37(9):582-8.

[60] Rousseau-Bussac G, Crequit P, Alifano M, Chouaid C. *Management of malignant pericardial effusion in lung cancer.* Rev Mal Respir 2014;31(8):746-53.

[61] Beauchamp KA. *Pericardial tamponade: an oncologic emergency*. Clin J Oncol Nurs 1998;2(3):85-95.

[62] Karam N, Patel P, deFilippi C. *Diagnosis and management of chronic pericardial effusions*. Am J Med Sci 2001;322(2):79–87.

[63] Wilkes JD, Fidias P, Vaickus L, Perez RP. *Malignancy-related pericardial effusion*. 127 cases from the Roswell Park Cancer Institute. Cancer 1995;76(8):1377-87.

[64] Adler Y, Charron P, Imazio M, Badano L, Barón-Esquivias G, Bogaert J, et al. *2015 ESC guidelines for the diagnosis and management of pericardial diseases: the task force for the diagnosis and management of pericardial diseases of the European society of cardiology (ESC)* Endorsed by: The European Association for Cardio-Thoracic Surgery (EACTS). Eur Heart J 2015;36(42):2921-64.

[65] Porte HL, Janecki-Delebecq TJ, Finzi L, Métois DG, Millaire A, Wurtz AJ. *Pericardioscopy for primary management of pericardial effusion in cancer patients.* Eur J Cardiothorac Surg 1999;16(3):287-91.

[66] Tsang TS, Enriquez-Sarano M, Freeman WK, Barnes ME, Sinak LJ, Gersh BJ, et al. *Consecutive 1127 therapeutic echocardiographically guided pericardiocenteses: clinical profile, practice patterns, and outcomes spanning 21 years*. Mayo Clin Proc 2002;77(5):429-36.

[67] Marcy PY, Bondiau PY, Brunner P. *Percutaneous treatment in patients presenting with malignant cardiac tamponade*. Eur Radiol 2005;15(9):2000-9.

[68] Allen KB, Faber LP, Warren WH, Shaar CJ. *Pericardial effusion: subxiphoid pericardiostomy versus percutaneous catheter drainage*. Ann Thorac Surg 1999;67 (2):437-40.

[69] Liu G, Crump M, Goss PE, Dancey J, Shepherd FA. *Prospective comparison of the sclerosing agents doxycycline and bleomycin for the primary management of malignant pericardial effusion and cardiac tamponade*. J Clin Oncol 1996;14(12): 3141-7.

[70] Kunitoh H, Tamura T, Shibata T, Imai M, Nishiwaki Y, Nishio M, et al. A randomised trial of intrapericardial bleomycin for malignant pericardial effusion with lung cancer (JCOG9811). Br J Cancer 2009;100(3):464-9.

[71] Gumrukcuoglu HA, Odabasi D, Akdag S, Ekim H. *Management of cardiac tamponade: a comparative study between echo-guided pericardiocentesis and surgery-a report of 100 patients*. Cardiol Res Pract 2011;2011:197838.

[72] Virk SA, Chandrakumar D, Villanueva C, Wolfenden H, Liou K, Cao C. *Systematic review of percutaneous interventions for malignant pericardial effusion*. Heart 2015;101(20):1619-26.

[73] Moriya T, Takiguchi Y, Tabeta H, Watanabe R, Kimura H, Nagao K, Kuriyama T. *Controlling malignant pericardial effusion by intrapericardial carboplatin administration in patients with primary non-small-cell lung cancer*. Br J Cancer 2000;83(7):858-62.

[74] Tomkowski WZ, Wiśniewska J, Szturmowicz M, Kuca P, Burakowski J, Kober J, Fijałkowska A. *Evaluation of intrapericardial cisplatin administration in cases with recurrent malignant pericardial effusion and cardiac tamponade*. Support Care Cancer 2004;12(1):53-7.

[75] Musch E, Gremmler B, Nitsch J, Rieger J, Malek M, Chrissafidou A. *Intrapericardial instillation of mitoxantrone in palliative therapy of malignant pericardial effusion*. Onkologie. 2003;26(2):135-9.

[76] Kawashima O, Kurihara T, Kamiyoshihara M, Sakata S, Ishikawa S, Morishita Y. *Management of malignant pericardial effusion resulting from recurrent cancer with local instillation of aclarubicin hydrochloride*. Am J Clin Oncol 1999;22(4):396-8.

[77] Martinoni A, Cipolla CM, Cardinale D, Civelli M, Lamantia G, Colleoni M, Fiorentini C. *Long-term results of intrapericardial chemotherapeutic treatment of malignant pericardial effusions with thiotepa*. Chest 2004;126(5):1412-6.

[78] Cullinane CA, Paz IB, Smith D, Carter N, Grannis FW Jr. *Prognostic factors in the surgical management of pericardial effusion in the patient with concurrent malignancy*. Chest 2004;125(4):1328-34.

[79] Jeon HW, Cho DG, Park JK, Hyun KY, Choi SY, Suh JH, et al. *Prognostic factors affecting survival of patients with cancer-related pericardial effusion managed by surgery*. World J Surg Oncol 2014;12:249.

[80] Jama GM, Scarci M, Bowden J, Marciniak SJ. *Palliative treatment for symptomatic malignant pericardial effusion*. Interact Cardiovasc Thorac Surg 2014;19(6):1019-26.

[81] Loblaw DA, Laperriere NJ, Mackillop WJ. *A population-based study of malignant spinal cord compression in Ontario*. Clin Oncol 2003;15(4):211-7.

[82] Mak KS, Lee LK, Mak RH, Wang S, Pile-Spellman J, Abrahm JL, et al. *Incidence and treatment patterns in hospitalizations for malignant spinal cord compression in the United States*, 1998-2006. Int J Radiat Oncol Biol Phys 2011;80(3):824-31.

[83] Schiff D, O'Neill BP, Wang CH, O'Fallon JR. *Neuroimaging and treatment implications of patients with multiple epidural spinal metastases*. Cancer 1998;83(8):1593-601.

[84] Schiff D, O'Neill BP, Suman VJ. *Spinal epidural metastasis as the initial manifestation of malignancy: clinical features and diagnostic approach*. Neurology 1997;49:452-6.

[85] Cole JS, Patchell RA. *Metastatic epidural spinal cord compression*. Lancet Neurol 2008;7(5):459-66.

[86] Spiller WG. *Rapidly progressive paralysis associated with carcinoma*. Arch Neurol Psychiatry 1925;13(4):471–77.

[87] Siegal T. *Spinal cord compression: from laboratory to clinic*. Eur J Cancer. 1995;31A(11):1748-53.

[88] Kato A, Ushio Y, Hayakawa T, Yamada K, Ikeda H, Mogami H. *Circulatory disturbance of the spinal cord with epidural neoplasm in rats*. J Neurosurg 1985;63(2):2605.

[89] Gabriel K, Schiff D. *Metastatic spinal cord compression by solid tumors*. Semin Neurol 2004;24(4):375-83.

[90] Tsukada Y, Nakamura N, Ohde S, Akahane K, Sekiguchi K, Terahara A. *Factors that delay treatment of symptomatic metastatic extradural spinal cord compression*. J Palliat Med 2015;18(2):107-13.

[91] Helweg-Larsen S, Sorenson PS. *Symptoms and signs in metastatic spinal cord compression: a study of progression from first symptoms until diagnosis in 153 patients*. Eur J Cancer 1994;30A(3):396-98.

[92] Husband DJ. *Malignant spinal cord compression: prospective study of delays in referral and treatment*. BMJ. 1998;317(7150):18-21.

[93] Kienstra GEM, Terwee CB, Dekker FW, Canta LR, Borstlap AC, Tijssen CC, et al. *Prediction of spinal epidural metastases*. Arch Neurol 2000;57(5):690-5.

[94] National Institute for Health and Care Excellence, 2008. *Metastatic spinal cord compression: diagnosis and management of patients at risk of or with metastatic spinal cord compression*. (CG75.) URL: www.nice.org.uk/guidance/CG75.

[95] Li KC, Poon PY. *Sensitivity and specificity of MRI in detecting malignant spinal cord compression and in distinguishing malignant from benign compression fractures of vertebrae*. Magn Reson Imaging 1988;6(5):547-56.

[96] Colletti PM, Siegal HJ, Woo MY, Young HY, Terk MR. *The impact on treatment planning of MRI of the spine in patients suspected of vertebral metastasis: an efficacy study*. Comput Med Imaging Graph 1996;20(3):159–62.

[97] Sorenson PS, Helweg-Larsen S, Mouridsen H, Hansen HH. *Effect of high-dose dexamethasone in carcinomatous metastatic spinal cord compression treated with radiotherapy: a randomized trial*. Eur J Cancer 1994;30A(1):22-7.

[98] Vecht CJ, Haaxma-Reiche H, van Putten WLJ, de Visser M, Vries EP, *Twijnstra A. Initial bolus of conventional versus high-dose dexamethasone in metastatic spinal cord compression*. Neurology 1989;39(9):1255-7.

[99] Graham PH, Capp A, Delaney G, Goozee G, Hickey B, Turner S, et al. *A pilot randomised comparison of dexamethasone 96 mg vs 16 mg per day for malignant spinal-cord compression treated by radiotherapy: TROG 01.05 Superdex study*. Clin Oncol (R Coll Radiol) 2006;18(1):70-6.

[100] Loblaw DA, Mitera G, Ford M, Laperriere NJ. *A 2011 updated systematic review and clinical practice guideline for the management of malignant extradural spinal cord compression*. Int J Radiat Oncol Biol Phys 2012 1;84(2):312-7.

[101] Rades D, Fehlauer F, Schulte R, Veninga T, Stalpers LJ, Basic H, et al. Prognostic factors for local control and survival after radiotherapy of metastatic spinal cord compression. J Clin Oncol 2006;24(21):3388–93.

[102] Rades D, Fehlauer F, Stalpers LJ, Wildfang I, Zschenker O, Schild SE, et al. *A prospective evaluation of two radiotherapy schedules with 10 versus 20 fractions for the treatment of metastatic spinal cord compression: Final results of a multicenter study*. Cancer 2004;101(11):2687-92.

[103] Maranzano E, Bellavita R, Rossi R, De Angelis V, Frattegiani A, Bagnoli R, et al. *Short-course versus split- course radiotherapy in metastatic spinal cord compression: Results of a phase III, randomized, multicenter trial*. J Clin Oncol 2005;23(15):3358-65.

[104] Maranzano E, Trippa F, Casale M, Costantini S, Lupattelli M, Bellavita R, et al. *8 Gy single-dose radiotherapy is effective in metastatic spinal cord compression: Results of a phase III randomized multicentre Italian trial*. Radiother Oncol 2009;93(2):174-9.

[105] Ryu S, Pugh SL, Gerszten PC, Yin FF, Timmerman RD, Hitchcock YJ, et al. *RTOG 0631 phase 2/3 study of image guided stereotactic radiosurgery for localized (1-3) spine metastases: phase 2 results*. Pract Radiat Oncol 2014;4(2):76-81.

[106] Patchell RA, Tibbs PA, Regine WF, Payne R, Saris S, Kryscio RJ, et al. *Direct decompressive surgical resection in the treatment of spinal cord compression caused by metastatic cancer: A randomised trial*. Lancet 2005;366(9486):643-8.

[107] Klimo P Jr., Thompson CJ, Kestle JR, Schmidt MH. *A meta-analysis of surgery versus conventional radiotherapy for the treatment of metastatic spinal epidural disease*. Neuro Oncol 2005;7(1):64-76.

[108] Wilson LD, Detterbeck FC, Yahalom J. Clinical practice. *Superior vena cava syndrome with malignant causes*. N Engl J Med 2007;356(18):1862-9.

[109] Eren S, Karaman A, Okur A. *The superior vena cava syndrome caused by malignant disease. Imaging with multi detector row CT*. Eur J Radiol 2006;59(1):93-103.

[110] Sculier JP, Evans WK, Feld R, DeBoer G, Payne DG, Shepherd FA, et al. *Superior vena cava obstruction syndrome in small cell lung cancer*. Cancer 1986;57(4):847–51.

[111] Perez-Soler R, McLaughlin P, Velasquez WS, Hagemeister FB, Zornoza J, Manning JT, et al. *Clinical features and results of management of superior vena cava syndrome secondary to lymphoma*. J Clin Oncol 1984;2(4):260–6.

[112] Kim HJ, Kim HS, Chung SH. *CT diagnosis of superior vena cava syndrome: importance of collateral vessels*. AJR Am J Roentgenol 1993;161(3):539–42.

[113] Rice TW, Rodriguez RM, Light RW. *The superior vena cava syndrome: clinical characteristics and evolving etiology*. Medicine (Baltimore) 2006;85(1):37-42.

[114] Schraufnagel DE, Hill R, Leech JA, Pare JA. *Superior vena caval obstruction.* Is it a medical emergency? Am J Med 1981;70(6):1169–74.

[115] Bell DR, Woods RL, Levi JA. *Superior vena caval obstruction: a 10-year experience.* Med J Aust 1986;145(11-12):566-8.

[116] Bechtold RE, Wolfman NT, Karstaedt N, Choplin RH. *Superior vena caval obstruction: detection using CT.* Radiology 1985;157(2):485–7.

[117] Schwartz EE, Goodman LR, Haskin ME. *Role of CT scanning in the superior vena cava syndrome.* Am J Clin Oncol 1986;9(1):71–8.

[118] Thornton MJ, Ryan R, Varghese JC, Farrell MA, Lucey B, Lee MJ. *A three-dimensional gadolinium-enhanced MR venography technique for imaging central veins.* AJR Am J Roentgenol 1999;173(4):999-1003.

[119] Uberoi R. *Quality assurance guidelines for superior vena cava stenting in malignant disease.* Cardiovasc Intervent Radiol 2006;29(3):319-22.

[120] YuJ B,Wilson LD, Detterbeck FC. *Superior vena cava syndrome–a proposed classification system and algorithm for management.* J Thorac Oncol 2008;3(8): 811–4.

[121] Wan FJ, Bezjak A. *Superior vena Cava syndrome.* Emerg Med Clin N Am 2009;27(2):243-55.

[122] Rowell NP, Gleeson FV. *Steroids, radiotherapy, chemotherapy and stents for superior vena caval obstruction in carcinoma of the bronchus.* Cochrane Database Syst Rev 2001;(4):CD001316.

[123] Otten TR, Stein PD, Patel KC, Mustafa S, Silbergleit A. *Thromboembolic disease involving the superior vena cava and brachiocephalic veins.* Chest 2003;123(3): 809-12.

[124] Pereira JR, Martins CJ, Ikari FK, Nikaedo SM, Gampel O. *Neoadjuvant chemotherapy vs. radiotherapy alone for superior vena cava syndrome (SVCS) due to non-small cell lung cancer (NSCLC): preliminary results of a randomized phase II trial.* Eur J Cancer 1999;35(Suppl 4):260.

[125] Lonardi F, Gioga G, Agus G, Coeli M, Campostrini F. *Double-flash, large-fraction radiation therapy as palliative treatment of malignant superior vena cava syndrome in the elderly.* Support Care Cancer 2002;10(2):156–60.

[126] Citron ML, Fossieck BE Jr, Krasnow SH, Johnston-Early A, Cohen MH. *Superior vena cava syndrome due to non-small-cell lung cancer. Resolution with chemotherapy alone.* JAMA 1983;250(1):71-2.

[127] Faivre-Finn C, Snee M, Ashcroft L, Appel W, Barlesi F, Bhatnagar A, et al. *Concurrent once-daily versus twice-daily chemoradiotherapy in patients with limited-stage small-cell lung cancer (CONVERT): an open-label, phase 3, randomised, superiority trial.* Lancet Oncol 2017;18(8):1116-25.

[128] Huang Z, Xu Z, Zhou Y. *Chemotherapy alone versus chemotherapy followed by consolidative radiotherapy for limited-stage aggressive non-Hodgkin's lymphoma: a meta-analysis of randomized controlled trials.* Cancer Radiother 2013;17(8):736-43.

[129] Bierdrager E, Lampmann LE, Lohle PN, Schoemaker CM, Schijen JH, Palmen FM, et al. *Endovascular stenting in neoplastic superior vena cava syndrome prior to chemotherapy or radiotherapy.* Neth J Med 2005;63(1):20–3.

[130] Kim YI, Kim KS, Ko YC, Park CM, Lim SC, Kim YC, et al. *Endovascular stenting as a first choice for the palliation of superior vena cava syndrome.* J Korean Med Sci 2004;19(4):519–2.

In: Cancer Management in Latin America II
Editors: Maurício F Silva et al.
ISBN: 978-1-53616-735-1

Chapter 12

MANAGEMENT OF CANCER PAIN

Víctor Manuel Silva Ortiz[1], MD, Jorge A Nájera Medellín[2], MD, Sarkis Horacio Adjounian Correa[2], MD, Jose Alberto Flores Cantisani[3,*], MD, PhD, Fiona Lim[4], MBBS, Bo Angela Wan[5], MD(C) and Mauricio F Silva[6,7,8], MD, PhD

[1]Department of Pain Medicine, School of Medicine and Health Sciences, Instituto Tecnológico de Monterrey, Mexico
[2]Palliative Medicine and Pain, School of Medicine and Health Sciences, Instituto Tecnológico de Monterrey, Mexico
[3]Instituto Mexicano del Seguro Social, Monterrey, Mexico
[4]Department of Oncology, Princess Margaret Hospital, Hong Kong, PR China
[5]Odette Cancer Centre, Sunnybrook Health Sciences Centre, Toronto, Ontario, Canada
[6]Radiation Oncology Unit, Santa Maria Federal University, Santa Maria, Brazil
[7]Radiation Oncology Unit, Hospital de Caridade Astrogildo de Azevedo, Santa Maria, Brazil
[8]Latin America Cooperative Oncology Group, Porto Alegre, Brazil

ABSTRACT

Pain is one of the most common symptoms in cancer patients and represents a great negative impact on their quality of life, being a multidimensional problem. About 59% of patients will experience pain regardless of their stage and more than 70% will experience pain in advanced stages of the disease. Multiple are the treatments that exist to manage pain in this type of patients being the opioid therapy considered the Gold standard. The

* Corresponding Author's Email: dr.florescantisani@gmail.com.

WHO analgesic ladder stipulates that there are three levels of therapy according to the intensity of pain (mild, moderate and severe), however, currently, the interventionist management of pain is being included as an additional therapy regardless of the severity of the pain, even in initial stages of disease. This chapter intends to make an updated review of the management of pain in its different modalities (pharmacological and interventional), to provide an optimal care of the oncological patient and thus improve their quality of life and treatment.

INTRODUCTION

Pain is one of the most common symptoms in cancer patients and it has the greatest impact on the quality of life on patients. Despite the existence of multiple treatment guidelines, oncological pain continues to be a challenge to offer adequate and effective treatment.

The inadequate management of oncological pain is a multidimensional problem; pain is a subjective symptom, its assessment and management can be affected by the patient, the physicians or the caregivers. Other factors that negatively affect the management and control of cancer pain is the availability and attitudes towards the use of opioids (1). Effective pain management needs a multidisciplinary approach.

"The aim of the wise is not to secure pleasure, but to avoid pain"

EPIDEMIOLOGY OF CANCER

Cancer was responsible for eight million deaths in 2013 worldwide. Cancer is the second cause of death, behind cardiovascular diseases (1). Cancer rates continues to increase due to the rapid growth of the population, the increase in life expectancy and the behaviors that increase the risk of cancer, such as smoking, diet and sedentary lifestyle (2).

It is estimated that in 2012 in Latin America there were about 1 million new cases of cancer and 500 thousand deaths related to cancer (3). In men, prostate cancer is the most common with an incidence adjusted for 54 cases and 17 deaths per 100,000 inhabitants, followed by lung cancer (19 cases and 17 deaths/100,000 inhabitants/year), stomach (13 cases and 11 deaths/100,000 inhabitants/year), liver (seven cases and six deaths/100,000 inhabitants/year). In women, the most common cancer in Latin America is breast cancer (47 cases and 13 deaths/100,000 inhabitants/year), cervical cancer is the second most common cancer with 22 cases and 9 deaths per 100,000 inhabitants per year, followed by colon cancer (13 cases and seven deaths/100,000 inhabitants/year), and stomach cancer (seven cases and six deaths/100,000 inhabitants/year) (4).

Pain is one of the most feared cancer symptoms by patients and their families. The prevalence of cancer pain ranges from 43 to 63% in all stages of the disease (5). Around 59% of patients on cancer treatment will experience pain, and even higher up to 70% of patients with advanced or terminal disease and 33% of cancer survivors will have pain (6).

In addition, 25% of patients reported pain to be associated with treatments and 10% developed painful syndromes related to the oncological process (7).

Almost 31% of patients will have two or three painful syndromes. 85% of patients will suffer pain from the oncological process the rest of the patients will present pain derived from the treatment and only 10% of the patients have pain not related to the oncological process (8). Breakthrough pain is one of the most prevalent symptoms among patients with cancer, affecting 40-80% of them (9).

Recent reports showed a decrease in the number of patients without oncological pain treatment of 25%. Despite improvement in the access to opioid treatment, up to one third of patients do not receive analgesics appropriate to the magnitude of pain (9).

In developing countries, more than 90% of patients die with pain related to cancer without receiving adequate treatment (10). About 84% of total opioid consumption occurs in developed countries. Countries such as Mexico, India or Afghanistan, despite being producers of opioids, their citizens do not have access to this type of medication (7).

CANCER PAIN

Cancer pain is the result of the cancer itself or its management. Pain is a subjective experience and varies among people. Therefore, its management and interventions must be individualized. The etiology of cancer pain is multifactorial, resulting from cellular tissue, tumor growth that invades adjacent structures like bones and nerves, or iatrogenic due to surgeries, chemotherapy, radiotherapy, etc. (7).

Cancer pain is classified into constant pain and breakthrough pain. Irruptive pain is defined as "an intermittent exacerbation that occurs in a patient who has a stable and persistent pain" (8-11).

Somatic pain originates in non-nervous or visceral structures such as skin or muscle and can be described as a localized, acute and superficial pain usually with no irradiation. Visceral pain originates from the viscera, it is usually diffuse and deep. Neuropathic pain is defined by The International Association for the Study of Pain (IASP) as "pain caused by an injury or disease of the somatosensory nervous system," characterized by numbness, paresthesia, or alterations in sensation and motor function.

The symptoms of cancer are a consequence of the systemic changes that occur due to uncontrolled cell proliferation, invasion and immune response. Cancer cells produce substances that affect homeostasis. Nociception involves dynamic changes which affect signal transduction pathways between tumor cells and the primary afferent nociceptor (12). The clinical features of cancer depend mainly on the histological type, the location of the primary tumors and metastases (12).

Management guidelines, including the World Health Organization and more recently the European Association for Palliative Care and the European Society of Medical Oncology, suggested that opioid-based therapy is effective in most cases (9, 13, 14). And it is recommended that analgesics should be administered through basal doses and extra doses for breakthrough pain.

Breakthrough pain

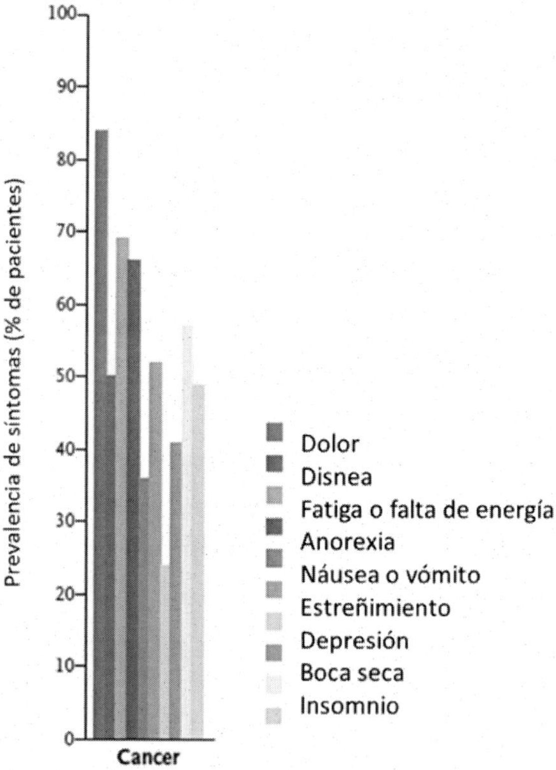

Modified from (11).

Figure 1. Symptom prevalence in cancer patients.

Breakthrough pain is a transient exacerbation of pain that occurs on top of chronic pain that is stable and relatively well controlled. It has a significant impact on the daily routine of cancer patients, causing psychological discomfort and negative effects on mood, work activity, social relationships, sleep and quality of life (14). Breakthrough pain can be classified as spontaneous or idiopathic (one the occur without an event, usually has slow onset and a longer duration), or as incidental (one that is triggered by some events, usually faster onset and a shorter duration; further sub-classified into predictable or unpredictable (15). Irruptive pain is related to the end of dose, its onset is more gradual and longer than the previous ones, and is possible to originate from two factors, an insufficient analgesic dose or a very prolonged administration interval (15).

The prevalence of oncologic breakthrough pain ranged from 39.9 to 53.8% in ambulatory patients. In hospices, the prevalence is almost 80%. The prevalence also varies depending on the patient clinical status, in which patients with metastasis had higher prevalence to near 70% (16).

Pain assessment

Cancer pain is multidimensional involving various types of cancer pain, each of them with own assessment tools and modalities of treatment (15). Pain can be assessed through simple and easy to apply tools such as visual, verbal, numerical or similar scales; or through long and complex questionnaires, which are more useful in the field of research. Visual, verbal, numerical or analogous scales are simple and easy to use, but have a limited sensitivity due to interindividual variation, idiosyncrasies and cultural differences of patients (15).

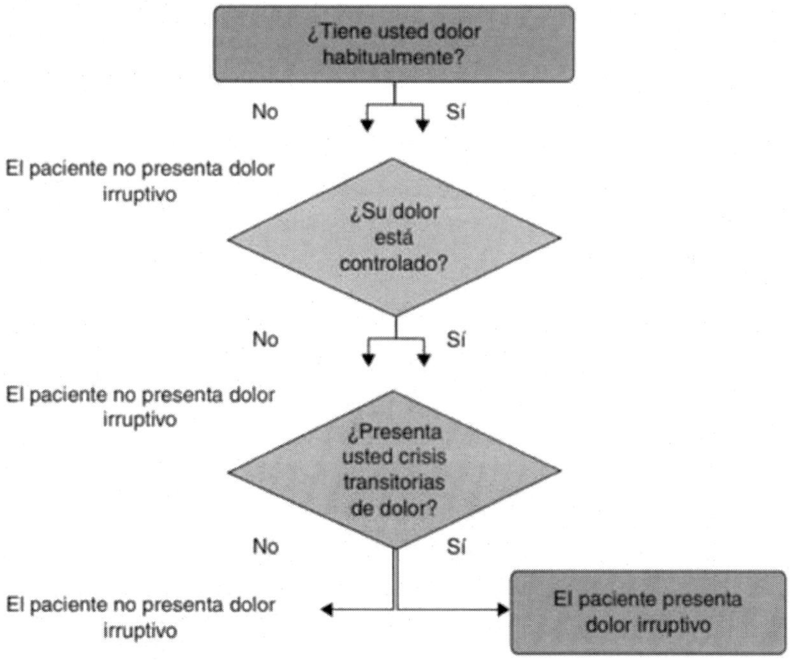

Modified from (79).

Figure 2. Davies algorithm.

The Edmonton classification system is a standard scale validated in Spanish for oncological pain and other symptoms (16). The ESAS score uses a visual analog scale from 0 to 10 to identify the severity of various symptoms including pain. This tool can be completed by patients or by health personnel or caregivers (17).

Multidimensional scales such as the McGill Questionnaire assess various aspects of pain such as emotional, temporal change in pain, aggravating factors and attitudes towards pain (18). Similar to other types of pain, neuropathic pain can also be related to the oncological process, treatments or comorbidities of the patient (19). Several assessment tools, such as NP questionnaire, PainDetect, and ID-Pain, help to identify up to 90% of cancer patients with neuropathic pain along with the physical examination that include touch, pressure, temperature, vibration and temporal summation (18).

Irruptive or breakthrough pain is a transient exacerbation of stable pain in a patient chronically treated with opioids. The assessment and diagnosis of breakthrough oncological pain are formulated according to the Davies algorithm (see Figure 2).

MANAGEMENT OF CANCER PAIN

In 1984 The World Health Organization (WHO) proposed the analgesic ladder for cancer pain management that proved to be an effective and safe tool with a success rate of up to 80% (see Figure 3) (19). The management of oncological pain is multidisciplinary and involves physical, psychological and spiritual elements (20, 21).

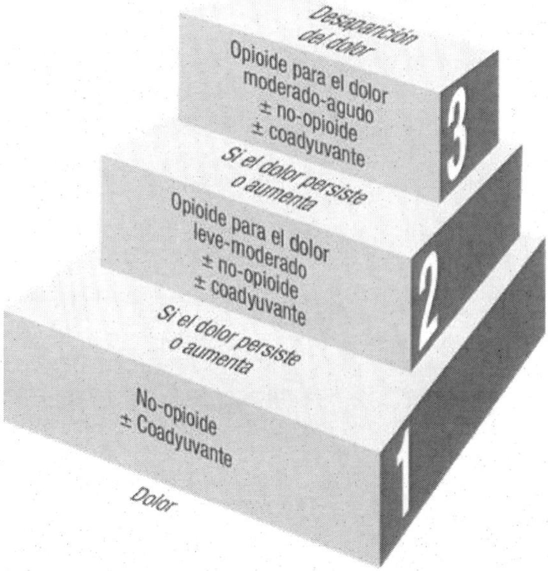

Modified from (80).

Figure 3. WHO analgesic ladder.

Pharmacotherapy

The current management of cancer pain is based on the analgesic ladder proposed by WHO, and treatments should be directed to address both basal and irruptive pain (22).

Opioids are the main part of cancer pain treatment. Its use is limited by adverse effects, which can be reversed by rotation to other opioids, by the use of analgesic adjuvants and interventional pain management (23). Lack of drug availability, as well as barriers in the health personnel (e.g., lack of knowledge of the pharmacology of opioids, lack of experience in the management of opioid) and society (e.g., abuse or misconception on opioids) are also factors that limit opioid use. Another limitation in the use of opioids are barriers in health personnel for several reasons (24).

Opioids

Opiates are derivatives of opium and are alkaloids of natural origin, while opioids are any substance, regardless of their origin, bind to opioid receptors and the effect of this union can be reversed with receptor antagonists such as naloxone. Synthetic opioids can be divided into four chemical groups: derivatives of morphine (levorphanol, butorphanol), diphenylheptane derivatives (methadone, propoxyphene), benzomorphan derivatives (pentazocine, phenazocine) and phenylpiperidine derivatives (fentanyl, sufentanil, remifentanil) (22).

They classified by their effects on the opioid receptors, namely agonists, partial agonists and antagonists. Opioids exert their action through binding on the receptors which are expressed in neurons of the central and peripheral nervous system, neuroendocrine cells and the immune system. There are three types of receptors in the central nervous system, the mu, delta and kappa receptors; other types of receptors like sigma, epsilon and the orphanin receptors have recently been proposed (20).

Generally, long-acting opioids are used for the treatment of basal pain and immediate release opioids are for breakthrough pain (25). Opioids can be administered by several routes, with oral route preferred over the parenteral route which is reserved for more advanced stages of cancer. The subcutaneous route has several advantages such as requirement of a lower dose, not required an injection site and specialized training is not necessary for its administration (25). On the other hand, the intravenous route offers advantages such as a rapid and predictable effect.

Opioid consumption in Latin America is below international levels. Argentina and Brazil have the highest opioid use rate in Latin America. Brazil, Argentina, Mexico, Cuba and Peru have good availability of immediate-release opioids but with limited availability of prolonged-release opioids and potent opioids (25).

Morphine

Morphine is the "Gold standard" for the management of mild to moderate cancer pain (24). It is a natural opioid derived from opium seeds and is available in presentations of immediate and prolonged release. It is metabolized in the liver by glucuronyl transferase. Its active metabolite is Morphine-6-glucuronide.

In 1986 WHO recommended the treatment of cancer pain with morphine every four hours; enteral morphine produces good pain relief for most patients with moderate or severe cancer pain (25).

A randomized study of morphine and weak opioid showed that almost 80% of patients treated with morphine initially responded with at least a 20% decrease in baseline pain, compared to the weak opioid group, which only 43% of Patients showed improvement (26).

Another study compared the efficacy of morphine with oxycodone, 62% of patients had a good response to the administration of morphine as a first-line treatment, and 67% of patients presented pain reduction with oxycodone, without being statistically significant (26).

Hydromorphone

Hydromorphone (dihydromorphinone) is a semisynthetic opioid, derived from morphine with similar chemical structure but with greater solubility and thus 5 to 7 times more potency (27). It is a μ receptor agonist with low affinity to κ receptors (27). Hydromorphone has multiple routes of administration including the spinal route.

A systematic review concluded that hydromorphone is effective for the treatment of cancer pain, but there is no evidence that it is better than morphine as the first line of treatment (28).

Oxycodone

It is a semisynthetic opioid derived from thebaine, is 1.5 times more potent than morphine, is a selective μ receptor agonist, and some studies suggest the activation of κ receptors (29).

Oxycodone offers similar levels of analgesia and adverse effects compared to other potent opioids such as morphine and can be used as first line treatment, or when inadequate pain relief or adverse effects with other types of opioids (30, 31). It has a better pharmacological profile in patients with renal impairment due to decreased production of metabolites that required renal excretion, but use of prolonged-release preparations is still not recommended and (31).

Fentanyl

Fentanyl is a synthetic opioid that is highly lipophilic and is 80 to 100 times more potent than morphine, with a rapid onset of action and short duration of the analgesic effect (32, 33). It is often used for management of acute and breakthrough pain (34). It has several formulations, with transdermal route more useful for stable pain; and oral transmucosal more useful for breakthrough pain.

The nasal formulation (Fentanyl Pectin Nasal Spray FPNS) for breakthrough pain is useful and well tolerated, with 70% patient-reported satisfaction as well as being convenient and easy to apply (35).

Methadone

Methadone is an important option in cancer patients and has an accessible cost. It had a long half-life that allows a dosing frequency of two or three times a day. It lacks active metabolites which makes it useful in patients with kidney disease (36).

Methadone is an opioid agonist that binds to the μ, δ and κ receptors, it is also an NMDA receptor antagonist (N-methyl-D-aspartate). Its onset of action is 30 minutes and has a variable half-life of 8-90 hours (36).

In patients with mixed cancer pain, methadone is as effective as prolonged-release morphine or transdermal fentanyl (37). Methadone is effective as a first line of treatment with analgesia and adverse effects similar to other opioids, also offers antihyperalgesic properties (38).

Buprenorphine

Buprenorphine has a high affinity for the μ receptor, it also binds to the δ receptor and is an antagonist for the κ receptor (39). It is safe for patients with mild or moderate hepatic failure and is safe in patients with chronic kidney disease on dialysis treatment (40, 41).

Transdermal buprenorphine is safe and effective in patients with cancer and severe neuropathic pain to be effective in combination with other adjuvant analgesics and can significantly improve quality of life (42).

Breakthrough pain treatment

The proper management of breakthrough pain is based on three aspects: prevention, anticipation and the use of drug of the correct potency for the type and severity of pain to decrease the frequency and intensity of episodes of breakthrough pain. The main pharmacological tool for the treatment of breakthrough pain are short-acting opioids.

Morphine has been the main approach in the prevention of anticipated breakthrough pain because of its onset of action of 30 to 45 minutes and so can be administered before starting any activity. Rapid onset opioids have better pain relief when compared to placebo in the first 30 minutes after the dose. Normal-release oral opioids have been the mainstay approach for patients who are receiving around the clock opioid regimen, but the onset and duration of action of oral opioids such as morphine may not be suitable for treating many breakthrough pains.

For the effective treatment of breakthrough pain in cancer it is necessary to find the adequate dose to provide sufficient analgesia to have mild to moderate pain in addition to the ideal administration route.

Intrathecal therapy for cancer pain management

Cancer pain is complex and difficult to manage. Almost 20% of patients treated with opioids for cancer pain will present severe adverse effects or failure to control pain. Intrathecal drug delivery systems can be effective in treating pain (43).

Intrathecal opioids are mainly reserved for use in oncological pain that is refractory to traditional treatment. It has been shown to be effective and does not have the magnitude of the adverse effects of parenteral opioids (44).

A retrospective study with intrathecal multimodal analgesia of morphine, Bupivacaine and clonidine demonstrated a reduction in pain in patients with nociceptive or mixed oncological pain (45).

Other retrospective study of patients treated with intrathecal drug delivery systems demonstrated the potential to improve pain in a variety of patients and types of cancer (43).

Non-Opioid drug for cancer pain management

Drugs non-related to opioids for the management of cancer pain include acetaminophen, NSAIDs, corticosteroids, antidepressants, anticonvulsive and bisphosphonates (46)

Drugs like antidepressants, anticonvulsive and corticosteroids are useful in treating neuropathic pain. Gabapentinoides reduce visceral and bone pain. Amitriptyline, a tricyclic antidepressant, improves neuropathic pain and reduce the opioids consumption (47).

A systematic revision found no good quality evidence to use and recommend the use of gabapentinoides like gabapentin or pregabalin or venlafaxine for the management of cancer pain (48).

Opioid-induced hyperalgesia

Opioid-induced hyperalgesia is a nociceptive sensitization caused by the use of opioids and could be related to opioid tolerance (49). The prevalence ranges from 14% to 28% in non-cancer patients (50). It's a paradoxical of opioid pain management in which larger opioid doses cause more pain. There is an increase in sensitivity to painful stimuli or allodynia. In general, there is an imbalance between pronociceptive and antinociceptive pathways (49).

In patients with terminal cancer, hyperalgesia can manifest as an exacerbation of baseline pain that coincides with the increase in the dose of opioid with intrathecal administration and that resolves with the decrease of opioids (51).

Opioid-induced hyperalgesia is demonstrated in animal models and by experiments in humans (52). Mechanisms for opioid-induced hyperalgesia are not yet known, which makes both diagnosis and treatment difficult. There are some clinical criteria for diagnosis, although they are not specific for patients with cancer pain (see Table 1) (51).

Table 1. Eisenberg criteria for the diagnosis of opioid-induced hyperalgesia

Increased pain during chronic treatment with opioids
Absence of disease progression
Absence of abstinence data
Elimination of tolerance to opioids (increase of pain with increase in dose)
Decreased pain with dose reduction
Elimination of addictive behaviors

Adapted from (51).

Perhaps the authors could consider giving some discussion on potential side effects of opioids and the strategies for managing that. And a short summary about pain management using various tools for assessment, various groups of medication for different types and severity of pain could be considered.

INTERVENTIONAL THERAPIES FOR ONCOLOGIC PAIN MANAGEMENT

Even though opioid analgesics are the gold standard for the treatment of oncologic pain and they provide relief of pain up to 80% of patients, in some cases, refractory pain is still present, diminishing quality of life in most cases. In this challenging clinical scenario, interventional therapies for the management of pain should be applied. These procedures should be selected according to severity, type and pain location. These therapies have been proposed by some authors (controvertibly) as the fourth analgesic step of the WHO analgesic ladder, and in some cases have been used in anticipated manner in early stages of disease, alone or together with other pharmacological approaches, to reduce the use of opioids and its adverse effects.

These techniques require a special training to be performed by pain physicians who should be aware of benefits, risks and complications about them (53).

Interventional procedures recommendations

Several safety recommendations must be taken in care before performing an interventional procedure to reduce incidence of complications (54). Patients should have received proper analgesic treatment according to WHO analgesic Ladder before the procedure. Proper interrogation and physical examination should be performed to establish etiology, and quality of pain. Proper evaluation of pain frequency, location and quality of life alteration should be assessed before and after the procedure and contraindications of performing the procedure must be taken in care. Injection site should be inspected to rule out local infections and patient's tolerability to stay in a proper position during procedure should be evaluated. Labs and imaging studies must be performed to diagnose tumor related anatomic and biochemical alterations that could hinder block realization. Patients should sign a written informed consent prior the procedure and this documentation must explain objectives, complications and alternatives of the procedure. Patient's choice should always be respected. Performing a diagnostic block before a therapeutic one is a reasonable choice.

Interventional therapy contraindications

Although these therapies are widely used in the management of pain in cancer patients, they are not exempt from complications, so there are relative and absolute contraindications applicable to all interventional procedures, which must be respected if complications are to be avoided (54).

Absolute contraindications

- Refusal of patient
- Local and systemic infection
- Coagulopathy (INR > 1.5, platelet count <50,000)
- Lack of operator technical experience
- Uncertain Diagnosis
- Poorly cooperative patient
- Opioid addictive patient
- Allergies to used drugs

Relative contraindications

- Concomitant Chemotherapy treatment
- Neutropenia.
- Neurological deficit prior the procedure

The performance of interventional procedures should be related to the anatomy to be blocked, so that the description of the different blocks according to the different anatomical areas of importance will be made in a didactic way

Interventions for head and neck cancer pain

Pain is one of the most common symptoms in head and neck cancer, reaching up to 85% of patients, of which up to 90% have a mixed pattern (neuropathic and nociceptive) (55).

The location of the pain can vary from dysphagia to pain of varying intensity in the head, face, mouth, ears, and cervical region. Pain in the head and neck can be particularly difficult to treat due to the extensive innervation and vascularization of the area, which also involves structures related to speech, swallowing, and breathing (56, 57).

The prevalence of refractory pain and intolerable adverse effects in oncological pathologies of the head and neck can reach up to 20%. Blocks that have been used successfully to relieve pain in this anatomical region are blockage of the trigeminal, glossopharyngeal, occipital, sphenopalatine ganglion and cervical plexus (58).

Interventions for thoracic wall cancer pain

The pain secondary to cancer in the thoracic region usually suggests bone invasion by metastasis, being its management in advanced cases palliatively. However, in these patients, interventions such as intercostal blocks, thoracic paravertebral, and erector spinal block can be performed depending on the location of the pain.

Regarding the intercostal block, the current recommendation is to perform the procedure through ultrasound guidance and avoid performing it purely from anatomical references on imaging to reduce the incidence of pneumothorax (59).

This procedure can be performed either with local anesthetic and steroid (Diagnostic and therapeutic) or with phenol (neurolytic block), the latter only reserved for cases of refractory pain in advanced stages of disease (terminal patients) where the blockage of the motility of the chest wall is no longer a concern. The pain relief rate reported for this procedure is close to 80% of the cases treated (59).

As for the erector blockage of the spine, it is a procedure of recent description, which has been used in multiple pathologies and clinical conditions (thoracic surgery, pain relief for herpes zoster in the thoracic area among others) despite the fact that good results have been reported in terms of its application for pain relief in both oncological and non-oncological patients (60-62). To date there are no systematic reviews, only case studies and case series.

Interventions in the upper abdomen

Celiac plexus block

The anatomical areas blocked with this technique include visceral organs (stomach, transverse colon, vesicle and pancreas.) The literature (randomized studies and meta-analysis) reports significant pain improvement in cancer patients undergoing this technique, which can be performed with local anesthetics and corticosteroids. (diagnostic and therapeutic technique) or with neurolytic substances The performance of this procedure (especially in advanced stages of pancreatic cancer) has shown a significant reduction in the intensity of pain (more than 50% reduction) and decrease in the need of analgesic rescue medicines, significantly improving the quality of life in the patients to whom it is performed (63-65).

Performing this block using phenol as a neurolytic agent is a frequent procedure and its effectiveness in relieving pain in pancreatic cancer has been demonstrated in multiple studies. A recent meta-analysis shows that there is significant improvement in pain with decreased opioid consumption at 2, 4, 6 and 8 weeks after the blockade with phenol in comparison to the group where it was performed with local anesthetic and steroids (65). However, a Cochrane review linked improvement of pain up to 4 weeks in patients undergoing celiac plexus block. Literature recommends the completion of this block early (although its duration of pain relief is approximately 3 to 6 weeks) (66) because it has been shown improvement in the quality of life of patients in the terminal stage and prolongation of the time of life (67, 68).

Interventions in pelvic and perineal cancer pain

About 75% of patients with cancer in the pelvic and perineal region will have pain at some point of their disease of which 30% will have severe pain. The performance of neurolytic blockade of the upper and lower hypogastric plexus are a useful tool to relieve pain in these patients (69).

Blocking of the upper hypogastric plexus

The sensory innervation of the bladder, uterus, vagina, prostate, testes, descending colon, and rectum is contributed by the superior hypogastric plexus, so that patients with tumors in these structures benefit from the performance of said procedure. The superior hypogastric plexus is a retroperitoneal structure that is located between L3 and S1 near the sacral promontory and the division of the bifurcation of the iliac veins (69).

The indications to perform this block are visceral, pelvic oncological, and refractory pain. The posterior approach is the most common. Plancarte and colleagues were the first to describe the classical technique in which needles are inserted bilaterally level L5 and S1, demonstrating between 70 to 90% pain relief (70) Complications inherent in this block are rare and are the injury to the common iliac veins, to the pelvic viscera to the nerve root of L5.

Inferior hypogastric plexus block

The inferior hypogastric plexus is in the presacral tissues ventral to the vertebrae S2-4 medial to the sacral foramen. This block is effective in terms of pain reduction and opioid use for pelvic perineal pain. Among its complications we can mention the appearance of transient paresthesia and lesion to the rectum. Although several studies report pain relief in patients with pelvic and perineal pain, more randomized studies evaluating their efficacy and safety are required (71).

Impar ganglion block

The impar ganglion or Walther's ganglion is a structure located in the bilateral union of the sympathetic chain, which provides nociceptive and sympathetic innervation to the perineum, distal rectum, perineal region, distal urethra, vulva, scrotum and to the distal third of the vagina (72) The indications for this block are rectal pain, coccygodinia, and tenesmoid pain (73) There are several approaches, the first one being described by Plancarte et al. of the anoccocigeal membrane of a bent needle Other approaches include the transcoccygeal route and the transdiscal route. The data reported on this blockade are scarce (report and series of cases), however, there is evidence of significant pain improvement in these studies.

Neuraxial analgesia

Neuraxial analgesia involves the administration of local anesthetics, opioids with or without the use of adjuvants in the epidural or intrathecal space using a percutaneous or implanted catheter (continuous intrathecal infusion system). The most frequent route of administration is intrathecal, and this is reserved for clinical situations where pain is refractory to conventional therapy or when the patient presents adverse effects intolerable to conventional pharmacological therapy. The main objective of intraneural drug therapy is to provide analgesia using very small doses of drugs, thus reducing their toxicity potential (74-76). Multiple drugs have been used to provide neuroaxial analgesia including morphine, hydromorphone, Fentanyl, Sufentanyl, Methadone, local anesthetics, alpha 2 agonists, baclofen, used as monotherapy or in combination, each with its specific indications, contraindications and complications (76). Regarding the use of these drugs as monotherapy or in combination, better analgesic results have been reported in the medium and long term when the drugs are used in combination, bearing in mind that there is a synergistic effect between them. Although this therapy is relatively safe, it requires trained personnel to perform it and is not exempt from complications, the most frequent being related to the catheter (infections, catheter blockage due to fibrosis, migration and rupture of the catheter, and cerebrospinal fluid fistula). Regarding the complications of neuraxial continuous administration systems, the most common complications are the failure of the battery and the internal mechanical system of the device (76). It must be taken into account when applying this type of therapy, that not all patients are candidates to receive these treatments and that as contraindications the literature describes the presence of systemic or local infection, anticoagulation or other bleeding conditions, endocranial hypertension and pathologies of the spinal canal. A multidisciplinary analysis prior to the application of these treatments is mandatory specially to assess the patient's motivation and adherence to treatment, it is also mandatory to make risk analysis benefit and discuss with the patient and their families the need to establish therapeutic goals and expectations (76).

OTHER INTERVENTIONIST PROCEDURES

Bone fixation with cement

Although the use of cement was initially described for the stabilization of vertebral body fractures, at present, it is used for the control of bone pain secondary to metastasis in multiple bones. Its mechanism of action is the mechanical stabilization of the fracture. The most performed procedures are vertebroplasty and kyphoplasty. Several studies have compared the effectiveness of the use of cement finding satisfactory results for the management of bone pain secondary to fractures, especially with the use of balloon technique compared to vertebroplasty without the balloon, however, there is no precise recommendation on this subject to date. A systematic review of the Cochrane library on the use of cement in vertebral body fractures concludes that this procedure is not routinely recommended since the effect of pain relief is short-lived compared to placebo which may be associated with adverse side effects as infiltration of the spinal cord with cement (77).

Injections of trigger points

In cancer patients, the prevalence of musculoskeletal pain due to various causes can be high, so the injection of local anesthetics and steroids is a useful and relatively safe tool to relieve this type of pain. However, its effectiveness to date has not been evaluated in oncological pain and only the results of non-oncological pain studies can be extrapolated, in addition, although several studies have been carried out, its effectiveness may be limited by the great anatomical variability and of location of trigger zones and by the heterogeneity of treatments (78).

References

[1] Global Burden of Disease Cancer Collaboration, Fitzmaurice C, Dicker D, Pain A, Hamavid H, Moradi-Lakeh M, et al. *The Global Burden of Cancer 2013*. JAMA Oncol 2015;1(4):505-27.

[2] Torre LA, Siegel RL, Ward EM, Jemal A. *Global cancer incidence and mortality rates and trends - an update*. Cancer Epidemiol Biomarkers Prev 2016;25(1):16-27.

[3] Sierra MS, Soerjomataram I, Antoni S, Laversanne M, Piñeros M, de Vries E, et al. *Cancer patterns and trends in Central and South America*. Cancer Epidemiol 2016;44(Suppl 1):S23-42.

[4] Curado MP, De Souza DLB. *Cancer burden in Latin America and the Caribbean*. Ann Glob Health 2014;80(5):370-7.

[5] van den Beuken-van Everdingen M, de Rijke J, Kessels A, Schouten H, van Kleef M, Patijn J. *Prevalence of pain in patients with cancer: a systematic review of the past 40 years.* Ann Oncol 2007;18(9):1437-49.

[6] Lara-Solares A, Ahumada Olea M, Basantes Pinos ALÁ, Bistre Cohén S, Bonilla Sierra P, Duarte Juárez ER, et al. *Pain management Latin-American guidelines for cancer pain management Practice points*. Pain Manag 2017;7(4):287-98.

[7] Are M, McIntyre A, Reddy S. *Global disparities in cancer pain management and palliative care.* J Surg Oncol 2017;115(5):637-41.

[8] Kumar S. *Cancer pain: A critical review of mechanism-based classification and physical therapy management in palliative care.* Indian J Palliat Care 2011;17(2):116-26.

[9] Greco MT, Roberto A, Corli O, Deandrea S, Bandieri E, Cavuto S, et al. *Quality of cancer pain management: An update of a systematic review of undertreatment of patients with cancer.* J Clin Oncol 2014;32(36):4149-54.

[10] *American Cancer Society.* Rising global cancer epidemic. URL: https://www.cancer.org/res earch/info graphics-gallery/rising-global-cancer-epidemic.html.

[11] Kelley AS, Morrison RS. *Palliative care for the seriously ill.* N Engl J Med 2015;373(8):747-55.

[12] Schmidt BL, Hamamoto DT, Simone DA, Wilcox GL. *Mechanism of cancer pain.* Mol Interv 2010;10(3):164-78.

[13] Regan JM, Peng P. *Neurophysiology of cancer pain.* Cancer Control 2000;7(2):111-9.

[14] World Health Organization. *Cancer pain relief: with a guide to opioid availability.* Geneva: WHO, 2014:1-70.

[15] Miró J. *Evaluación de la intensidad del dolor en el paciente con cáncer.* Psicoon-cología 2013;9(2-3):129-40.

[16] Ngamkham S, Vincent C, Finnegan L, Holden JE, Wang ZJ, Wilkie DJ. *The McGill pain questionnaire as a multidimensional measure in people with cancer: an integrative review.* Pain Manag Nurs 2012;13(1):27-51.

[17] Mulvey MR, Rolke R, Klepstad P, Caraceni A, Fallon M, Colvin L, et al. *Confirming neuropathic pain in cancer patients: Applying the NeuPSIG grading system in clinical practice and clinical research.* Pain 2014;155(5):859-63.

[18] Esin E, Yalcin S. *Neuropathic cancer pain: What we are dealing with? How to manage it?* Onco Targets Ther. 2014;7:599-618.

[19] Vargas-Schaffer G. *Is the WHO analgesic ladder still valid?* Twenty-four years of experience. Can Fam Physician 2010;56(6):514-7.

[20] Scott-Warren J, Bhaskar A. *Cancer pain management-Part I: General principles.* CEACCP 2014;14(6):278-84.

[21] Grant M, Ugalde A, Vafiadis P, Philip J. *Exploring the myths of morphine in cancer: views of the general practice population.* Support Care Cancer 2014;23(2):483-9.

[22] Mercadante S, Vitrano V. *Pain in patients with lung cancer: Pathophysiology and treatment.* Lung Cancer 2010;68(1):10-5.

[23] Mercadante S. *Intravenous morphine for management of cancer pain.* Lancet Oncol 2010;11(5):484-9.

[24] Wiffen PJ, McQuay HJ. *Oral morphine for cancer pain.* Cochrane Database Syst Rev 2007;4:CD003868.

[25] Bandieri E, Romero M, Ripamonti CI, Artioli F, Sichetti D, Fanizza C, et al. Randomized trial of low-dose morphine versus weak opioids in moderate cancer pain. J Clin Oncol 2016;34(5):436-42.

[26] Riley J, Branford R, Droney J, Gretton S, Sato H, Kennett A, et al. Morphine or oxycodone for cancer-related pain ? a randomized, open-label, controlled trial. J Pain Symptom Manage 2015;49(2):161-72.

[27] Bao YJ, Hou W, Kong XY, Yang L, Xia J, Hua BJ, et al. Hydromorphone for cancer pain. Cochrane Database Syst Rev 2016;10:CD011108.

[28] Pigni A, Brunelli C, Caraceni A. *The role of hydromorphone in cancer pain treatment: A systematic review.* Palliat Medicine 2010;25(5):471-7.

[29] Pergolizzi J V., Seow-Choen F, Wexner SD, Zampogna G, Raffa RB, Taylor R. *Perspectives on intravenous oxycodone for control of postoperative pain.* Pain Pract 2016;16(7):924-34.

[30] Schmidt-Hansen M, Bennett MI, Arnold S, Bromham N, Hilgart JS. *Oxycodone for cancer-related pain.* Cochrane Database Syst Rev 2015;(2):CD003870.

[31] Leppert W. *Role of oxycodone and oxycodone/naloxone in cancer pain management.* Pharmacol Rep 2010;62(4):578-91.

[32] Sukcharoen K, Jeffery Z, Ratcliffe L, Miller J, Mulgrew C. *Prescribing analgesia for patients with impaired renal function.* Br J Hosp Med (Lond) 2018;79(5):C74-7.

[33] Hadley G, Derry S, Moore RA, Wiffen PJ. *Transdermal Fentanyl for Cancer Pain.* Cochrane Database Syst Rev 2013;10:CD010270.

[34] Mercadante S. *Pharmacotherapy for breakthrough cancer pain - the author's reply.* Drugs 2012;72(2):181-90.

[35] Portenoy RK, Burton AW, Gabrail N, Taylor D. *A multicenter, placebo-controlled, double-blind, multiple-crossover study of Fentanyl Pectin Nasal Spray (FPNS) in the treatment of breakthrough cancer pain.* Pain 2010;151(3):617-24.

[36] McPherson ML, Costantino RC, McPherson AL. *Methadone: Maximizing Safety and Efficacy for Pain Control in Patients with Cancer.* Hematol Oncol Clin North Am 2018:32(3):405-51.

[37] Mercadante S, Porzio G, Ferrera P, Fulfaro F, Aielli F, Verna L, et al. *Sustained-release oral morphine versus transdermal fentanyl and oral methadone in cancer pain management.* Eur J Pain 2008;12(8):1040-6.

[38] Mercadante S, Bruera E. *Methadone as a first-line opioid in cancer pain management: a systematic review.* J Pain Symptom Manage 2018;55(3):998-1003.

[39] Prommer E. *Buprenorphine for cancer pain: is it ready for prime time?* Am J Hosp Palliat Med 2015;32(8):881-9.

[40] Davis MP. *Twelve reasons for considering buprenorphine as a frontline analgesic in the management of pain.* J Support Oncol 2012;10(6):209-19.

[41] Pergolizzi J, Aloisi AM, Dahan A, Filitz J, Langford R, Likar R, et al. *Current knowledge of buprenorphine and its unique pharmacological profile.* Pain Pract 2010;10(5):428-50.

[42] Leppert W, Kowalski G. *Long-term administration of high doses of transdermal buprenorphine in cancer patients with severe neuropathic pain.* Onco Targets Ther 2015;8:3621-7.

[43] Sayed D, Monroe F, Orr WN, Phadnis M, Khan TW, Braun E, et al. *Retrospective analysis of intrathecal drug delivery: Outcomes, efficacy, and risk for cancer-related pain at a high volume academic medical center.* Neuromodulation 2018;21(7):660-4.

[44] Huang Y, Li X, Zhu T, Lin J, Tao G. Efficacy and safety of ropivacaine addition to intrathecal morphine for pain management in intractable cancer. Mediators Inflamm 2015;2015:439014.

[45] Mastenbroek TC, Kramp-Hendriks BJ, Kallewaard JW, Vonk JM. *Multimodal intrathecal analgesia in refractory cancer pain.* Scand J Pain 2017;14:39-43.

[46] Vardy J, Agar M. *Nonopioid drugs in the treatment of cancer pain.* J Clin Oncol 2014;32(16):1677-90.

[47] Shinde S, Gordon P, Sharma P, Gross J, Davis MP. *Use of non-opioid analgesics as adjuvants to opioid analgesia for cancer pain management in an inpatient palliative unit: does this improve pain control and reduce opioid requirements*? Support Care Cancer 2014;23(3):695-703.

[48] van den Beuken-van Everdingen MHJ, de Graeff A, Jongen JLM, Dijkstra D, Mostovaya I, Vissers KC. *Pharmacological treatment of pain in cancer patients: the role of adjuvant analgesics, a systematic review.* Pain Pract 2016;17(3):409-19.

[49] Roeckel LA, Le Coz GM, Gavériaux-Ruff C, Simonin F. *Opioid-induced hyperalgesia: Cellular and molecular mechanisms.* Neuroscience 2016;338:160-82.

[50] Arout CA, Edens E, Petrakis IL, Sofuoglu M. *Targeting opioid-induced hyperalgesia in clinical treatment: neurobiological considerations.* CNS Drugs 2015;29(6):465-86.

[51] Eisenberg E, Suzan E, Pud D. *Opioid-Induced hyperalgesia (OIH): a real clinical problem or just an experimental phenomenon*? J Pain Symptom Manage 2015;49(3):632-6.

[52] Sandkühler J. *Models and mechanisms of hyperalgesia and allodynia.* Physiol Rev 2009;89(2):707-58.

[53] Vayne-Bossert P, Afsharimani B, Good P, Gray P, Hardy J. *Interventional options for the management of refractory cancer pain - What is the evidence?* Support Care Cancer 2016;24(3):1429-38.

[54] Bhatnagar S, Gupta M. *Evidence-based clinical practice guidelines for interventional pain management in cancer pain.* Indian J Palliat Care 2015;21(2): 137-47.

[55] Kou P, Williams JE. *Pain control in head and neck cancer.* In: Agulnik M, ed. Head and Neck Cancer. London: InTech, 2012:351-71.

[56] Potter J, Higginson IJ, Scadding JW, Quigley C. *Identifying neuropathic pain in patients with head and neck cancer: Use of the leeds assessment of neuropathic symptoms and signs scale*. J R Soc Med 2003;96(8):379-83.

[57] Silva VM, Flores JA, Arechiga GE, Reyes JI, Cantu F. *Interventional techniques for head and neck cancer pain*. Diagnosis and management of head and neck cancer. IntechOpen 2017. URL: https://www.intechopen.com/chapter/pdf-downloa d/56045.

[58] Sist T. *Head and neck nerve blocks for cancer pain management*. Tech Reg Anesth Pain Manage 1997;1(1):3-10.

[59] Wong FC, Lee TW, Yuen KK, Lo SH, Sze WK, Tung SY. *Intercostal nerve blockade for cancer pain: Effectiveness and selection of patients*. Hong Kong Med J 2007;13(4):266-70.

[60] Forero M, Adhikary S, Lopez H, Tsui C, Chin K. *The erector spinae plane block*. A novel analgesic technique in thoracic neuropathic pain. Reg Anesth Pain Med 2016;41(5):621-7.

[61] Ramos J, Peng P, Forero M. *Long-term continuous erector spinae plane block for palliative pain control in a patient with pleura mesothelioma*. Can J Anaesth 2018;65(7):852-3.

[62] Forero M, Rajarathinam M, Adhikary SD, Chin KJ. *Erector spinae plane block for the management of chronic shoulder pain: a case report*. Can J Anesth 2018;65(3): 288-93.

[63] Chambers WA. Nerve blocks in palliative care. Br J Anaesth 2008;101(1):95-100.

[64] Wong GY, Schroeder DR, Carns PE, Wilson JL, Martin DP, Kinney MO, et al. *Effect of neurolytic celiac plexus block on pain relief, quality of life, and survival in patients with unresectable pancreatic cancer: a randomized controlled trial*. JAMA 2004;291(9):1092-9.

[65] Staats PS, Hekmat H, Sauter P, Lillemoe K. *The effects of alcohol celiac plexus block, pain, and mood on longevity in patients with unresectable pancreatic cancer: a doubleblinded, randomized, placebo-controlled study*. Pain Med 2001;2(1):28-34.

[66] Zhong W, Yu Z, Zeng JX, Lin Y, Yu T, Min XH, et al. *Celiac plexus block for treatment of pain associated with pancreatic cancer: a meta-analysis*. Pain Pract 2014;14(1):43-51.

[67] Arcidiacono PG, Calori G, Carrara S, McNicol ED, Testoni PA. *Celiac plexus block for pancreatic cancer pain in adults*. Cochrane Database Syst Rev 2011;3:CD007519.

[68] Lillemoe KD, Cameron JL, Kaufman HS, Yeo CJ, Pitt HA, Sauter PK. *Chemical splanchnicectomy in patients with unresectable pancreatic cancer*. A prospective randomized trial. Ann Surg 1993;217(5):447-55.

[69] Schmidt AP, Schmidt SR, Ribeiro SM. *Is superior hypogastric plexus block effective for treatment of chronic pelvic pain*? Rev Bras Anestesiol 2005;55(6):669-79.

[70] Plancarte R, Amescua C, Patt RB, Aldrete JA. *Superior hypogastric plexus block for pelvic cancer pain*. Anesthesiology 1990;73(2):236-9.

[71] Schultz DM. *Inferior hypogastric plexus blockade: A transsacral approach*. Pain Physician 2007;10(6):757-63.

[72] Plancarte R, Amescua C, Patt RB, Allende S. *Presacral blockade of the ganglion of Walther (ganglion impar)*. Anesthesiology 1990;73:A751.

[73] Eker HE, Cok OY, Kocum A, Acil M, Turkoz A. *Transsacrococcygeal approach to ganglion impar for pelvic cancer pain: a report of 3 cases*. Reg Anesth Pain Med 2008;33(4):381-2.

[74] Afsharimani B, Kindl K, Good P, Hardy J. *Pharmacological options for the management of refractory cancer pain-what is the evidence*? Support Care Cancer 2015;23(5):1473-81.

[75] Deer TR, Prager J, Levy R, Rathmell J, Buchser E, Burton A, et al. *Polyanalgesic consensus conference 2012: recommendations for the management of pain by intrathecal (intraspinal) drug delivery: report of an interdisciplinary expert panel*. Neuromodulation 15(5):436-64.

[76] Myers J, Chan V, Jarvis V, Walker-Dilks C. *Intraspinal techniques for pain management in cancer patients: a systematic review*. Support Care Cancer 2010;18(2):137-49.

[77] Buchbinder R, Golmohammadi K, Johnston RV, Owen RJ, Homik J, Jones A, et al. *Percutaneous vertebroplasty for osteoporotic vertebral compression fracture.* Cochrane Database Syst Rev 2015;4:CD006349.

[78] Scott NA, Guo B, Barton PM, Gerwin RD. Trigger point injections for chronic non-malignant musculoskeletal pain: a systematic review. Pain Med 2009;10(1):54-69.

[79] Escobar Álvarez Y, Biete i Solà A, Camba Rodríguez M, Gálvez Mateos RM, *Mañas Rueda A, Rodríguez Sánchez CA, et al. Diagnóstico y tratamiento del dolor irruptivo oncológico: recomendaciones de consenso.* Rev Soc Esp Dolor 2013;20(2):61-8.

[80] World Health Organization. *WHO's cancer pain ladder for adults*. Geneva: World Health Organization. URL: http://www.who.int/cancer/palliative/painladder/en.

In: Cancer Management in Latin America II
Editors: Maurício F Silva et al.
ISBN: 978-1-53616-735-1

Chapter 13

MANAGEMENT OF PALLIATIVE CARE

Tania Zertuche-Maldonado[1,*], MD,
Sofía Velasco Figueroa[1], MD,
Alberto Flores Cantisani[2], Fiona Lim[3], MBBS,
Bo Angela Wan[4], MD(C) and Mauricio F Silva[5,6,7], MD, PhD
[1]Tecnologico de Monterrey, Escuela de Medicina y Ciencias de la Salud, Monterrey, N.L, México
[2]Instituto Mexicano del Seguro Social, UMAE, Monterrey, N.L. México,
[3]Princess Margaret Hospital, Hong Kong, PR China,
[4]Odette Cancer Centre, Sunnybrook Health Sciences Centre, Toronto, Ontario, Canada,
[5]Radiation Oncology Unit, Santa Maria Federal University, Santa Maria, Brazil,
[6]Radiation Oncology Unit, Hospital de Caridade Astrogildo de Azevedo, Santa Maria, Brazil
[7]Latin America Cooperative Oncology Group, Porto Alegre, Brazil

ABSTRACT

Palliative care is characterized by having an integral and multidisciplinary approach with multiple benefits for patients with advanced disease. Its development in Latin America continues to be heterogeneous, based on individual or group willingness. Nonetheless, it is slowly advancing with government led strategies. The present chapter reviews the published peer reviewed and gray literature on the development, current state and idiosyncrasy of palliative care in this region. Overall, there is a progressive increase in palliative care with efforts to increase the implementation of clinical programs, education, opioid availability and investigation. However, many countries still have

[*] Corresponding Author's Email: taniazm@itesm.mx.

scarce access to services, let alone education. Efforts must be made to expand the current availability in a collaborative and interdisciplinary manner since future needs will be overwhelming for our countries' healthcare capacities.

INTRODUCTION

Latin America consists of 19 countries with a common cultural tradition in an area of approximately 21,069 km^2, though there are vast differences regarding geography, ethnicity and political background (1). Latin America has the highest income gap in the world, having mostly developed in social and economically unstable centrally-led governments. Latin America has approximately 56.5 million inhabitants, with Spanish as the official language in most countries (2). In low- and middle-income economies, health care has limited infrastructure and functions. Chronic degenerative diseases continue to increase in Latin America, causing pressure on the healthcare system (3). It is estimated that around 2,588,117 people in Latin America need end of life care, of which around 40% are cancer patients. By 2030, there will be around 1.7 million cancer cases, and more than 1 million deaths will be attributed to cancer per year (4). In general, Latin America is not ready to confront the increasing incidences in cancer and its disproportionately high mortality (5); one of the most troubling challenges in Latin America is inequality in healthcare provision including that in palliative care (PC) (6-8). The care of patients in these circumstances must be a fundamental task of the healthcare system, and health workers must be sensible to the psychosocial and cultural aspects of disease (9). Palliative care needs are estimated to be involved with 37% of all deaths in general, varying according to each country (10).

Palliative care is "an approach that improves the quality of life of patients and their families facing the problems associated with life-threatening illness through the prevention and relief of suffering by means of early identification and impeccable assessment and treatment of pain and other problems, physical, psychosocial, and spiritual" (11). The main objectives of PC are to achieve the best quality of life for patients and families. PC aims to "humanize" care at the end of life, based on honest and open communication with patients, participation of patients in decision making, and responsible use of technology in this process. According to the World Health Organization, illnesses that should receive end of life care include: Alzheimer's and other neurodegenerative disease, cancer, cardiovascular, chronic obstructive pulmonary disease, diabetes, HIV and AIDS, chronic kidney disease, resistant tuberculosis, rheumatoid arthritis, multiple sclerosis and Parkinson's disease (10). PC seeks to help patients and families adjust to new coping strategies when facing chronic advanced disease. This can be achieved through impeccable symptom management, excellent communication, psychosocial support, and collaborative and coordinated care (12). Although palliative care is an essential part of the universal health coverage, and excellent strategies exist for low-middle income countries, the need for palliative care and pain relief has largely been neglected for the most vulnerable populations (5).

BENEFITS OF PALLIATIVE CARE

As mentioned before, major obstacles in provision of care that have been extensively identified include lack of integrated national healthcare laws that include palliative care, lack of infrastructure and adequate training, and lack of research and publications (7, 13, 14). Most cases of cancer in Latin America present with advanced disease, with few opportunities for patients to be diagnosed during early preclinical stages. Currently, PC seeks to care for patients in early stages since it has been shown that not only does it improve quality of life, but also decrease depression and increase survival (15). Different studies have shown the cost-benefit of palliative care and end-of-life care, finding that costs of care are reduced even when quality of life is better (16-19).

There is robust evidence that PC improves symptoms, quality of life, patient satisfaction and reduces caregiver burden (20-23). PC involvement leads to higher hospice use and less aggressive care at the end of life. Since 2012, the American Oncology Society recommends early inclusion of palliative care in parallel to achieve holistic integral care of patients with advanced disease or high symptom burden. It is also recommended that caregivers or family have access to PC intervention. It has been observed that reference to a multidisciplinary care leads to better results with the patient and family and higher treatment adherence. None of the research suggest that PC causes harm or excessive costs.

In countries such as ours, where there is usually a late diagnosis of disease and treatments give few positive results, it is of special interest to implement strategies such as PC, which might reduce healthcare costs. A Cochrane review showed that home palliative care in oncological patients increases the likelihood of home deaths, with less symptom burden and without higher grief impact in caregivers (24).

PALLIATIVE CARE DEVELOPMENT IN LATIN AMERICA

In general, it may be said that PC has until recently been considered by governments as low priority and its development has been motivated by local pioneers with some contact with PC in Europe and United States (1,25). There are around 922 palliative care services and 600 PC physicians according to ALCP surveys (26). Weaknesses detected from PC professionals and experts in Latin America include lack of national PC programs, limited connection between policymakers and professionals, limited number of specialists, isolated services provision, and barriers to opioid access (2). Prioritizing PC in the formulation of health care policies would improve quality of care from providers for advanced cancer patients (27); organizations such as the WHO and PAHO (Pan American Health Organization) have created initiatives to help promote PC concepts and bring changes to legislations to incorporate PC as a public health issue (28). Expert opinion and different cross-sectional surveys have shown that Latin America is quite heterogeneous in relation to levels of PC development. Until 2012, when a multinational project was promoted to identify the level of development of PC in Latin America, there were 1.63 services per million, almost half of which were in Argentina and Chile, which accounted for only 10% of the Latin American population (1). Consistent increases in PC in recent years have taken place in Latin America, but integration of services is still incomplete. A successful example is Costa Rica: though a small country, its universal health care and strong recognition in PC for patients with advanced cancer has helped achieve a ratio of 1:109,000 for PC services (compared to Mexico and Brazil 1:7.8 million and 1:8.8 million respectively).

Efforts have been made to identify factors that predict quality of care for advanced cancer patients, which found that perspectives are highly heterogenous depending on the country analyzed. Specifically, access to care most predicted the quality of advanced cancer care (27). After the index development, countries such as Costa Rica, Chile and Mexico show a higher development rate, while countries such as Bolivia, Honduras and Dominican Republic have lower development rate. Having a national policy does not necessarily imply better access to PC (29) (Table 2). According to the Wright classification, Argentina and Chile are at a 4a level, where specialized services are in preliminary integration with standard services (30). On the other hand, Bolivia, El Salvador, Ecuador, Nicaragua, Perú and Honduras are in level 3a, with isolated services. In Bolivia for example, until 2012 there was only one hospice, one home service, and no hospital service at the 2nd and 3rd levels; there was no law that regulated PC provision. Countries such as México, Venezuela and Uruguay, although categorized as level 3a, have consistently grown, seeking to achieve a generalized service available to all the population.

An important caveat in PC development measurement is the difficulty of homogenizing indicators and its quantification as well as its validity; certain macro indicators help infer the magnitude of development, but nonetheless may neglect certain micro level assessments. The systematic and regular inclusion of measures are necessary to improve accessibility to PC and indexes such as the ACLP index may aid in this mission (29).

In 2012, the Latin America Association of Palliative Care (ALCP) in collaboration with the International Association for Hospice and Palliative Care (IAHPC) developed certain indicators to measure PC development in Latin America (31). These indicators include:

Table 1. Level of palliative care in Latin American countries

	First level services: Home care	First level services: community centers	Hospice-type residences	Multilevel services	Hospital support services	Second level services	Third level services	Services hospital support	Levels of development of palliative care
Argentina	21	0	11	16	80	2	21	80	3b
Bolivia	1	0	1	3	1	0	0	1	2
Brazil	24	0	6	26	21	0	16	21	3a
Chile	83	0	3	57	74	32	28	74	4a
Colombia	2	0	4	3	0	1	13	0	3a
Costa Rica	0	17	2	43	1	0	0	1	4a
Cuba	40	7	0	0	1	0	3	1	3
Ecuador	2	0	3	3	2	0	2	2	3
El Salvador	0	0	0	3	0	0	1	0	3
Guatemala	1	0	3	0	0	0	3	0	3a
Honduras	0	0	0	1	1	0	0	1	2
Mexico	47	17	7	4	0	34	10	0	3
Nicaragua	1	0	0	5	7	0	0	7	2
Panama	2	3	0	0	1	2	1	1	3a
Paraguay	0	0	1	0	2	0	1	2	3a
Perú	0	0	0	4	0	1	7	0	3a
Dominican Republic	0	0	1	2	2	0	3	2	3a
Uruguay	0	1	1	14	0	1	6	0	4a
Venezuela	0	23	1	3	0	8	10	0	3a

2: early development; 3a: isolated provision; 3b (generalized provision); 4a: preliminary integration.

1. Existence of a national program in palliative care that includes a designated strategy to integrate services in the public system.
2. Proportion of schools that include case concepts of palliative care such as evaluation and approach of symptoms, social aspects, psychological evaluation, communication and coordination with patient and family.
3. Number of programs for doctors, including subspecialties, master's degrees or certificates.
4. Access to palliative care in the first level of care.
5. Ratio of PC services per million inhabitants.
6. Ratio of doctors working in PC per million inhabitants, including assistance of patients with progressive or incurable diseases.
7. Opioid consumption in relation to cancer deaths.
8. Opioid consumption per capita.
9. Relation of pharmacies with opioid dispension per million inhabitants.

Development of PC in Different Countries in Latin America

Mexico

In Mexico, the emergence of "pain medicine" proposed by Dr Vicente García Olivera in the early 1960s and the founding of Pain Clinics in the 1970s motivated numerous anesthesiologists to commit to the management of chronic pain and to develop specialized centers. A prominent example includes the National Institute of Cancerology (INCan). Pain clinics specialized and grew in the states of Jalisco (General De Occidente Hospital Zoquipan, Guadalajara, Jal 1990), Nuevo León (Medical Unit of High Specialty No. 25 IMSS, 1992) by Dr José Alberto Flores Cantisani, as well as that of the Medical Center of the ISSSTE, by Dr. Rafael Hernández Santos. In 1989 the first PC academic program was created at the National Institute of Cancerology, which not only taught the physical aspects of care, but also emphasized the psychological, social and spiritual aspects of a dying patient (32). The Mexican statement of pain relief in cancer was signed, and in 1990, it was recognized as an official policy within public health. The first palliative care unit was created at the Civil Hospital of Guadalajara (Juan I Menchaca) by Dr Gustavo Montejo Rosas. In the year 2000, the PALIA Institute was created by Dr Guillermo Aréchiga Órnelas. In 2002, "Hospice Cristina" opens its doors, founded by Beatriz Montes de Oca, a first-of-its-kind private institution that uses the hospices movement created by Cicely Saunders (33).

In 2009, the general health law stated that all terminal patients have the right to receive palliative care. To make it possible, general practitioners were now allowed access to the narcotics recipe book. However, education for doctors at the university level continues to be scarce. Of the 111 national medicine programs, only 17 taught palliative care and 2 had palliative care as optional topics (5).

Previously, COFEPRIS, the agency in Mexico in charge of access to controlled substances required the use of narcotics prescription with bar codes. In order to obtain them, doctors had had to travel to the main cities of the country. In 2014, after exhaustive analysis and interviews with palliative care pioneers, an important Humans Rights Watch research was published. It identified the gap existing between opioid access in the urban versus rural populations. The lack of access to these drugs is due not only to a shortage but also the availability of licenses that enabled doctors to prescribe them (34). In recent years there has been an intensive and extensive strategy to promote access to palliative care. This includes the benefit of palliative care through Seguro Popular, a large-scale training of first-level doctors and nurses, but above all, the transition to electronic prescription of narcotics since 2015, which facilitated greater opioid availability. This allowed for prescription to be made with greater ease and effectiveness (5).

Argentina

Argentina has one of the highest rates of deaths caused by noncommunicable diseases (467.3 per 100,000 inhabitants). These changes in the demographic and epidemiological profile make the PC an important strategy. PC began in the 80's in isolation through home visits by Dr Roberto Wenk. A subsequent regulatory framework of integration to basic health services was implemented in 2000, and the current state of PC in Argentina is of category 4a (30,35). Although there is a national program of a right to access PC, the autonomy of each province limits the incorporation of PC services according to the priority granted. Out of 24 provinces in Argentina, only 10 have provincial legislation on PC.

The most readily available PC services in Argentina are hospital-based, including both specific units designed for PC, and also hospital support services (30). In 2015, PCs are recognized as a specialty. A strong aspect for Argentina is its leadership in the research and dissemination of CP. Various meetings and scientific congresses are generated, with at least 5 research groups and a significant number of professionals being members of the ALCP.

Opioid Use and Availability

Pain is a public health issue; access to analgesics is a recognized fundamental human right. Every person with pain should be valued and able to receive an appropriate treatment. The prevalence of chronic pain ranges from 1 to 60%. It has a significant economic impact since up to 3% of the health budget stems directly from this issue. Latin

America is characterized by scarce and heterogeneous availability of opioids. An important cause of this is the opiophobia of physicians and health personnel with misperceptions about opioids (36).

According to the World Health Organization, more than 3.5 million persons die of terminal cancer and HIV each year without any access to opioids. It is estimated that up to 80% of terminal cancer patients and 50% of patients with advanced HIV/AIDS experience pain of moderate-severe intensity (5).

The Committee on Economic, Social, and Cultural Rights (CESCR) has held that a fundamental one obligation of the state is to provide essential drugs including those defined under the WHO Action Programme on Essential Drugs. Morphine and codeine are on the WHO list of essential medicines making them a core obligation under the right to health (37). These drugs must be readily available within reach for all the population. Of the 298.5 metric tonnes of morphine-equivalent doses of opioids distributed in the world per year, only 0.1 metric tonne is distributed to low income countries (5).

5,500 million people (83% of the world's population) live in countries with limited access to medications for moderate to severe pain; only 15% of patients needing palliative care have access to sufficient pain medication (38). In 2015, 45% of global deaths were associated with suffering from serious diseases, 80% of which were in developing countries. Of the 298 metric tons of morphine-equivalent doses of opioids were distributed annually in the world, only 0.1 metric tons were distributed to developing countries. Countries like Bolivia or Haiti consume an average of 74 and 5 mg respectively of opioids per patient in need of palliative care annually (5). In contrast, countries such as the United States and Canada have a much larger distribution than those required by patients in palliative care. This is a problem of justice and morality. These patients of limited resources with palliative needs do not have access to essential interventions that are low cost but highly effective (5).

Although moderate levels of opioid consumption in Latin America are reported (1-10 mg of morphine equivalents per capita per year), consumption remains far below international standards. WHO guidelines for chronic cancer pain have helped justify the role of opioids to local governments, as well as to help educate health care professionals about pain management. Latin American experts still consider that adequate pain management in Latin America continues to be a matter to be resolved (36). According to Cleary et al., despite increases in opioid consumption, many countries in Latin America continue to have impaired widespread opioid availability. Certain restrictions were identified that contribute to such phenomena, including patient registrations, special prescription forms, maximum numbers of prescription days, special designated pharmacies and nearly no availability of opioids in emergency settings.

Most countries analyzed have a concerning low opioid consumption, defined as a daily dose of <200 mg/day/100,000 people. It has been observed that certain opioids with more economical incentives such as fentanyl transdermal patch have less barriers for availability (39). It is also observed that there is lack of pharmaceutical industry interest in opioid medications (2). Another important contributor is the emphasis media places on opioid diversion and abuse (2).

In 1994, the Florianópolis declaration succeeded in raising awareness about the accessibility and availability of opioids in the Latin America. In 2000, the Latin American Association of Palliative Care was created. In order to eliminate the barriers of opioid availability and the advance of palliative care, it is necessary to improve factors including limited education in pain control and palliative care and political will. Having strategies to evaluate and eliminate such factors will be important for the country's progress in PC. Workshops with the most relevant players, including the leaders in each country, worked towards eliminating such barriers, but are not enough to produce a difference in opium availability thus far. Actions plans generated in such workshops are useful to eliminate barriers, but the high political barrier limits their implementation. One case of success has been the implementation of the electronic prescription of opioids in Mexico, which has allowed a greater number of opioid prescriptions.

Table 2. Essential package for pain relief and palliative care services (5)

Medications	**Medical Equipment**	**Staff**
• Amitriptyline • Bisacodile • Dexamethasone • Diazepam • Difenhidramine • Fluconazole • Fluoxetine • Furosemide • Hyoscina • Haloperidol • Ibuprofen • Lactose • Loperamide • Metoclopramide • Metronidazole • Morphine • Naloxona • Omeprazole • Ondansetron • Acetaminophen	• Pneumatic mattress • Nasogastric tubes • Urinary catheters • Safety box for opioids • Flashlight with rechargeable batteries • Adult diapers • Oxygen	• Doctors • Nurses • Social workers • Psychiatrist, psychologist • Physical therapist • Pharmacist • Staff for clinical support • Staff for administrative support

According to the Lancet commission, one of the most important recommendations is to have oral morphine or injectable morphine with immediate release in patients with moderate pain or in a terminal state that is not relieved by other means. In 2015, the cost of the actual opioids would be 0.009% of the total health expenditure if the deficit were to be covered (5). Another one of the 5 recommendations are the use of an essential package of services for an adequate delivery of palliative care for those most needed (see Table 1). The cost per year of universal access to the essential package, as a total percentage of public expenditure is 0.8% in Mexico ($694 per patient with SHS, or $2.50 per capita). In Mexico, the price of injectable morphine in the public sector registered in 2014 is much higher than the lowest price reported internationally. Although the cost of medications in Mexico includes administration of the medicine, oral morphine has a much higher price compared to the international market.

Authorities in charge of opioid availability in most Latin American countries have limited staff and multiple responsibilities, which might limit their attention to its lack of availability to patients. Some of their major concerns include risk of diversion, abuse and misuse (39, 40). Open ongoing communication between health care professionals and government officials is an important priority in order to achieve sustained improvement (41). The INCB (International Narcotics Control Board) is a body responsible for the monitoring of international control treaties of countries that are part of the United Nations Organization; its annual report provides information on the current situation of narcotics worldwide and is responsible for identifying dangerous trends and helps propose measures to be adopted. In the case of Mexico, since June 2015 the number of prescriptions has increased following the introduction of an electronic platform as well as greater control of substances for the treatment of pain and palliative care. In Mexico there is currently a decree that allows the minister of health to regulate research on pharmacological derivatives of cannabis and its use for medical purposes. In Argentina, Colombia, Paraguay and Peru, they launched initiatives to regulate the sale of cannabis for medical purposes.

In Argentina, morphine consumption is 7.30 mg/per capita, one of the highest in the Americas. Since 2014, the Pilot program of Opioids has been implemented in Argentina, a collaboration between government authorities, palliative care specialists and pharmacists, with the purpose of designing pharmacological presentations that would be useful for management of chronic and severe pain. The program was implemented in nine public hospitals where medicines were supplied for the high-quality public sector (42). In 2015, a group of pain doctors held an expert panel to discuss and create general recommendations for the use of opioids in Latin America, creating relevant clinical guidelines available to health personnel at all levels of care (36).

EDUCATION AND TRAINING

A study by Pastrana et al. (29) through analysis of ACLP macro indicators showed that there was a positive, statistically significant correlation between the proportion of medical schools with PC in undergraduate curriculum and the number of PC services per million inhabitants (29). Among 19 countries, only nine have at least one post-graduate program. Low prioritization of palliative care education has been identified as a barrier for better quality of care in advanced cancer patients (27).

PC is not included in the majority of undergraduate curriculum and postgraduate programs are limited (2). Only 30% of nations in Latin America offer PC courses in the region, with lack of training opportunities in many parts. A caveat of existing program is that few showed any evaluation of structure and feedback, most had a classroom-led course, with little opportunity to learn in a clinical environment. Programs identified are mainly postgraduate and focused on interdisciplinary teams (43).

In Cuba and Uruguay, PC is offered as an individual subject or in a few non-mandatory hours. In Bolivia, El Salvador, Honduras and Nicaragua, there is no curriculum for PC (1). PC certification is available in various countries, with increased research and participation in international conferences; PC is increasingly recognized by other disciplines, and in general, the number of professionals in palliative care is increasing. Postgraduate courses are offered in only 10 countries, the majority offered only to physicians. In 2012, PC was recognized as a specialty in four countries and as a certificate in six countries (1).

According to an index of the level of development of the PC program, Costa Rica, Chile and Mexico have a higher development index, while Bolivia, Honduras, Dominican Republic and Guatemala have a lower level development. Although several countries have generated national policies, having one does not reflect a higher accessibility to PC services (29).

In 2010 Argentina, procedures for recognition before the Ministry of Health of the Nation were initiated to issue a Medical Specialist in Palliative Care in Adult or Pediatric Care certification. It is given by the board of medical professionals of the National Academy of Medicine (30). In Bolivia, there is no postgraduate or undergraduate training and teachers of Palliative Care were not identified. The Palliative Care Association is in the process of being developed. In 2006-2009 Chile, the Ministry of Health, in agreement with the university, formed two promotions of Specialists in Palliative Medicine. There are postgraduate training programs in different universities as well as undergraduate training programs and 27 clinical research centers (26). Colombia and Costa Rica have recognized PC as a specialty with the title of Specialist in Pain Medicine and Palliative Care.

A study by Dalpai et al. showed that undergraduate students show lack of theoretical knowledge regarding palliative care patients, and lack of knowledge regarding symptom control in 80% of cases. Pain was perceived as difficult to handle despite having theoretical knowledge on the subject (44). Regarding education or perception of what PC is, Brazilian ICU doctors perceive PC as a type of care appropriate for the final stages of life, in which futile measures are avoided and comfort is provided to patient and family;

they also perceived a need to improve communication among the healthcare professionals in order to standardise patient care, with need for training in PC (45).

In general, the number of health professionals trained in PC is constantly growing, with certification in several countries and greater attendance at international conferences. Less than 10% of PC practitioners in a 2006 survey had full participation in research within 5 years. About half of PC practitioners received some training in research and had some mentorship from an expert. The main barriers identified to doing research in Latin America include lack of funding, insufficient knowledge and expertise and lack of interest (46).

ADVANCED CARE PLANNING AND INFLUENCE IN DECISION MAKING

Advance care planning (ACP) is a process that allows patients to identify their goals for medical care, and to have tailored-made decisions when the patient is not able to speak for himself. Yennurajalingam et al. (47) found that compared to Hispanic USA caregivers, Latin American caregivers preferred a more passive decisional role in advanced cancer patients; nevertheless, both groups sought a shared decisional control among the patient-physician-family triad (47). Being younger and with higher educational levels also correlates with wanting a more active decision role. An important finding is that independent of type of decision preference control, cancer patients want to know their diagnosis and prognosis (48).

Kelley et al. (49) surveyed older Latinos living in the United States and found that the majority expressed preferences for comfort focused and non-aggressive end of life care. Interestingly, most wanted family to be involved in decision making, and very few wanted to make decisions on their own or with help from only one family member. Although the majority of seniors had a conversation about advance care planning with family or physicians, less than one quarter of them had completed advanced directives which reflects an opportunity to enhance EOL care in the United States (49).

Advance directives are more prevalent in Latino patients who received interventions by home support teams of palliative care compared to those who did not receive this type of care (50). An interesting finding by Torres-Vigil et al. (51) is regarding parenteral hydration at the end of life. Compared to physicians from countries like Japan and Canada, most Latin American physicians consider this treatment as essential and a minimum standard of care (51). Compared to Japanese, Latin American PC physicians feel they would be criticized by their colleagues if they withheld parenteral hydration (61% vs 9-10%).

Palliative Care in Specific Populations

Regarding palliative care in geriatric population, Cruz et al. conducted a literature review which found that Latin American seniors prefer a family approach in decision making, less aggressive treatments, but are less likely to have advanced directives, and are more likely to die in the hospital.

The level of acculturation does not correlate with the use of home health care services and factors such as lack of awareness, availability, and language barriers have more influence on the underutilization of resources (52). Latin American geriatric patients with advanced dementia receive more mechanical ventilation, less use of nursing homes or DNR orders compared to non-Latin American Caucasian patients. A review by Cruz-Oliver et al. showed that this might be due to geographical variables more so than to race or ethnicity as areas with larger Hispanic population demonstrated higher hospice use.

A study by Pereira et al. (53) identified that the predominant referrals of geriatric patients in Brazil were for: advanced dementia (45%), cancer (38%), and congestive heart failure (25%), with an in-hospital mortality of 50% (53).

Palliative care in non-oncologic diseases

Patients with non-oncological diseases such as dementia or chronic kidney disease often suffer levels of symptoms equal to or greater than cancer patients. However, they often do not receive adequate symptomatic treatment and sometimes receive more aggressive levels of care at end of life (52). A study in northern Mexico found that in an internal medicine unit, around 16% of patients with advanced non-oncological disease would benefit from a strategy focused on palliative care (54). In a study by Cervantes et al. (55), patients on hemodialysis prefer to discuss their symptoms and quality of life while they are physically stable and prefer routine conversations about end-of-life care; however, most would opt for cardiopulmonary resuscitation in case of cardiac arrest (55).

Pediatric patients

98% of patients who die with serious diseases associated with suffering occur in developing countries; a great majority of them could be avoidable (5). Pediatric patients also require palliative care; the majority of these patients have conditions secondary to congenital anomalies, neonatal conditions, protein malnutrition, meningitis, or cardiovascular diseases. Latin Americas has one of the highest needs of pediatric oncological palliative care (11.6%) (30). According to a survey of pediatricians in Latin America, the main barriers identified include lack of access to: psychosocial support for children, pastoral care, nursing care at home and hospice care (56). Pediatric palliative care help children and their family throughout their illness trajectory, not only near death.

A study in Mexico City showed that up to 88% of adolescents with cancer die in the hospital and 40% continue to receive chemotherapy treatments with healing purposes even at the end of life. This highlights the prevailing need for palliative care services targeted to this population (57). Pediatric patients are considered a vulnerable population due to their neurodevelopment, their pattern of response before the terminal illness goes hand in hand with chronological and mental age. In the children of 1-5 years there will be anguish of separation, anxiety before the unknown, they experience separation aggression during hospitalizations, injections, etc. From 2-6 years, this can manifest as a fear of death, pain, mourning due to the absence of parents or relatives, and can show regressions to early stages of development, phobias, aggression, depression or sleep disturbances. At the ages of 13-18 years, fear is based on the idea of being rejected by friends, and the loss of independence and control. Palliative care in pediatrics helps the child and family members not only close to death, but throughout the disease and its symptoms. The defensive reactions of the family of children and adolescents to situations at end of life such as guilt, overprotection, rejection, denial of illness, dependence, denial is frequent. It is necessary during advanced stages to provide psychiatric-psychological support to prepare families through empathy, communication, and management of emotions and thoughts for an adequate decision making (58).

Despite advances in the study of mixed pain in the pediatric population, there is still a lack of scientific research on new pharmacological treatments. One of the strategies in this age group is use of the biphasic strategy, with the modification of the WHO analgesic ladder proposed in 2012, the use of NSAIDs and potent opioids, such as morphine in cases of moderate-severe pain. The use of both have been proposed with their respective adjuvants (dexamethasone + gabapentin). These must be administered according to a schedule, an appropriate route of administration, and individualized treatment in each case (59).

SUFFERING ASSOCIATED WITH HEALTHCARE

Knowing the possible course of a patient's trajectory allows professionals to ensure that patients and their families become aware of the imminence of death. Suffering is defined by Cassell as a "state of severe distress associated with events that threaten the intactness of person" (60). Suffering is health related when associated with illness or injury and becomes serious when it affects physical, social or emotional functioning (5). A threat identified by palliative care experts includes the possible legalization of euthanasia and assisted suicide in Colombia, Mexico and other countries (2). The view and decision about palliative sedation is not influenced by the physician's religion and is considered ethically as a different and independent process from euthanasia by Latin American doctors. It is interesting to note that doctors consider palliative sedation more for existential suffering than for symptoms such as refractory dyspnea or terminal pain (61). When comparing Latin American guidelines with European guidelines, there are few federal laws in general devoted to PC patients, but none of the guidelines differ significantly from European approaches regarding palliative sedation (62).

Spirituality seems to be an important theme regarding end of life care among Latinos in the US. A focus led group by Born et al. aimed at identifying important end of life issues among minorities found that Latino communities valued maintaining dignity and being with family, and placed emphasis on compassionate communication (63). This reflects a well-known cultural dimension, where Hispanics tend to help family members to a greater degree than their individual needs.

A review on the integration of Latin cultural values into PC identified that little research has been done to outline the cultural values in Latin America towards facing end of life care. Five core values of Latin American patients were identified:

1. Familisimo (family-centered socialization with considerable connectedness and interdependence),
2. Personalismo (according to Falicov, when establishing relationships with professionals, Latin Americans require rapport building that includes warmth, informality and regard),
3. Respeto (reveals the hierarchical structures that may exist in Latin communities),
4. Confianza (trust; regarding to when someone expresses his or her deeper feelings only to an inner circle of familiar confidants, and establishing relationships with reciprocal trust),
5. Dignidad (dignity; associated with worthiness and feeling valued)(64).

Important factors observed in Latino families include cautious initial interactions with the healthcare team; such is normal, and an expected part of strategies employed by minorities to cope with a history of oppression or discrimination. In a study on Brazilian PC patients, there was higher quality of life and higher score in brief spiritual-religious coping scale, which leads to the belief that religion is useful for quality of life in patients facing difficult times (65). A study by Reyes et al. in PC patients from Chile found that spiritual symptoms may be evaluated and their intensity observed through the ENESE instrument (66).

Conclusion

Palliative care is an ongoing matter that healthcare personnel and governments are progressively becoming more aware of. Although there have been progressive increases in PC, its growth may not be enough for the exponential increase in chronic degenerative disease prevalence in South American countries. In certain countries, efforts are beginning to be made, including the development of structured national policies. In addition, implementation is crucial to achieve homogeneity in the provision of care across the country. Education is important not only academically, but also socially. Research and investigation will remain to be the most effective strategy to generalize the benefits of palliative care, an essential specialty deep-rooted in benevolence.

References

[1] Pastrana T, Eisenchlas J, Centeno C, De Lima L. *Status of palliative care in Latin America: looking through the Latin America Atlas of Palliative Care.* Curr Opin Support Palliat Care 2013;7(4):411-6.

[2] Pastrana T, Centeno C, De Lima L. *Palliative care in Latin America from the professional perspective: a SWOT analysis.* J Palliat Med 2015;18(5):429-37.

[3] Albala C, Vio F, Yáñez M. *Epidemiological transition in Latin America: a comparison of four countries.* Rev Med Chil 1997;125(6):719-27.

[4] Ferlay J, Soerjomataram I, Ervik M, Dikshit R, Eser S, Mathers C, et al. *Cancer incidence and mortality worldwide.* IARC 2012,10:11.

[5] Knaul FM, Farmer PE, Krakauer EL, De Lima L, Bhadelia A, Jiang Kwete X, et al. *Alleviating the access abyss in palliative care and pain relief-an imperative of universal health coverage: the Lancet Commission report.* Lancet 2018;391(1012 8):1391-1454.

[6] Strasser-Weippl K, Chavarri-Guerra Y, Villarreal-Garza C, Bychkovsky BL, Debiasi M, Liedke PER, et al. *Progress and remaining challenges for cancer control in Latin America and the Caribbean.* Lancet Oncol 2015;16(14):1405-38.

[7] Basu A, Mittag-Leffler BN, Miller K. Palliative care in low- and medium-resource countries. Cancer J 2013;19(5):410-3.

[8] Dachs JNW, Ferrer M, Florez CE, Barros AJD, Narváez R, Valdivia M. *Inequalities in health in Latin America and the Caribbean: descriptive and exploratory results for self-reported health problems and health care in twelve countries.* Rev Panam Salud Publica 2002;11(5-6):335-55.

[9] The Illness Narratives. *Suffering, eealing, and the human condition.* URL: http://psycnet.apa.org/re cord/1988-97187-000.

[10] WHO. *Global atlas of palliative care at the end of life.* URL: http://www.who.i nt/nmh/Glo bal_Atlas_of_Palliative_Care.pdf.

[11] WHO. WHO definition of palliative care 2012. URL: http://www.who.int/cancer/palliative/definiti on/en/

[12] Organización Panamericana de la Salud. Cuidados Paliativos: Guía para el Manejo Clínico. Organización Mundial de la Salud 1992. [*Panamerican healt organization. Palliative Care: Guide for clinical managment. World health organization 1992*]. URL:https://www.paho.org/hq/dmdocumen ts/2012/PAHO-Guias-Manejo-Clinico-2002-Spa.pdf.

[13] Soto-Perez-de-Celis E, Chavarri-Guerra Y, Pastrana T, Ruiz-Mendoza R, Bukowski A, Goss PE. *End-of-life care in Latin America.* J Glob Oncol 2017;3(3): 261-70.

[14] Von Roenn JH. *Palliative care and the cancer patient: Current state and state of the art.* J Pediatr Hematol Oncol 2011;33(Suppl 2):S87-9.

[15] Temel JS, Greer JA, Muzikansky A, Gallagher ER, Admane S, Jackson VA, et al. *Early palliative care for patients with metastatic non-small-cell lung cancer.* N Engl J Med 2010;363(8):733-42.

[16] May P, Garrido MM, Cassel JB, Kelley AS, Meier DE, Normand C, et al. *Prospective cohort study of hospital palliative care teams for inpatients with advanced cancer: earlier consultation is associated with larger cost-saving effect.* J Clin Oncol 2015;33(25):2745-52.

[17] Morrison RS, Penrod JD, Cassel JB, Caust-ellenbogen M, Litke A, Spragens L, et al. *Cost savings associated with us hospital palliative care consultation programs.* Arch Intern Med 2008;168(16):1783-90.

[18] Hartjes TM. *Making the case for palliative care in critical care.* Crit Care Nurs Clin North Am 2015;27(3):289-95.

[19] Zalenski RJ, Jones SS, Courage C, Waselewsky DR, Kostaroff AS, Kaufman D, et al. *Impact of palliative care screening and consultation in the icu: a multihospital quality improvement project.* J Pain Symptom Manage 2017;53(1):5-12.

[20] Higginson IJ, Bs BM, Finlay IG, Goodwin M, Hood K, Edwards AGK, et al. *Is there evidence that palliative care teams alter end-of-life experiences of patients and their caregivers?* J Pain Symptom Manage 2003;25(2):150-68.

[21] of Clinical Oncology AS, Others. *The integration of palliative care into standard oncology care.* J Clin Oncol 2012;30:880-8.

[22] Hui D, Bruera E. *Integrating palliative care into the trajectory of cancer care.* Nat Rev Clin Oncol 2016;13(3):159-71.

[23] Ferrell BR, Temel JS, Temin S, Smith TJ. *Integration of palliative care into standard oncology Care: ASCO clinical practice guideline update summary.* J Oncol Pract 2017;13(2):119-21.

[24] Gomes B, Calanzani N, Curiale V, McCrone P, Higginson IJ. *Effectiveness and cost-effectiveness of home palliative care services for adults with advanced illness and their caregivers.* Cochrane Database Syst Rev 2013;6:CD007760.

[25] Wenk R, Bertolino M. *Palliative care development in South America: a focus on Argentina.* J Pain Symptom Manage 2007;33(5):645-50.

[26] Pastrana T, De Lima L, Pons JJ, Centeno C. *Atlas de Cuidados Paliativos de Latinoamérica. Edición cartográfica 2013.* [*Palliative Care Atlas of Latin America. Cartographic edition 2013. Houston: IAHPC Press, 2013*]. Houston: IAHPC Press, 2013.

[27] Torres Vigil I, Aday LA, De Lima L, Cleeland CS. *What predicts the quality of advanced cancer care in Latin America*? A look at five countries: Argentina, Brazil, Cuba, Mexico, and Peru. J Pain Symptom Manage 2007;34(3):315-27.

[28] De Lima L, Bruera E. *The Pan American Health Organization: its structure and role in the development of a palliative care program for Latin America and the Caribbean.* J Pain Symptom Manage 2000;20(6):440-8.

[29] Pastrana T, Torres-Vigil I, De Lima L. *Palliative care development in Latin America: an analysis using macro indicators.* Palliat Med 2014;28(10):1231-8.

[30] Pastrana T, De Lima L, Pons JJ, Centeno C. *Atlas de Cuidados Paliativos de Latinoamérica. Edición cartográfica 2013.* [*Palliative Care Atlas from Latin America. Cartographic edition 2013. Houston: IAHPC Press. 2013*]. Houston, TX: IAHPC Press, 2013.

[31] De Lima L, Perez-Castells M, Berenguel M, Monti C, Aguilar A, Ahumada M, Ramirez L, TorresVigil I, Vargas Y, Herrera E. Indicadores de Cuidado Paliativo ALCP. Primera edición. Houston, TX: IAHPC Press, 2013. [Palliative Care indicatorscadores ALCP. First edition. Houston, TX: IAHPC Press, 2013].

[32] Covarrubias-Gómez A. Las clínicas del dolor en México. Revista Mexicana de Anestesiología 2008;31(1):66-70. [*Pain Clinics in Mexico. Mexican Journal of Anesthesiology 2008;31(1):66-70*].

[33] De Oca Lomelí GM. Historia de los cuidados paliativos. Revista Digital Universitaria. URL: http://www.revista.unam.mx/vol.7/num4/art23/abr_art23.pdf. [History of the Palliative Care. University Digital Magazine].

[34] Secretaria de Salud M. *Solicitud de Permiso para Utilizar Recetarios Especiales con Códigos de Barras para Prescribir Estupefacientes.* Sistema Electrónico de Trámites Sanitario. URL: http://www.cofepris.gob.mx/Documents/RecetariosLib ros/ManualRecetarios.pdf. [*Mynistry of Health M. Application form to use special prescriptions with barcodes to prescribed drugs. Electronic system of sanitary procedures.*]

[35] Wright M, Wood J, Lynch T, Clark D. Mapping levels of palliative care development: a global view. J Pain Symptom Manage 2008;35(5):469-85.

[36] Lara-Solares A, Aguayo Zamora C, Amescua García C, Garcia JBS, Berenguel Cook MDR, Bonilla Sierra P, et al. *Latin-American guidelines for opioid use in chronic nononcologic pain.* Pain Manag 2017;7(3):207-15.

[37] Thomas L. *Global State of Pain Treatment.* Humans Right Watch 2011. URL:https://www.hrw.org.

[38] Public health dimension of the world drug problem including in the context of the Special session of the United Nations General Assembly on the world drug problem, to be held in 2016. *World Health Organization* 2016. URL: http://apps. who.int/

[39] Cleary J, De Lima L, Eisenchlas J, Radbruch L, Torode J, Cherny NI. *Formulary availability and regulatory barriers to accessibility of opioids for cancer pain in Latin America and the Caribbean: a report from the Global Opioid Policy Initiative (GOPI).* Ann Oncol 2013;24 Suppl 11:xi41-50.

[40] De Lima L, Pastrana T. *Evaluation of the effectiveness of workshops on the availability and rational use of opioids in Latin America.* J Palliat Med 2016;19(9):964-71.

[41] Leon MX, De Lima L, Florez S, Torres M, Daza M, Mendoza L, et al. *Improving availability of and access to opioids in Colombia: description and preliminary results of an action plan for the country.* J Pain Symptom Manage 2009;38(5):758-66.

[42] Arana IP. Cuidados paliativos: abordaje de la atención en salud desde un enfoque de derechos humanos [*Palliative Care: approach to health care from a human rights point of view.*]. URL: http://www.cuidadospaliativosdh.org/archivos/Infor me.pdf.

[43] Vindrola-Padros C, Mertnoff R, Lasmarias C, Gómez-Batiste X. *Palliative care education in Latin America: A systematic review of training programs for healthcare professionals.* Palliat Support Care 2017;11:1-11.

[44] Dalpai D, Mendes FF, Asmar JAVN, Carvalho PL, Loro FL, Branco A. *Pain and palliative care: the knowledge of medical students and the graduation gaps.* Revista Dor 2017;18(4):307-10.

[45] Gulini JEHM de B, Nascimento ERP do, Moritz RD, Rosa LM da, Silveira NR, Vargas MA de O. *Intensive care unit team perception of palliative care: the discourse of the collective subject.* Rev Esc Enferm USP 2017;51:e03221.

[46] Wenk R, De Lima L, Eisenchlas J. *Palliative care research in Latin America: results of a survey within the scope of the Declaration of Venice.* J Palliat Med 2008;11(5):717-22.

[47] Yennurajalingam S, Parsons HA, Duarte ER, Palma A, Bunge S, Palmer JL, et al. *Decisional control preferences of Hispanic patients with advanced cancer from the United States and Latin America.* J Pain Symptom Manage 2013;46(3):376-85.

[48] Noguera A, Yennurajalingam S, Torres-Vigil I, Parsons HA, Duarte ER, Palma A, et al. *Decisional control preferences, disclosure of information preferences, and satisfaction among Hispanic patients with advanced cancer.* J Pain Symptom Manage 2014;47(5):896-905.

[49] Kelley AS, Wenger NS, Sarkisian CA. *Opiniones: end-of-life care preferences and planning of older Latinos.* J Am Geriatr Soc 2010;58(6):1109-16.

[50] Fischer SM, Cervantes L, Fink RM, Kutner JS. *Apoyo con Cariño: a pilot randomized controlled trial of a patient navigator intervention to improve palliative care outcomes for Latinos with serious illness*. J Pain Symptom Manage 2015;49(4):657-65.

[51] Torres-Vigil I, Mendoza TR, Alonso-Babarro A, De Lima L, Cárdenas-Turanzas M, Hernandez M, et al. *Practice patterns and perceptions about parenteral hydration in the last weeks of life: a survey of palliative care physicians in Latin America*. J Pain Symptom Manage 2012;43(1):47-58.

[52] Cruz-Oliver DM, Talamantes M, Sanchez-Reilly S. *What evidence is available on end-of-life (EOL) care and Latino elders?* A literature review. Am J Hosp Palliat Care 2014 Feb;31(1):87-97.

[53] Arcanjo SP, Saporetti LA, Curiati JA, Jacob-Filho W, Avelino-Silva TJ. *Clinical and laboratory characteristics associated with referral of hospitalized elderly to palliative care*. Einstein (São Paulo) 2018;16(1):eAO4092.

[54] Zertuche-Maldonado T, Tellez-Villarreal R, Pascual A, Valdovinos-Chavez SB, Barragan-Berlanga AJ, Sanchez-Avila MT, et al. *Palliative care needs in an acute internal medicine ward in Mexico*. J Palliat Med 2018;21(2):163-8.

[55] Cervantes L, Linas S, Keniston A, Fischer S. *Latinos with chronic kidney failure treated by dialysis: understanding their palliative care perspectives*. Am J Kidney Dis 2016;67(2):344-7.

[56] Varela AMS, Dussel V, Barfield R, Bidegain M, Delima L, Dellon E. *Perceived resources and barriers to pediatric palliative care among healthcare practitioners attending the Latin American palliative care association (ALCP) meeting (755)*. J Pain Symptom Manage 2011;41(1):306.

[57] Cicero-Oneto CE, Mata-Valderrama G, Valdez-Martínez E. *Mortality of young people with cancer: clinical-epidemiological characteristics of death and emerging ethical aspects*. Gac Med Mex 2018;154(1):8-15.

[58] González C, Méndez J, Romero JI, Bustamante J, Castro R, Jiménez J. *Cuidados paliativos en México*. [*Palliative Care in Mexico*.] Rev Med Hosp Gen 2012;75(3):173-9.

[59] Yazde MLP, Gómez KV, Majdalani A, Pigliapoco V, Santos GC. *Opioid treatment for mixed pain in pediatric patients assisted by the Palliative Care team*. Five years of experience. Arch Argent Pediatr 2018;116(1):62-4.

[60] Eric C. *The Relief of Suffering*. Archives of Internal Medicine 1983. URL: http://www.ericcassell.com/download/ReliefOfSuffering.pdf.

[61] Moyano J, Zambrano S, Ceballos C, Santacruz CM, Guerrero C. *Palliative sedation in Latin America: survey on practices and attitudes*. Support Care Cancer 2008;16(5):431-5.

[62] Manzini JL. *Palliative sedation: ethical perspectives from Latin America in comparison with European recommendations*. Curr Opin Support Palliat Care 2011;5(3):279-84.

[63] Born W, Greiner KA, Sylvia E, Butler J, Ahluwalia JS. *Knowledge, attitudes, and beliefs about end-of-life care among inner-city African Americans and Latinos*. J Palliat Med 2004;7(2):247-56.

[64] Adames HY, Chavez-Dueñas NY, Fuentes MA, Salas SP, Perez-Chavez JG. *Integration of Latino/a cultural values into palliative health care: a culture centered model*. Palliat Support Care 2014;12(2):149-57.

[65] Matos TD de S, Meneguin S, Ferreira M de L da S, Miot HA. *Quality of life and religious-spiritual coping in palliative cancer care patients*. Rev Lat Am Enfermagem 2017;25:e2910.

[66] Reyes MM, de Lima L, Taboada P, Villarroel L, Vial J de D, Blanco O, et al. *Escala numérica para evaluar síntomas espirituales en cuidados paliativos*. [*Numerical scale to evaluate spiritual symtoms in palliative care*.] Rev méd Chile 2017;145(6):747-54.

In: Cancer Management in Latin America II
Editors: Maurício F Silva et al.

ISBN: 978-1-53616-735-1

Chapter 14

COST-EFFECTIVENESS IN CANCER CARE

Wendel Mombaque dos Santos[1,*]***, PhD,***
Fiona Lim[2]***, MBBS, Bo Angela Wan***[3]***, MD(C),***
Beatriz Amendola[4]***, MD, Jessica Yumi Matuoka***[1]***, MD,***
Silvia Regina Secoli[1]***, PhD and Mauricio F Silva***[5,6,7]***, MD, PhD***

[1]University of São Paulo, São Paulo, Brazil
[2]Department of Oncology, Princess Margaret Hospital, Hong Kong, PR China
[3]Odette Cancer Centre, Sunnybrook Health Sciences Centre, Toronto, Ontario, Canada
[4]Innovative Cancer Institute, South Miami, Florida, United States of America
[5]Radiation Oncology Unit, Santa Maria Federal University, Santa Maria, Brazil
[6]Radiation Oncology Unit, Hospital de Caridade Astrogildo de Azevedo, Santa Maria, Brazil
[7]Latin America Cooperative Oncology Group, Porto Alegre, Brazil

ABSTRACT

The economic burden of cancer treatment has increased rapidly over the past few years. In this context, health workers and policy makers need to understand the concept of cost-effectiveness in order to optimize budget distribution among different diseases. We aimed to present the Health Technologies Assessment (HTA) for conducting economic evaluation research on cancer treatment through conducting a narrative literature review. HTA has implications for the selection of technologies to be financed, the identification of conditions or subgroups in which technologies should be used, and the promotion of efficiency and quality in a healthcare system. In HTA, analytical techniques including cost minimization, cost-benefit, cost-utility, and cost-effectiveness analysis are utilised.

[*] Corresponding Author's Email: wendel@usp.br.

The cost-effectiveness analysis is important to evaluate the best treatment on different healthcare contexts. We conclude that health professionals and policy makers should include the resulting information from HTA in oncology guidelines to ensure that cost-effectiveness ratios will be taken into account in treatment choice.

INTRODUCTION

The prevalence of cancer is expected to increase worldwide. In 2017, there were 1,688,780 new cancer cases and 600,920 cancer deaths in the United States of America (USA) (1). Therefore, cancer treatments are becoming one of the most expensive expenditures in healthcare, especially in low or middle-income countries (2-3).

The economic impact of cancer treatments has been increasing rapidly over the last few years, with costs estimated to double every four years (2-3). For instance, in the European Union, cost of cancer care increased stably from €35.7 billion in 1995 to €83.2 billion in 2014, tripling over the past 20 years (4). When considering the economic burden of cancer, costs can be even higher after taking into account the productivity loss and other indirect costs. In 2009, this was an estimated €126 billion, accounting for 51% of overall health care costs (5).

In the USA, the estimated total direct medical cost was US $124.5 billion, with expenditures estimated to be US $160 billion in 2010 (6). In a recent analysis of expenditures in oncology, the authors presented a projection of US $158 billion by 2020, and even this estimation was thought to be conservative by the authors based on the increases observed in the previous years (7).

The increase of health expenditures and the constant budget constraints result in the need to come up with strategies to make more efficient use of the budget while providing the best available care (6). In this context, health workers and police makers can directly or indirectly impact the costs of cancer care according to different kinds of treatments available (8-9). Therefore, the concept of cost effectiveness needs to be further discussed, given its impact on the overall budget (8, 10).

Globally, the economy has a problematic relationship with health professionals and policy makers. Economists focus more on social perspectives, while health professionals focus more on individualistic ones in which they value health as priceless, and a life saved justifies any effort and cost (11). It is important to determine whose point of view will be considered and who are the stakeholders involved (i.e., decision makers, patients, industry) (12). A correct articulation between these fields is required for a more efficient allocation of resources to healthcare (13).

Health economics plays an indispensable role, especially in countries with public sector as the main healthcare provider to the population. In this regard, robust tools are needed to systemically and critically appraise the available information to guide the decision making for the best treatment in different health contexts. Our objective in this article is to present the HTA for conducting economic evaluation research on cancer treatment, especially in Latin America.

LITERATURE REVIEW

This article contains opinions based on a narrative literature review of the publications including books and peer-reviewed journal articles. This method was utilized to describe and discuss the state of economic evaluation in cancer treatment However, this review is not designated to describe the methodological way that permits reproduction of data nor answer specific quantitative research questions. The objective of this paper is to introduce the reader to the HTA process and its main concepts, and to highlight the importance of this tool to the sustainability of the health care system.

Health technologies assessment: Definitions and general notions

The HTA consists of a systematic and multidisciplinary process of evaluation of the effects, properties, and impacts of health technology. HTA is a multidisciplinary area in which different professionals use analytical models designed from a variety of methods to compare these technologies (14-15).

HTA aims to support decision making regarding the rational use of resources, to present alternative treatments to clinicians, patients or managers (14). The HTA has implications for the selection of technologies to be financed and for the identification of the conditions or subgroups in which they should be used, to make the health system more efficient to promote, protect and recover the health of the population (16).

In several countries, the conduction of economic analyses is mandatory in order to approve the introduction of financed technologies and any reimbursements. Even though the first report dated from the 60s, not until the late 80's that its importance began to be recognized (17).

HTA is defined as a device or method used to promote health, prevent death, treat diseases, improve rehabilitation and care at the individual or population level. Health technologies include medicine, equipment, care procedures, and techno-assistance models (18). These technologies can be assembled into three categories: hard, light-hard and light technology. Hard technology is represented by concrete material such as equipment, permanent furniture and consumer materials; light-hard technology includes structured knowledge represented by disciplines that act in health; and light technology is expressed as the production process of communication and links that lead to the meeting of the users with health action needs.

In oncological settings, health technologies involve diagnostic tools, imaging modalities, genetic or general laboratory tests, and treatment options (e.g., radiotherapy machines, drugs, surgical procedures) (18-19).

Efforts have been made to improve outcomes of some types of cancer by increasing overall survival and improving quality of life. The diverse prognosis, treatments and procedures that are targeted to specifically defined cancer patient populations have resulted in higher final costs (19).

In this context, the use of HTA can contribute to the transparency in decision making, which is based on objective, reproducible and comparable clinical and economic criteria (20-22).

Economic analysis

In the HTA, analytical techniques are used, namely: cost minimization (ACM), cost-benefit (CBA), cost-effectiveness analysis (ACE), and cost-utility analysis (ACU), (18, 23).

ACM aims to demonstrate the clinical effectiveness and equivalencies of comparative interventions. Therefore, it only focuses on the costs of preparing different interventions, and not on the final clinical outcomes. Consequently, the "best" intervention would have the lowest cost. ACM consists of description of costs and impacts associated with diseases from the perspectives of patients, society or institutions, and includes information on prevalence, incidence, lethality, and cure rate (24-25).

In CBA, the costs and benefits (outcomes) are both measured in monetary units and cost-benefit ratios. It contemplates the aspects of allocative efficiency and is a fundamental tool in the evaluation of programs with different outcomes to determinate which of them presents the best benefit (26).

In ACE, the ratio between the costs of the technology and the outcomes are evaluated in a natural health unit. The results are provided as cost per outcome, and as an incremental cost-effectiveness ratio (ICR). This analysis compares interventions in which the effects are measured in the same unit (25-27).

When comparing the outcomes and costs of a new intervention to the standard treatment, four scenarios can be obtained: greater costs and lower effectiveness, lower costs and higher effectiveness, lower costs and lower effectiveness, higher costs and higher effectiveness. For these possibilities, the incremental cost-effectiveness ratio of the current intervention to the new intervention helps to determine the additional cost required to obtain an incremental of a benefit unit (25-27).

Due to the limitations of the ACE, it is not possible to compare results from studies with different units, therefore, it is not appropriate to combine reductions in morbidity and mortality in a single index. To address this, a new form of measurement called "utility," was created, and this analysis is termed ACU. This is a quantitative measure that evaluates the patient's preference for a specific health condition (25-27).

Evaluating cost-effectiveness of cancer treatments in the United States health care systems

Traditionally, after a medication has a demonstrated effectiveness in a clinical trial, the government organization evaluates its benefits and risks regardless of its cost to grant approval (12). However, nowadays, health institutions need to use various tools to balance the growing cost of technologies with restricted healthcare budgets and the challenging societal priorities in order to address efficiency and equity in the healthcare system (28-29). The cost of cancer treatment is increasingly being used as the deciding factor on whether a new technology should be incorporated into the preventive, diagnostic, or therapeutic repertoire of a health system. As such, it is increasingly important to define the value of cancer care in different clinical scenarios (10, 30-31).

In 2007, the American Society of Clinical Oncology (ASCO) published the results of their *Cost of Cancer Care Task Force* in which they posited that the challenges related to the cost of cancer care should be identified and addressed using various strategies (10). In 2009, ASCO published their guidance statement regarding this issue (30). It was reported that oncology policy makers, who are directly or indirectly responsible for the costs of cancer care, should consider the costs of the treatment, adopt strategies that are based on the best available evidence, improve communication with the institution and their patients on cost matters to maximize patient education strategies, and finally, stimulate agencies to conduct their own analyses. Different authors suggested ways to minimize costs and optimize expenditures in cancer care (10, 30). Some of these ideas include the following:

1. Changes in practice: the oncologists should evaluate if a particular procedure will be beneficial for patients (e.g., Will *BRCA* screening make any difference for thyroid cancer? Will it be beneficial to start chemotherapy for advanced pancreatic cancer?);
2. Changes of attitude: Acknowledge limitations in practice, and that some changes are needed. Oncologists should openly communicate with their patients and families;
3. Make decisions based on reliable criteria: Specialists can and should include evidence-based medicine concepts in their practice and rely their decisions on comparative effectiveness and cost-effectiveness analysis;
4. Regularly discuss costs with patients and managers with the objective of providing the best available care, while optimizing resource use;
5. Offer oncologists education and training to conduct economic analyses.

In the context of HTA, two parameters were utilized to perform ACE. The first parameter uses the quality-adjusted-life-years (QALYs), which refers to the number of years of life that would be gained by an intervention, adjusted for quality of life. The second parameter uses the incremental cost-effectiveness ratio (ICER), which is defined as the ratio of additional cost to incremental benefit of an intervention and is expressed as the cost per a clinical outcome (10,30-31).

The use of ICER must the compared against a willingness to pay threshold (WTP), and this WTP is different in each country (32). There is no consensus regarding what threshold values are acceptable, but references suggest that the WTP can be between 0.5 to 3 times the per capita gross domestic product (GDP) of a country. However, in the case of cancer treatment, this threshold may be higher (33).

Despite the different incidences of cancer around different areas of the USA, the mortality-to-incidence ratio is greater than 0.35. However, the overall mean expenditure per new cancer patient is from US $700.92 to US $24400.00 (34). This factor represents the direct impact on WTP on that country, primarily because of the high-cost of cancer treatment (35).

Additionally, several anticancer drugs are more expensive in low-to-medium income countries (LMIC) than in high-income countries, showing that no relationship exists between pharmaceutical prices in LMICs and national GDP (36, 37). The access to health is recognized as a constitutional right in most Latin American countries (38). Based on this legislated perspective, citizens are unable to access therapies through regular channels of the health system increasingly resort to filing legal suits against the government, citing their constitutional right to health care (39-40).

The judiciary recurrently finds itself ruling on funding a specific drug for a specific patient. This trend toward judicialization of medicine has various grades and has an impact in most Latin American countries, and judicial authorities tend to rule in favor of patients' claims. These litigations, steadily overruling national funding policies, can undermine the sustainability of public health care systems by diverting resources away from rational use that provides collective benefit to the general society (39, 40).

Some may say that by relying on economic studies to inform healthcare practice, we are "rationing health care". The essence is that health professionals and policy makers should be conscious of costs, because our resources are finite and should cover as many patients as possible, especially given the increasing incidences of most diseases, not only cancers.

Although we witnessed the growing importance of economic analysis in oncology, represented by the increasing number of economic studies, mostly cost-effectiveness and cost-utility analyses are developed in academic settings or conducted with the objective to include treatments financed by the payer (37-39).

Healthcare professionals involved in cancer care rarely conduct this type of study and many of them find it difficult to interpret (40). There is a need to address this issue in a gradate course, to introduce this language to discuss costs and to offer training to develop healthcare professionals to conduct their own analyses.

Discussion

The cost of cancer care is a major concern considering the budgetary constraints we have been witnessing. Strategies to reduce costs and avoid bankruptcy are needed (30). The knowledge of health economics can support the use of cost-effective treatments in oncology. In addition, this knowledge can improve the redistribution of budget for cancer care and the collective negotiation can create resource funds, provide evidence-based adaptations of treatment plans, and enhance participation in clinical research (11, 29, 34). The use of cost-effectiveness analyses and health technology assessments help to assign the limited budget to the best value for patients without abandoning other significant interventions (34, 36).

The redistribution of the budget for cancer care is necessary to make subsidies accessible for expensive treatments when they are essential (34, 36, 40). Also, the collective negotiation and the creation of resource funds can increase the chance of drugs becoming available at lower fixed prices.

Evidence-based adaptation of schemes of treatment must be used when the clinical guidelines applicable in high-income settings may not be financially feasible in middle or low-income countries (13, 34). Therefore, a scientific evidence-based approach to those costly and therapeutically optimal alternatives is desirable. This factor is related to the participation in clinical research, usually because clinical trials rarely respond to the real public health priorities of a specific region (11, 28, 33, 40).

Technological advances in improving technology can decrease cost. On one hand, major technological progress certainly comes at a higher cost, and there are many concerns regarding the value of that progress. On the other hand, newer equipment and resource costs associated with technologies such as in cutting-edge radiation oncology can be partly mitigated by shorter treatment courses. Better tumor control, reduced toxicity, and fewer treatment courses decrease the indirect costs of cancer care, including lost time and economic productivity secondary to treatment-related and cancer-related illness and death (41).

Specifically, new technologies in radiation therapy will have tremendous impact in Latin America. It would be easier to treat large numbers of patients in shorter treatment schedules and facilitate access for distant patients to treatment centers. Some specific examples of how new technologies in radiation therapy are cost effective include radiation therapy technique include Stereotactic Body Radiation Therapy (SBRT) and Stereotactic Radiosurgery (SRS). Improved cost effectiveness can also be the result of treatment hypofractionation such as partial-breast irradiation in breast cancer and shorter treatment schemes for prostate and lung cancer (41).

The cost effectiveness of cancer care is dependent on a multitude of factors and has implications that reach multiple populations. Health professionals, patients, and policy makers must be aware that guaranteeing access to high-cost drugs is questionable in reducing cancer mortality rates (11, 29, 30, 33, 40). Professionals involved with cancer care should conduct economic studies in their daily practice to make their work more efficient. Policy makers should also conduct cost-effectiveness analyses to determine the best treatment on different healthcare contexts. As a result, cancer treatments with the most advantageous cost-effectiveness ratios will be the first choice of treatment. Moreover, the participation in discussions of economic priorities in health care and consideration of the impact of new technologies is warranted.

REFERENCES

[1] Siegel RL, Miller KD, Jemal A. *Cancer statistics, 2016*. CA Cancer J Clin 2016;66(1):7-30.

[2] Eagle D. *The cost of cancer care: Part I*. Oncology 2012;26(10):918-24.

[3] Eagle D. *The cost of cancer care: Part II*. Oncology 2012;26(11):1104-8.

[4] Jonsson B, Hofmarcher T, Lindgren P, Wilking N. *The cost and burden of cancer in the European Union 1995-2014*. Eur J Cancer 2016;66(1):162-70.

[5] Luengo-Fernandez R, Leal J, Gray A, Sullivan R. *Economic burden of cancer across the European Union: a population-based cost analysis*. Lancet Oncol 2013;14(12):1165-74.

[6] Miller JD, Foley KA, Russell MW. *Current challenges in health economic modeling of cancer therapies: a research inquiry*. Am Health Drug Benefits 2014;7(3):153-62.

[7] Scalo JF, Rascati KL. *Trends and issues in oncology costs*. Expert Rev Pharmacoecon Outcomes Res 2014;14(1):35-44.

[8] Siddiqui M, Rajkumar SV. *The high cost of cancer drugs and what we can do about it*. Mayo Clinic Proceedings 2012;87(10):935-43.

[9] Good M, Good CB. *Bending the cost curve in cancer care*. N Engl J Med 2011;365(7):674-5.

[10] Meropol NJ, Schrag D, Smith TJ, Mulvey TM, Langdon RM, Jr., Blum D, et al. *American Society of Clinical Oncology guidance statement: The cost of cancer care*. J Clin Oncol 2009;27(23):3868-74.

[11] Greenberg D, Hammerman A, Vinker S, Shani A, Yermiahu Y, Neumann PJ. *Which is more valuable, longer survival or better quality of life?* Israeli oncologists' and family physicians' attitudes toward the relative value of new cancer and congestive heart failure interventions. Value Health 2013;16(5):842-7.

[12] Wallner PE, Konski A. *A changing paradigm in the study and adoption of emerging health care technologies: coverage with evidence development*. J Am Coll Radiol 2008;5(11):1125-9.

[13] Schrag D, Hanger M. *Medical oncologists' views on communicating with patients about chemotherapy costs: a pilot survey*. J Clin Oncol 2007;25(2):233-7.

[14] Cruz LN, Filha NTS, Miguel SRPS, Kelles SMB. *Dicionário de Avaliação de Tecnologias em Saúde. Healthcare. Porto Alegre: Instituto de Avaliação de Tecnologia em Saúde (IATS)* [*Health Technology Assessment Dictionary. Healthcare. Porto Alegre: Institute of Health Technology Assessment (IATS)*], 2014.

[15] Gomes RM, Jd C, Lemos LL, Faleiros D, Caires AL, Dias G, et al. *Análise da produção de avaliação de tecnologias em saúde do centro colaborador do sistema único de Saúde (SUS)* [*Analysis of the production of health technology assessment at the collaborating center of the Unified Health System (SUS)*], Brasil - Uma Parceria Entre o Governo E A Academia. Value Health 2015;18(7):A848.

[16] Gomes MP, Nunes AA, Sarti FM, Netto AR. *Análise de custo-efetividade do tratamento diretamente observado da tuberculose* [*Cost-effectiveness analysis of the directly observed treatment of tuberculosis.*] Value Health 2017:20(9):A888-9.

[17] Soárez PCd, Soares MO, Novaes HMD. *Modelos de decisão para avaliações econômicas de tecnologias em saúde* [*Decision models for economic assessments of health technologies*]. Ciência Saúde Coletiva 2014;19:4209-22.

[18] Nita ME, Secoli SR, Nobre MRC, Ono-Nita SK, Campino ACC, Santi FM, et al. *Avaliação de tecnologias em saúde: Evidência clínica, análise econômica e análise de decisão* [*Health technology assessment: Clinical evidence, economic analysis and decision analysis*]. Healthcare. São Paulo: Artmed Editora, 2009.

[19] Buffery D. *Health economics in oncology: A necessary tool for value-based patient care.* Am Health Drug Benefits 2015;8(4):184.

[20] Nita ME, Secoli SR, Nobre M, Ono-Nita SK. *Métodos de pesquisa em avaliação de tecnologia em saúde* [*Research methods in health technology assessment*]. Arquivos Gastroenterologia 2009;46(4):252-5.

[21] Barbosa EC. 25 *Anos do sistema único de Saúde: Conquistas e desafios* [*Years of the Single Health System: Achievements and challenges*]. Revista de Gestão em Sistemas de Saúde 2013;2(2):85-102.

[22] Whittington M, Atherly A, Van Raemdonck L, Lampe S. *Strategic methodologies in public health cost analyses.* J Public Health Manag Pract 2016;23(6):e10-6.

[23] Silva EN, Silva MT, Pereira MG. *Health economic evaluation studies: definition and applicability to health systems and services.* Epidemiol Serv Saúde 2016;25(1):205-7.

[24] Smith M. *Custo em saúde, qualidade e desfechos: O livro de termos da ISPOR* [*Health costs, quality and outcomes: ISPOR's terms book*]. Healthcare. São Paulo: Associação Brasileira de Farmacoeconomia e Pesquisa de Desfechos, 2009.

[25] Secoli SR, Padilha KG, Litvoc J, Maeda ST et al. *Farmacoeconomia: perspectiva emergente no processo de tomada de decisão* [*Pharmacoeconomics: an emerging perspective in the decision-making process*]. Ciência Saúde Coletiva 2005;10 (Suppl):287-96.

[26] Drummond MF, McGuire A. *Economic evaluation in health care: Merging theory with practice.* New York: Oxford University Press, 2001.

[27] Mariotto AB, Yabroff KR, Shao Y, Feuer EJ, Brown ML. *Projections of the cost of cancer care in the United States: 2010-2020.* J Natl Cancer Inst 2011;103(2):117-28

[28] Berry SR, Bell CM, Ubel PA, Evans WK, Nadler E, Strevel EL, et al. *Continental Divide? The attitudes of US and Canadian oncologists on the costs, cost-effectiveness, and health policies associated with new cancer drugs.* J Clin Oncol 2010;28(27):4149-53.

[29] Neumann PJ, Palmer JA, Nadler E, Fang C, Ubel P. *Cancer therapy costs influence treatment: a national survey of oncologists.* Health Aff (Millwood) 2010;29(1):196-202.

[30] Meropol NJ, Schulman KA. *Cost of cancer care: issues and implications.* J Clin Oncol 2007;25(2):180-6.

[31] Tirelli U. *Access to cancer care: the cost of treatment matters.* Recenti Prog Med 2014;105(5):181-3.

[32] Pavel MS, Chakrabarty S, Gow J. *Assessing willingness to pay for health care quality improvements.* BMC Health Serv Res 2015;15(2):43-7.

[33] Cuffe S, Hon H, Qiu X, Tobros K, Wong CK, De Souza B, et al. *Cancer patients acceptance, understanding, and willingness-to-pay for pharmacogenomic testing.* Pharmacogenet Genomics 2014;24(7):348-55.

[34] Ruiz R, Strasser-Weippl K, Touya D, Herrero Vincent C, Hernandez-Blanquisett A, St Louis J, et al. *Improving access to high-cost cancer drugs in Latin America: Much to be done.* Cancer 2017;123(8):1313-23.

[35] Kingham TP, Alatise OI. *Establishing translational and clinical cancer research collaborations between high- and low-income countries.* Ann Surg Oncol 2015;22(3):741-6.

[36] Chalkidou K, Marquez P, Dhillon PK, Teerawattananon Y, Anothaisintawee T, Gadelha CA, et al. *Evidence-informed frameworks for cost-effective cancer care and prevention in low, middle, and high-income countries.* Lancet Oncol 2014;15(3):e119-31.

[37] Horton S, Gauvreau CL. *Cancer in low- and middle-income countries: An economic overview.* In: Gelband H, Jha P, Sankaranarayanan R, Horton S, eds. Cancer: Disease Control Priorities, Third Edition (Volume 3). Washington DC: World Bank, 2015:263-80.

[38] Espinosa M. *The Caribbean origins of the National Public Health System in the USA: A global approach to the history of medicine and public health in Latin America.* Hist Cienc Saude Manguinhos 2015;22(1):241-53.

[39] Ramos Rde S, Gomes AM, de Oliveira DC, Marques SC, Spindola T, Nogueira VP. *Access the Unified Health System actions and services from the perspective of judicialization.* Rev Lat Am Enfermagem 2016;24:e2689.

[40] Vargas-Pelaez CM, Rover MR, Leite SN, Rossi Buenaventura F, Farias MR. *Right to health, essential medicines, and lawsuits for access to medicines-a scoping study.* Soc Sci Med 2014;121(4):48-55.

[41] Amendola B. *Cost effectiveness in new technologies.* Rep Pract Oncol Radiother 2013;18(2):S9-11.

SECTION TWO: ACKNOWLEDGMENTS

In: Cancer Management in Latin America II
Editors: Maurício F Silva et al.
ISBN: 978-1-53616-735-1

Chapter 15

ABOUT THE EDITORS

Maurício F Silva, MD, PhD, is a clinical and academic specialist in radiation oncology, with a number of internationally recognised senior positions dedicated to clinical practice and research in this field. Head of Radiation Oncology, Assistant Professor of Radiation Oncology at Santa Maria Federal University, in South Brazil and the Head of Education for the Brazilian Society of Radiotherapy, with extensive international clinical research experience across academic centres of excellence, in Brazil, Spain (in 2007), Australia (in 2009) and Canada. Chair of the Radiation Oncology (advisory) arm at the Latin America Cooperative Oncology Group (LACOG), a contract research organization responsible for the development and oversight of all steps involved with clinical trials development. These unique work experiences, at the interface of clinical oncology, academia and contract research organisations, have resulted in extensive ongoing input to the design and implementation of large oncology clinical trials, and co-authorship of critical documents in the field of radiation oncology, such as the updated systematic review in hypofractionated radiotherapy in patients suffering from bone metastases, published in the Radiotherapy and Oncology Journal – the official journal of the European Society of Radiotherapy and Oncology. Currently the Chief Investigator (international PI) of a phase 3 multi-centre international randomised clinical trial (involving eight countries in five continents), evaluating the safety of radiation therapy on bone metastases, and its effects on patient reported clinical outcomes, such as pain control and quality of life. Main academic interests include: Exploring the potential interaction between radiotherapy and drug therapies (with focus on novel immunotherapies). It is likely that the net therapeutic effect is stronger than the sum of their parts, and this is a largely unexplored field of oncology. Currently investigating possible academic collaborations with industry and other partners to implement trials in this field. Understanding the effects of radiation therapy on patient reported outcomes (PROs)/clinical outcome assessments (COAs). Email: mauricio.f.silva@ufsm.br

Gustavo Nader Marta, MD, PhD, is a clinical and academic specialist in radiation oncology working at the Hospital Sírio Libanês and University of Sao Paulo Medicine School - Sao Paulo State Cancer Institute in Brazil. Professor of Oncology (postgraduate level) and Head of research for the Brazilian Society of Radiotherapy. Vice-chair of the Radiation Oncology (advisory) arm at the Latin America Cooperative Oncology Group (LACOG). Member of the Board of Directors for International Education Committee – American Society for Radiation Oncology (ASTRO). Email: gustavo.marta@hc.fm.usp.br

Luis CM Antunes, MD, MSc, PhD, is a clinical and academic specialist in oncology. He received his medical degree and completed his residence in oncology at the University of Santa Maria (UFSM), in South Brazil. He completed his Masters (MSc) in gastroenterology and hepatology at the Federal University of Rio Grande do Sul (UFRGS) in Porto Alegre, Brazil. He them obtained his PhD in Health Science from the UFRGS. He is head oncologist of multi-professional Team Care of Hematology-Oncology Service of the University Hospital of Santa Maria and Professor of Oncology at Franciscan University in Santa Maria, Brazil. He is a principal investigator in studies of immunotherapy drugs for cancer. Investigator at the Cancer and Neurobiology Laboratory, Experimental Research Center, Porto Alegre Clinical Hospital, in Porto Alegre, Brazil. His main areas of interest include signal pathways cancer, immunotherapy, gastrointestinal tumors and melanoma. He has served on the editorial board member of a number of journals. He is member of the American Society of Clinical Oncology (ASCO), Brazilian Gastrointestinal Tumors Group (GTG), Brazilian Group of Melanoma (GBM) and of the Brazilian Society of Clinical Oncology (SBOC). Email: luisantunes@clinicaviversm.com.br

Fiona Lim, MBBS (HKU) FRCR(UK) FHKCR FHKAM (Radiology) DipPallMed (Wales), graduated from The University of Hong Kong in 2006. She received residency training in clinical oncology in the Department of Oncology, Princess Margaret Hospital. She obtained the fellowship in the Royal College of Radiologist in Clinical Oncology and Diploma with Merit in Palliative Medicine (Cardiff University) in 2014. She is also the honorary clinical assistant professor at the Department of Oncology (The University of Hong Kong), Department of Medicine and Therapeutics (The Chinese University of Hong Kong), School of Pharmacy (The Chinese University of Hong Kong) and visiting lecturer for Department of Health Technology and Informatics (The Hong Kong Polytechnic University). She received further overseas training in stereotactic body radiotherapy and image-guided brachytherapy in Sunnybrook Health Sciences Center, Toronto and Mount Vernon Hospital, United Kingdom in 2016. Dr Lim also actively participated in various clinical researches and was appointed as panel member in Research Ethics Committee of Kowloon West Cluster. Her current interest is in lung cancer, gynecological cancer, stereotactic body radiotherapy and palliative medicine. Email: lmy084@ha.org.hk

Bo Angela Wan, MD(C), is a third year medical student from Canada. Her interests are in oncology, hematology and palliative care. Email: iamangelawan@gmail.com

Beatriz Amendola, MD, DABR, FACR, FASTRO, FACRO, completed her residency in Radiation Oncology at the Medical College of Virginia in Richmond, Virginia with Board Certification in Therapeutic Radiology by the American Board of Radiology in 1980. She has held several academic positions, including Acting Chairman of the Department of Radiation Oncology at the University of Michigan and Associate Professor and Director of Residency Training at the University of Miami, Department of Radiation Oncology. Founder and Director of Innovative Cancer Institute and the Brachytherapy Institute of South Florida presently. She has edited a textbook on radiation oncology and published more than 60 scientific articles in peer-reviewed medical journals of the specialty. She has been awarded Fellowship from the American Society of Radiation Oncology (ASTRO), from the American College of Radiation Oncology (ACRO) and from The American College of Radiology (ACR). Her main areas of interest include breast, lung, head/neck and prostate cancer as well as brain tumors. Extensive knowledge in the field of radiation therapy, with expertise in brachytherapy, as well as in radiosurgery using gamma knife and LINAC based radiosurgery. Delivered more than 500 scientific presentations, scientific exhibits, and lectures nationally and internationally. She has received multiple honors and awards including the Gold Medal from CRILA (Circulo de Radioterapeutas Ibero Latino Americano). In 2015 awarded Honorary Membership in the Spanish Society of Radiation Oncology (SEOR) because of her multiple contributions to the specialty of radiation oncology in Spain. She is a volunteer faculty member of eCancer since 2015 and Lacort Medical since 2018. Email: bamendola@innovativecancer.com

Joav Merrick, MD, MMedSci, DMSc, born and educated in Denmark is professor of pediatrics, Division of Pediatrics, Hadassah Hebrew University Medical Center, Mt Scopus Campus, Jerusalem, Israel and Kentucky Children's Hospital, University of Kentucky, Lexington, Kentucky United States and professor of public health at the Center for Healthy Development, School of Public Health, Georgia State University, Atlanta, United States, the former medical director of the Health Services, Division for Intellectual and Developmental Disabilities, Ministry of Social Affairs and Social Services, Jerusalem, the founder and director of the National Institute of Child Health and Human Development in Israel. Numerous publications in the field of pediatrics, child health and human development, rehabilitation, intellectual disability, disability, health, welfare, abuse, advocacy, quality of life and prevention. Received the Peter Sabroe Child

Award for outstanding work on behalf of Danish Children in 1985 and the International LEGO-Prize ("The Children's Nobel Prize") for an extraordinary contribution towards improvement in child welfare and well-being in 1987. In 2017 appointed a Kentucky Colonel by the Commonwealth of Kentucky, the highest honor the governor can bestow to a person. Email: jmerrick@zahav.net.il

In: Cancer Management in Latin America II
Editors: Maurício F Silva et al.
ISBN: 978-1-53616-735-1

Chapter 16

ABOUT THE RADIATION ONCOLOGY UNIT, SANTA MARIA UNIVERSITY HOSPITAL (UFSM), SANTA MARIA, BRAZIL

The Santa Maria Federal University in Brazil is a public university with almost 40.000 students under the auspices of the Ministry of Education. It is a Brazilian public university located in Santa Maria in the state of Rio Grande do Sul and funded by the federal government of Brazil. It was founded in 1960 by Professor José Mariano da Rocha Filho (1915-1998), a physician, educator and the first Dean.

UFSM's presence in the municipality of Santa Maria is one of the reasons why the city is sometimes called "university city" or "culture city". It is located in western Rio Grande do Sul, approximately 290 km far from the capital city of the state, Porto Alegre, thus being set in the heart of the pampas of Brazil.

As a public university, students do not pay tuition fees. It is the oldest federal university not located in a Brazilian state capital city and the largest in number of undergraduate courses offered in Rio Grande do Sul state. As for 2015, the university was ranked at position 15 at national ranking from MEC (Wikipedia).

The university is divided into nine academic centers, which administer and organize the undergraduate and postgraduate courses offered. The Centro de Ciências da Saúde (CCS) or Centre of Health Sciences provides undergraduate courses at the Campus of Santa Maria in nursing, pharmacy and biochemistry, physical therapy, speech and language therapy, occupational therapy, medicine and dentistry, but with some classes offered in downtown Santa Maria.

The Radiation Oncology Unit at Santa Maria University Hospital is a reference center for the South of Brazil, assisting about 500 new patients a year with excellence. The unit is involved in teaching activities in several under- and graduate courses, local and international research and collaborations.

Contact

Maurício F Silva, MD, PhD
Director, Radiation Oncology Unit
Santa Maria Federal University
Santa Maria, Brazil
Email: mauricio.filva@ufsm.br

In: Cancer Management in Latin America II
Editors: Maurício F Silva et al.
ISBN: 978-1-53616-735-1

Chapter 17

About the National Institute of Child Health and Human Development in Israel

The National Institute of Child Health and Human Development (NICHD) in Israel was established in 1998 as a virtual institute under the auspices of the Medical Director, Ministry of Social Affairs and Social Services in order to function as the research arm for the Office of the Medical Director. In 1998 the National Council for Child Health and Pediatrics, Ministry of Health and in 1999 the Director General and Deputy Director General of the Ministry of Health endorsed the establishment of the NICHD.

Mission

The mission of a National Institute for Child Health and Human Development in Israel is to provide an academic focal point for the scholarly interdisciplinary study of child life, health, public health, welfare, disability, rehabilitation, intellectual disability and related aspects of human development. This mission includes research, teaching, clinical work, information and public service activities in the field of child health and human development.

Service and academic activities

Over the years many activities became focused in the south of Israel due to collaboration with various professionals at the Faculty of Health Sciences (FOHS) at the Ben Gurion University of the Negev (BGU). Since 2000 an affiliation with the Zusman Child Development Center at the Pediatric Division of Soroka University Medical Center has resulted in collaboration around the establishment of the Down Syndrome Clinic at that center. In 2002 a full course on "Disability" was established at the Recanati School for Allied Professions in the Community, FOHS, BGU and in 2005 collaboration was started with the Primary Care Unit of the faculty and disability became part of the master of public health course on "Children and society". In the academic year 2005-2006 a one semester course on "Aging with disability" was started as part of the master of science program in gerontology in our collaboration with the Center for Multidisciplinary Research in Aging. In 2010 collaborations with the Division of Pediatrics, Hadassah Hebrew University Medical Center, Jerusalem, Israel around the National Down Syndrome Center and teaching students and residents about intellectual and developmental disabilities as part of their training at this campus.

Research activities

The affiliated staff have over the years published work from projects and research activities in this national and international collaboration. In the year 2000 the International Journal of Adolescent Medicine and Health and in 2005 the International Journal on Disability and Human Development of De Gruyter Publishing House (Berlin and New York) were affiliated with the National Institute of Child Health and Human Development. From 2008 also the International Journal of Child Health and Human Development (Nova Science, New York), the International Journal of Child and Adolescent Health (Nova Science) and the Journal of Pain Management (Nova Science) affiliated and from 2009 the International Public Health Journal (Nova Science) and Journal of Alternative Medicine Research (Nova Science). All peer-reviewed international journals.

National collaborations

Nationally the NICHD works in collaboration with the Faculty of Health Sciences, Ben Gurion University of the Negev; Department of Physical Therapy, Sackler School of Medicine, Tel Aviv University; Autism Center, Assaf HaRofeh Medical Center; National Rett and PKU Centers at Chaim Sheba Medical Center, Tel HaShomer; Department of Physiotherapy, Haifa University; Department of Education, Bar Ilan University, Ramat Gan, Faculty of Social Sciences and Health Sciences; College of Judea and Samaria in Ariel and in 2011 affiliation with Center for Pediatric Chronic Diseases and National Center for Down Syndrome, Department of Pediatrics, Hadassah Hebrew University Medical Center, Mount Scopus Campus, Jerusalem.

International collaborations

Internationally with the Department of Disability and Human Development, College of Applied Health Sciences, University of Illinois at Chicago; Strong Center for Developmental Disabilities, Golisano Children's Hospital at Strong, University of Rochester School of Medicine and Dentistry, New York; Centre on Intellectual Disabilities, University of Albany, New York; Centre for Chronic Disease Prevention and Control, Health Canada, Ottawa; Chandler Medical Center and Children's Hospital, Kentucky Children's Hospital, Section of Adolescent Medicine, University of Kentucky, Lexington; Chronic Disease Prevention and Control Research Center, Baylor College of Medicine, Houston, Texas; Division of Neuroscience, Department of Psychiatry, Columbia University, New York; Institute for the Study of Disadvantage and Disability, Atlanta; Center for Autism and Related Disorders, Department Psychiatry, Children's Hospital Boston, Boston; Department of Pediatric and Adolescent Medicine, Western Michigan University Homer Stryker MD School of Medicine, Kalamazoo, Michigan, United States; Department of Paediatrics, Child Health and Adolescent Medicine, Children's Hospital at Westmead, Westmead, Australia; International Centre for the Study of Occupational and Mental Health, Düsseldorf, Germany; Centre for Advanced Studies in Nursing, Department of General Practice and Primary Care, University of Aberdeen, Aberdeen, United Kingdom; Quality of Life Research Center, Copenhagen, Denmark; Nordic School of Public Health, Gottenburg, Sweden, Scandinavian Institute of Quality of Working Life, Oslo, Norway; The Department of Applied Social Sciences (APSS) of The Hong Kong Polytechnic University Hong Kong.

Targets

Our focus is on research, international collaborations, clinical work, teaching and policy in health, disability and human development and to establish the NICHD as a permanent institute in Israel in order to conduct model research and policy.

Contact

Professor Joav Merrick, MD, MMedSci, DMSc
Director, National Institute of Child Health and Human Development, Jerusalem, Israel.
E-mail: jmerrick@zahav.net.il

In: Cancer Management in Latin America II
Editors: Maurício F Silva et al.
ISBN: 978-1-53616-735-1

Chapter 18

ABOUT THE BOOK SERIES "HEALTH AND HUMAN DEVELOPMENT"

Health and human development is a book series with publications from a multidisciplinary group of researchers, practitioners and clinicians for an international professional forum interested in the broad spectrum of health and human development.

- Merrick J, Omar HA, eds. *Adolescent behavior research.* International perspectives. New York: Nova Science, 2007.
- Kratky KW. *Complementary medicine systems: Comparison and integration.* New York: Nova Science, 2008.
- Schofield P, Merrick J, eds. *Pain in children and youth.* New York: Nova Science, 2009.
- Greydanus DE, Patel DR, Pratt HD, Calles Jr JL, eds. *Behavioral pediatrics*, 3 ed. New York: Nova Science, 2009.
- Ventegodt S, Merrick J, eds. *Meaningful work: Research in quality of working life.* New York: Nova Science, 2009.
- Omar HA, Greydanus DE, Patel DR, Merrick J, eds. *Obesity and adolescence.* A public health concern. New York: Nova Science, 2009.
- Lieberman A, Merrick J, eds. *Poverty and children.* A public health concern. New York: Nova Science, 2009.
- Goodbread J. *Living on the edge.* The mythical, spiritual and philosophical roots of social marginality. New York: Nova Science, 2009.
- Bennett DL, Towns S, Elliot E, Merrick J, eds. *Challenges in adolescent health: An Australian perspective.* New York: Nova Science, 2009.
- Schofield P, Merrick J, eds. *Children and pain.* New York: Nova Science, 2009.

- Sher L, Kandel I, Merrick J, eds. *Alcohol-related cognitive disorders: Research and clinical perspectives*. New York: Nova Science, 2009.
- Anyanwu EC. *Advances in environmental health effects of toxigenic mold and mycotoxins.* New York: Nova Science, 2009.
- Bell E, Merrick J, eds. *Rural child health. International aspects*. New York: Nova Science, 2009.
- Dubowitz H, Merrick J, eds. *International aspects of child abuse and neglect.* New York: Nova Science, 2010.
- Shahtahmasebi S, Berridge D. *Conceptualizing behavior: A practical guide to data analysis*. New York: Nova Science, 2010.
- Wernik U. *Chance action and therapy*. The playful way of changing. New York: Nova Science, 2010.
- Omar HA, Greydanus DE, Patel DR, Merrick J, eds. *Adolescence and chronic illness*. A public health concern. New York: Nova Science, 2010.
- Patel DR, Greydanus DE, Omar HA, Merrick J, eds. *Adolescence and sports.* New York: Nova Science, 2010.
- Shek DTL, Ma HK, Merrick J, eds. *Positive youth development: Evaluation and future directions in a Chinese context*. New York: Nova Science, 2010.
- Shek DTL, Ma HK, Merrick J, eds. *Positive youth development: Implementation of a youth program in a Chinese context*. New York: Nova Science, 2010.
- Omar HA, Greydanus DE, Tsitsika AK, Patel DR, Merrick J, eds. *Pediatric and adolescent sexuality and gynecology: Principles for the primary care clinician.* New York: Nova Science, 2010.
- Chow E, Merrick J, eds. *Advanced cancer. Pain and quality of life*. New York: Nova Science, 2010.
- Latzer Y, Merrick, J, Stein D, eds. *Understanding eating disorders*. Integrating culture, psychology and biology. New York: Nova Science, 2010.
- Sahgal A, Chow E, Merrick J, eds. *Bone and brain metastases: Advances in research and treatment.* New York: Nova Science, 2010.
- Postolache TT, Merrick J, eds. *Environment, mood disorders and suicide*. New York: Nova Science, 2010.
- Maharajh HD, Merrick J, eds. *Social and cultural psychiatry experience from the Caribbean Region*. New York: Nova Science, 2010.
- Mirsky J. *Narratives and meanings of migration*. New York: Nova Science, 2010.
- Harvey PW. *Self-management and the health care consumer*. New York: Nova Science, 2011.
- Ventegodt S, Merrick J. *Sexology from a holistic point of view*. New York: Nova Science, 2011.

- Ventegodt S, Merrick J. *Principles of holistic psychiatry: A textbook on holistic medicine for mental disorders*. New York: Nova Science, 2011.
- Greydanus DE, Calles Jr JL, Patel DR, Nazeer A, Merrick J, eds. *Clinical aspects of psychopharmacology in childhood and adolescence*. New York: Nova Science, 2011.
- Bell E, Seidel BM, Merrick J, eds. *Climate change and rural child health*. New York: Nova Science, 2011.
- Bell E, Zimitat C, Merrick J, eds. *Rural medical education: Practical strategies*. New York: Nova Science, 2011.
- Latzer Y, Tzischinsky. *The dance of sleeping and eating among adolescents: Normal and pathological perspectives*. New York: Nova Science, 2011.
- Deshmukh VD. *The astonishing brain and holistic consciousness: Neuroscience and Vedanta perspectives*. New York: Nova Science, 2011.
- Bell E, Westert GP, Merrick J, eds. *Translational research for primary healthcare*. New York: Nova Science, 2011.
- Shek DTL, Sun RCF, Merrick J, eds. *Drug abuse in Hong Kong: Development and evaluation of a prevention program*. New York: Nova Science, 2011.
- Ventegodt S, Hermansen TD, Merrick J. *Human Development: Biology from a holistic point of view*. New York: Nova Science, 2011.
- Ventegodt S, Merrick J. *Our search for meaning in life*. New York: Nova Science, 2011.
- Caron RM, Merrick J, eds. *Building community capacity: Minority and immigrant populations*. New York: Nova Science, 2012.
- Klein H, Merrick J, eds. *Human immunodeficiency virus (HIV) research: Social science aspects*. New York: Nova Science, 2012.
- Lutzker JR, Merrick J, eds. *Applied public health: Examining multifaceted Social or ecological problems and child maltreatment*. New York: Nova Science, 2012.
- Chemtob D, Merrick J, eds. *AIDS and tuberculosis: Public health aspects*. New York: Nova Science, 2012.
- Ventegodt S, Merrick J. *Textbook on evidence-based holistic mind-body medicine: Basic principles of healing in traditional Hippocratic medicine*. New York: Nova Science, 2012.
- Ventegodt S, Merrick J. *Textbook on evidence-based holistic mind-body medicine: Holistic practice of traditional Hippocratic medicine*. New York: Nova Science, 2012.
- Ventegodt S, Merrick J. *Textbook on evidence-based holistic mind-body medicine: Healing the mind in traditional Hippocratic medicine*. New York: Nova Science, 2012.

- Ventegodt S, Merrick J. *Textbook on evidence-based holistic mind-body medicine: Sexology and traditional Hippocratic medicine*. New York: Nova Science, 2012.
- Ventegodt S, Merrick J. *Textbook on evidence-based holistic mind-body medicine: Research, philosophy, economy and politics of traditional Hippocratic medicine*. New York: Nova Science, 2012.
- Caron RM, Merrick J, eds. *Building community capacity: Skills and principles.* New York: Nova Science, 2012.
- Lemal M, Merrick J, eds. *Health risk communication.* New York: Nova Science, 2012.
- Ventegodt S, Merrick J. *Textbook on evidence-based holistic mind-body medicine: Basic philosophy and ethics of traditional Hippocratic medicine*. New York: Nova Science, 2013.
- Caron RM, Merrick J, eds. *Building community capacity: Case examples from around the world.* New York: Nova Science, 2013.
- Steele RE. *Managed care in a public setting*. New York: Nova Science, 2013.
- Srabstein JC, Merrick J, eds. *Bullying: A public health concern*. New York: Nova Science, 2013.
- Pulenzas N, Lechner B, Thavarajah N, Chow E, Merrick J, eds. *Advanced cancer: Managing symptoms and quality of life*. New York: Nova Science, 2013.
- Stein D, Latzer Y, eds. *Treatment and recovery of eating disorders*. New York: Nova Science, 2013.
- Sun J, Buys N, Merrick J. *Health promotion: Community singing as a vehicle to promote health*. New York: Nova Science, 2013.
- Pulenzas N, Lechner B, Thavarajah N, Chow E, Merrick J, eds. *Advanced cancer: Managing symptoms and quality of life*. New York: Nova Science, 2013.
- Sun J, Buys N, Merrick J. *Health promotion: Strengthening positive health and preventing disease*. New York: Nova Science, 2013.
- Merrick J, Israeli S, eds. *Food, nutrition and eating behavior*. New York: Nova Science, 2013.
- Shahtahmasebi S, Merrick J. *Suicide from a public health perspective*. New York: Nova Science, 2014.
- Merrick J, Tenenbaum A, eds. *Public health concern: Smoking, alcohol and substance use*. New York: Nova Science, 2014.
- Merrick J, Aspler S, Morad M, eds. *Mental health from an international perspective*. New York: Nova Science, 2014.
- Merrick J, ed. *India: Health and human development aspects*. New York: Nova Science, 2014.

- Caron R, Merrick J, eds. *Public health: Improving health via inter-professional collaborations*. New York: Nova Science, 2014.
- Merrick J, ed. *Pain Management Yearbook 2014*. New York: Nova Science, 2015.
- Merrick J, ed. *Public Health Yearbook 2014*. New York: Nova Science, 2015.
- Sher L, Merrick J, eds. *Forensic psychiatry: A public health perspective*. New York: Nova Science, 2015.
- Shek DTL, Wu FKY, Merrick J, eds. *Leadership and service learning education: Holistic development for Chinese university students*. New York: Nova Science, 2015.
- Calles JL, Greydanus DE, Merrick J, eds. *Mental and holistic health: Some international perspectives*. New York: Nova Science, 2015.
- Lechner B, Chow R, Pulenzas N, Popovic M, Zhang N, Zhang X, Chow E, Merrick J, eds. *Cancer: Treatment, decision making and quality of life*. New York: Nova Science, 2016.
- Lechner B, Chow R, Pulenzas N, Popovic M, Zhang N, Zhang X, Chow E, Merrick J, eds. *Cancer: Pain and symptom management*. New York: Nova Science, 2016.
- Lechner B, Chow R, Pulenzas N, Popovic M, Zhang N, Zhang X, Chow E, Merrick J, eds. *Cancer: Bone metastases, CNS metastases and pathological fractures*. New York: Nova Science, 2016.
- Lechner B, Chow R, Pulenzas N, Popovic M, Zhang N, Zhang X, Chow E, Merrick J, eds. *Cancer: Spinal cord, lung, breast, cervical, prostate, head and neck cancer*. New York: Nova Science, 2016.
- Lechner B, Chow R, Pulenzas N, Popovic M, Zhang N, Zhang X, Chow E, Merrick J, eds. *Cancer: Survival, quality of life and ethical implications*. New York: Nova Science, 2016.
- Davidovitch N, Gross Z, Ribakov Y, Slobodianiuk A, eds. *Quality, mobility and globalization in the higher education system: A comparative look at the challenges of academic teaching*. New York: Nova Science, 2016.
- Henry B, Agarwal A, Chow E, Omar HA, Merrick J, eds. *Cannabis: Medical aspects*. New York: Nova Science, 2017.
- Henry B, Agarwal A, Chow E, Merrick J, eds. *Palliative care: Psychosocial and ethical considerations*. New York: Nova Science, 2017.
- Furfari A, Charames GS, McDonald R, Rowbottom L, Azad A, Chan S, Wan BA, Chow R, DeAngelis C, Zaki P, Chow E, Merrick J, eds. *Oncology: The promising future of biomarkers*. New York: Nova Science, 2017.
- O'Hearn S, Blake A, Wan BA, Chan S, Chow E, Merrick J, eds. *Medical cannabis: Clinical practice*. New York: Nova Science, 2017.

- Lui LC, Wong K, Yeung R, Merrick J, eds. *Palliative care: Oncology experience from Hong Kong*. New York: Nova Science, 2017.
- Shek DTL, Leung JTY, Lee T, Merrick J, eds. *Psychosocial needs: Success in life and career planning*. New York: Nova Science, 2017.
- Kopytin A, Lebedev A. *Clinical art psychotherapy with war veterans*. New York: Nova Science, 2017.
- Malek L, Lim F, Wan BA, Diaz PL, Chow E, Merrick J, eds. *Cancer and exercise*. New York: Nova Science, 2018.

Contact

Professor Joav Merrick, MD, MMedSci, DMSc
Director, National Institute of Child Health and Human Development, Jerusalem, Israel
E-mail: jmerrick@zahav.net.il

SECTION THREE: INDEX

INDEX

D

E

F

G

H

I

L

M

R

S

T

V

Z